Household Safety Sourcebook
Hypertension Sourcebook
Immune System Disorders Sourcebook
Infant & Toddler Health Sourcebook
Infectious Diseases Sourcebook
Injury & Trauma Sourcebook
Kidney & Urinary Tract Diseases & Disorders Sourcebook
Learning Disabilities Sourcebook, 2nd Edition
Leukemia Sourcebook
Liver Disorders Sourcebook
Lung Disorders Sourcebook
Medical Tests Sourcebook, 2nd Edition
Men's Health Concerns Sourcebook, 2nd Edition
Mental Health Disorders Sourcebook, 3rd Edition
Mental Retardation Sourcebook
Movement Disorders Sourcebook
Muscular Dystrophy Sourcebook
Obesity Sourcebook
Osteoporosis Sourcebook
Pain Sourcebook, 2nd Edition
Pediatric Cancer Sourcebook
Physical & Mental Issues in Aging Sourcebook
Podiatry Sourcebook
Pregnancy & Birth Sourcebook, 2nd Edition
Prostate Cancer
Public Health Sourcebook
Reconstructive & Cosmetic Surgery Sourcebook
Rehabilitation Sourcebook
Respiratory Diseases & Disorders Sourcebook
Sexually Transmitted Diseases Sourcebook, 2nd Edition
Skin Disorders Sourcebook
Sleep Disorders Sourcebook, 2nd Edition
Smoking Concerns Sourcebook
Sports Injuries Sourcebook, 2nd Edition
Stress-Related Disorders Sourcebook
Stroke Sourcebook
Substance Abuse Sourcebook
Surgery Sourcebook
Thyroid Sourcebook
Transplantation Sourcebook
Traveler's Health Sourcebook
Vegetarian Sourcebook
Women's Health Concerns Sourcebook, 2nd Edition
Workplace Health & Safety Sourcebook
Worldwide Health Sourcebook

Teen Health Series

Alcohol Information for Teens
Asthma Information for Teens
Cancer Information for Teens
Diet Information for Teens
Drug Information for Teens
Eating Disorders Information for Teens
Fitness Information for Teens
Mental Health Information for Teens
Sexual Health Information for Teens
Skin Health Information for Teens
Sports Injuries Information for Teens
Suicide Information for Teens

Dermatological Disorders SOURCEBOOK

Second Edition

Health Reference Series

Second Edition

Dermatological Disorders SOURCEBOOK

Basic Consumer Health Information about Conditions and Disorders Affecting the Skin, Hair, and Nails, Such as Acne, Rosacea, Rashes, Dermatitis, Pigmentation Disorders, Birthmarks, Skin Cancer, Skin Injuries, Psoriasis, Scleroderma, and Hair Loss, Including Facts about Medications and Treatments for Dermatological Disorders and Tips for Maintaining Healthy Skin, Hair, and Nails

Along with Information about How Aging Affects the Skin, a Glossary of Related Terms, and a Directory of Resources for Additional Help and Information

Edited by
Amy L. Sutton

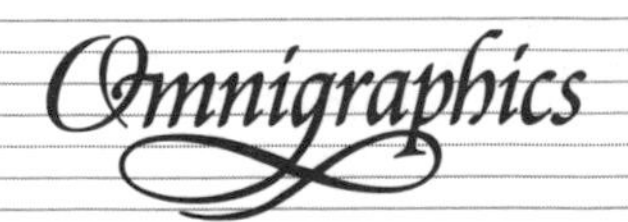

615 Griswold Street • Detroit, MI 48226

Bibliographic Note

Because this page cannot legibly accommodate all the copyright notices, the Bibliographic Note portion of the Preface constitutes an extension of the copyright notice.

Edited by Amy L. Sutton

Health Reference Series

Karen Bellenir, *Managing Editor*
David A. Cooke, M.D., *Medical Consultant*
Elizabeth Barbour, *Permissions and Research Coordinator*
Dawn Matthews, *Verification Assistant*
Laura Pleva Nielsen, *Index Editor*
Cherry Stockdale, *Permissions Assistant*
EdIndex, Services for Publishers, *Indexers*

* * *

Omnigraphics, Inc.

Matthew P. Barbour, *Senior Vice President*
Kay Gill, *Vice President—Directories*
Kevin Hayes, *Operations Manager*
Leif Gruenberg, *Development Manager*
David P. Bianco, *Marketing Director*

* * *

Peter E. Ruffner, *Publisher*

Frederick G. Ruffner, Jr., *Chairman*

ISBN 0-7808-0795-2

Library of Congress Cataloging-in-Publication Data

Dermatological disorders sourcebook : basic consumer health information about conditions and disorders affecting the skin, hair, and nails, such as acne, rosacea, rashes, dermatitis, pigmentation disorders, birthmarks, skin cancer, skin injuries, psoriasis, scleroderma, and hair loss, including facts about medications and treatments for dermatological disorders and tips for maintaining healthy skin, hair, and nails; along with information about how aging affects the skin, a glossary of related terms, and a directory of resources for additional help and information / edited by Amy L. Sutton. -- 2nd ed.
p. cm. -- (Health reference series)
Summary: "Provides basic consumer health information about the skin, hair, and nails and related conditions and disorders. Includes index, glossary of related terms, and other resources"--Provided by publisher.
Includes index.
ISBN 0-7808-0795-2 (hardcover : alk. paper)
1. Skin--Diseases--Popular works. 2. Hair--Diseases--Popular works. 3. Nails--Diseases--Popular works. I. Sutton, Amy L. II. Series: Health reference series (Unnumbered)
RL85.D47 2005
616.5--dc22
2005024956

This book is printed on acid-free paper meeting the ANSI Z39.48 Standard. The infinity symbol that appears above indicates that the paper in this book meets that standard.

Printed in the United States

Table of Contents

Visit www.healthreferenceseries.com to view *A Contents Guide to the Health Reference Series*, a listing of more than 10,000 topics and the volumes in which they are covered.

Part III: Rashes, Skin Signs of Systemic Diseases, and Allergic Skin Conditions

Part IV: Pigmentation Disorders, Vascular Skin Changes, and Benign Skin Growths

Part V: Malignant Skin Growths and Dermatological Side Effects of Cancer Treatment

Part VI: Skin Trauma, Ulcering, and Blistering Disorders

Part VII: Infectious, Inflammatory, and Other Skin Conditions

Part VIII: Hair and Nail Disorders

Part IX: Dermatological Medications and Treatments

Part X: Skin Hygiene, Care, and Protection

Part XI: Additional Help and Information

Preface

About This Book

The skin—the body's outer covering and largest organ—shields us from injury and infection. Along with the hair, it helps to regulate body temperature. The nails provide support and protection for the sensitive ends of the fingers and toes. Although the skin, hair, and nails serve to protect the body, they are not immune to injuries, infections, or congenital disorders.

Disorders that affect the skin, hair, and nails are common but can be costly to diagnose and treat. In some cases, skin disorders are becoming more prevalent across the United States. Consider these facts:

- Acne, a skin condition that produces pimples on the face and upper body, is the most common skin disorder. It affects 17 million Americans. Nearly 85 percent of people between the ages of 12 and 24 develop acne.
- More than 15 million people in the United States have symptoms of atopic dermatitis, a condition that causes skin inflammation and is linked to allergic conditions, such as hay fever and asthma. This condition accounts for 10 to 20 percent of all annual visits to dermatologists.
- Psoriasis, a chronic disorder that causes inflammation and scaling skin, affects between 5 and 8 million people in the United States. The overall costs of treating psoriasis are estimated at about $3 billion annually.

- Every year in the United States, more than a million people learn they have nonmelanoma skin cancer (most commonly basal cell and squamous cell carcinoma) and more than 50,000 are diagnosed with melanoma, the deadliest form of skin cancer. In the last 30 years, the percentage of people who have developed melanoma has doubled.

Fortunately, many skin, hair, and nail problems can be prevented or effectively treated when people take precautions, learn to recognize early symptoms, and know when to seek professional care.

This *Sourcebook* describes the structure and function of the skin, hair, and nails and explains how lifestyle choices and aging affect them. It offers information about the diagnosis and treatment of acne, rosacea, rashes, allergic skin conditions, and skin problems caused by trauma, infection, and inflammation, including psoriasis and scleroderma. Chapters about pigmentation disorders, vascular skin changes, and benign skin growths are also included, along with comprehensive information about the diagnosis, treatment, and prevention of malignant skin conditions, such as basal cell carcinoma, squamous cell carcinoma, and melanoma. A glossary and a directory of resources provide further help and information.

How to Use This Book

This book is divided into parts and chapters. Parts focus on broad areas of interest. Chapters are devoted to single topics within a part.

Part I: Understanding the Skin, Hair, and Nails provides general information about the function and structure of the skin, hair, and nails. It describes how skin changes from adolescence to old age and highlights specific age-related concerns.

Part II: Acne, Rosacea, and Sweat Gland Disorders offers detailed information about acne, including risk factors, causes, diagnostic tests, and treatments. It also describes rosacea—a chronic disease that causes pimples, redness, and thickened skin—and sweat gland disorders, including hyperhidrosis, dyshidrosis, and hidradenitis suppurativa.

Part III: Rashes, Skin Signs of Systemic Diseases, and Allergic Skin Conditions begins with overview information about rashes in general. Additional chapters describe the specific skin signs of systemic diseases, such as dermatitis herpetiformis and dermatomyositis, and allergic skin conditions, including atopic dermatitis (eczema), contact dermatitis, diaper rash, seborrheic dermatitis, and rashes related to drug allergies and water exposure.

Part IV: Pigmentation Disorders, Vascular Skin Changes, and Benign Skin Growths includes detailed information about disorders that affect the skin's pigment, such as acanthosis nigricans, progressive pigmentary purpura, albinism, and vitiligo. Facts about the symptoms, diagnosis, and treatment of pigmented birthmarks and vascular skin changes are also included, as is information about skin tags, moles, dysplastic nevi, and the neurocutaneous syndromes, including neurofibromatosis and Sturge-Weber syndrome.

Part V: Malignant Skin Growths and Dermatological Side Effects of Cancer Treatment contains chapters about actinic keratoses, the precursors to skin cancer, as well as information about common types of skin cancer, such as basal cell carcinoma, squamous cell carcinoma, and melanoma. Facts about other types of cancers that involve the skin—including mycosis fungoides, Kaposi sarcoma, and Merkel cell carcinoma—and tips about caring for your skin, hair, and nails during cancer treatment are also included.

Part VI: Skin Trauma, Ulcering, and Blistering Disorders includes chapters about common skin injuries, such as bites, stings, corns, calluses, blisters, burns, and cuts. It also provides information on scarring and conditions that cause blistering and skin ulcers, such as epidermolysis bullosa and pemphigus.

Part VII: Infectious, Inflammatory, and Other Skin Conditions includes chapters on other common dermatological disorders, including warts, cold sores, chickenpox, shingles, head and pubic lice, scabies, psoriasis, and scleroderma.

Part VIII: Hair and Nail Disorders describes the causes and treatments for hair problems, such as hair loss and excess hair growth. Facts about disorders that affect the structure and function of the nail are also included.

Part IX: Dermatological Medications and Treatments provides information about nonsurgical and surgical dermatological treatments, including Botox, cosmetic laser surgery, chemical peels, dermabrasion, and hair loss treatments.

Part X: Skin Hygiene, Care, and Protection explains the basics of skin care with suggestions for special concerns related to the summer and winter seasons. It also discusses skin care needs of people with health conditions such as diabetes or lupus. Facts about health risks related to indoor tanning, tattoos, permanent makeup, body piercings, and hair-care products are also included, along with tips for nail care and safe hair removal.

Part XI: Additional Help and Information offers a glossary of important terms and a directory of government agencies and private organizations that provide help and information to patients with dermatological concerns.

Bibliographic Note

This volume contains documents and excerpts from publications issued by the following U.S. government agencies: Agency for Healthcare Research and Quality (AHRQ); Centers for Disease Control and Prevention (CDC); National Cancer Institute (NCI); National Institute of Allergy and Infectious Diseases (NIAID); National Institute of Arthritis and Musculoskeletal and Skin Diseases (NIAMS); National Institute of Child Health and Human Development; National Institute of Diabetes and Digestive and Kidney Diseases (NIDDK); National Institute of Neurological Disorders and Stroke (NINDS); National Institutes of Health (NIH); National Women's Health Information Center (NWHIC); U.S. Food and Drug Administration (FDA); and the Wisconsin Department of Health and Family Services.

In addition, this volume contains copyrighted documents from the following organizations and individuals: A.D.A.M., Inc.; American Academy of Dermatology; American College of Allergy, Asthma and Immunology; American Podiatric Medical Association; American Porphyria Foundation; American Pregnancy Association; American Osteopathic College of Dermatology (AOCD); American Social Health Association; American Society for Dermatologic Surgery; Camino Medical Group; Cleveland Clinic Foundation; Gale Group; Gluten Intolerance Group of North America; International Pemphigus Foundation; Lyme Disease Foundation; Heino F. L. Meyer-Bahlburg, M.D.; The Myositis Association; National Jewish Medical and Research Center; National Organization for Albinism and Hypopigmentation; National Women's Health Resource Center; Nemours Center for Children's Health Media; Marie New, M.D.; Skin Cancer Foundation; and University of Iowa's Virtual Hospital.

Full citation information is provided on the first page of each chapter. Every effort has been made to secure all necessary rights to reprint the copyrighted material. If any omissions have been made, please contact Omnigraphics to make corrections for future editions.

Acknowledgements

Thanks go to the many organizations, agencies, and individuals who have contributed materials for this *Sourcebook* and to medical consultant Dr. David Cooke, verification assistant Dawn Matthews, and document engineer Bruce Bellenir. Special thanks go to managing editor Karen Bellenir and permissions and research coordinator Liz Barbour for their help and support.

About the Health Reference Series

The *Health Reference Series* is designed to provide basic medical information for patients, families, caregivers, and the general public. Each volume takes a particular topic and provides comprehensive coverage. This is especially important for people who may be dealing with a newly diagnosed disease or a chronic disorder in themselves or in a family member. People looking for preventive guidance, information about disease warning signs, medical statistics, and risk factors for health problems will also find answers to their questions in the *Health Reference Series*. The *Series*, however, is not intended to serve as a tool for diagnosing illness, in prescribing treatments, or as a substitute for the physician/patient relationship. All people concerned about medical symptoms or the possibility of disease are encouraged to seek professional care from an appropriate health care provider.

Locating Information within the Health Reference Series

The *Health Reference Series* contains a wealth of information about a wide variety of medical topics. Ensuring easy access to all the fact sheets, research reports, in-depth discussions, and other material contained within the individual books of the *Series* remains one of our highest priorities. As the *Series* continues to grow in size and scope, however, locating the precise information needed by a reader may become more challenging.

A Contents Guide to the Health Reference Series was developed to direct readers to the specific volumes that address their concerns. It presents an extensive list of diseases, treatments, and other topics of general interest compiled from the Tables of Contents and major index headings. To access *A Contents Guide to the Health Reference Series*, visit www.healthreferenceseries.com.

Medical Consultant

Medical consultation services are provided to the *Health Reference Series* editors by David A. Cooke, M.D. Dr. Cooke is a graduate of Brandeis University, and he received his M.D. degree from the University of Michigan. He completed residency training at the University of Wisconsin Hospital and Clinics. He is board-certified in Internal Medicine. Dr. Cooke currently works as part of the University of Michigan Health System and practices in Ann Arbor, MI. In his free time, he enjoys writing, science fiction, and spending time with his family.

Our Advisory Board

We would like to thank the following board members for providing guidance to the development of this *Series*:

- Dr. Lynda Baker,
  Associate Professor of Library and Information Science,
  Wayne State University, Detroit, MI
- Nancy Bulgarelli,
  William Beaumont Hospital Library, Royal Oak, MI
- Karen Imarisio,
  Bloomfield Township Public Library, Bloomfield Township, MI
- Karen Morgan,
  Mardigian Library, University of Michigan-Dearborn,
  Dearborn, MI
- Rosemary Orlando,
  St. Clair Shores Public Library, St. Clair Shores, MI

Health Reference Series *Update Policy*

The inaugural book in the *Health Reference Series* was the first edition of *Cancer Sourcebook* published in 1989. Since then, the *Series* has been enthusiastically received by librarians and in the medical community. In order to maintain the standard of providing high-quality health information for the layperson the editorial staff at Omnigraphics felt it was necessary to implement a policy of updating volumes when warranted.

Medical researchers have been making tremendous strides, and it is the purpose of the *Health Reference Series* to stay current with the most recent advances. Each decision to update a volume is made on an individual basis. Some of the considerations include how much new information is available and the feedback we receive from people who use the books. If there is a topic you would like to see added to the update list, or an area of medical concern you feel has not been adequately addressed, please write to:

Editor
Health Reference Series
Omnigraphics, Inc.
615 Griswold Street
Detroit, MI 48226
E-mail: editorial@omnigraphics.com

Part One

Understanding the Skin, Hair, and Nails

Chapter 1

Skin, Hair, and Nails: Their Structure and Function

The skin is our largest organ. If the skin of a typical 150-pound (68-kilogram) adult male were stretched out flat, it would cover about 2 square yards (1.7 square meters) and weigh about 9 pounds (4 kilograms). Our skin protects the network of muscles, bones, nerves, blood vessels, and everything else inside our bodies. Our eyelids have the thinnest skin, the soles of our feet the thickest.

Hair is actually a modified type of skin. Hair grows everywhere on the human body except the palms of the hands, soles of the feet, eyelids, and lips. Hair grows more quickly in summer than winter, and more slowly at night than during the day.

Like hair, nails are a type of modified skin—and they're not just for beauty. Nails protect the sensitive tips of our fingers and toes. Human nails aren't necessary for living, but they do provide support for the tips of the fingers and toes, protect them from injury, and aid in picking up small objects. Without them, we'd have a hard time scratching an itch or untying a knot. Nails can be an indicator of a person's general health, and illness often affects their growth.

This information was provided by KidsHealth, one of the largest resources online for medically reviewed health information written for parents, kids, and teens. For more articles like this one, visit www.KidsHealth.org, or www.Teens Health.org. © 2003 The Nemours Center for Children's Health Media, a division of The Nemours Foundation. Reviewed by Wayne Ho, M.D., June 2003.

What Is the Skin and What Does It Do?

Skin is essential to a person's survival. It forms a barrier that prevents harmful substances and microorganisms from entering the body. It protects body tissues against injury. Our skin also controls the loss of life-sustaining fluids like blood and water, helps us regulate body temperature through perspiration, and protects us from the sun's damaging ultraviolet rays. Without the nerve cells in our skin, we couldn't feel warmth, cold, or other sensations. The erector pili muscles contract to make the hairs on our skin stand up straight when we're cold or frightened.

Every square inch of skin contains thousands of cells and hundreds of sweat glands, oil glands, nerve endings, and blood vessels. Skin is made up of three layers: the epidermis (pronounced: eh-puh-**dur**-mis), dermis, and the subcutaneous (pronounced: sub-kyoo-**tay**-nee-us) tissue.

The upper layer of our skin, the epidermis, is the tough, protective outer layer. It's about as thick as a sheet of paper over most parts of the body. The epidermis has four layers of cells that are constantly flaking off and being renewed. In these four layers are three special types of cells:

- Melanocytes (pronounced: meh-**lah**-nuh-sites) produce melanin, the pigment that gives skin its color. All people have roughly the same number of melanocytes; those of dark-skinned people produce more melanin. Exposure to sunlight increases the production of melanin, which is why people get suntanned or freckled.
- Keratinocytes (pronounced: ker-uh-**tih**-no-sites) produce keratin, a type of protein that is a basic component of hair and nails.
- Langerhans (pronounced: **lahng**-ur-hanz) cells help protect the body against infection.

Because the cells in the epidermis are completely replaced about every 28 days, cuts and bruises heal quickly.

Below the epidermis is the next layer of our skin, the dermis, which is made up of blood vessels, nerve endings, and connective tissue. The dermis nourishes the epidermis. Without certain molecules in the dermis, our skin wouldn't stretch when we bend nor reposition itself when we straighten up. These two types of molecules, collagen (pronounced: **kah**-luh-jen) and elastin (pronounced: ih-**las**-tin), combine in fibers in the dermis to give us our ease of movement. Collagen is strong and hard to stretch and elastin, as its name suggests, is elastic. In older people, some of the elastin-containing fibers disappear, which is one reason why the skin looks wrinkled.

The dermis also contains a person's sebaceous glands. These glands, which surround and empty into our hair follicles and pores, produce an oil called sebum (pronounced: **see**-bum) that lubricates the skin and hair. Sebaceous glands are found mostly in the skin on the face, upper back, shoulders, and chest.

Most of the time, the sebaceous glands make the right amount of sebum. As a person's body begins to mature and develop during the teenage years, though, hormones stimulate the sebaceous glands to make more sebum. When pores become clogged by too much sebum and too many dead skin cells, this causes acne. Later in life, these glands produce less sebum, which contributes to dry skin.

The bottom layer of our skin, the subcutaneous tissue, is made up of connective tissue, sweat glands, blood vessels, and cells that store fat. This layer helps protect the body from blows and other injuries and helps it hold in body heat.

There are two types of sweat-producing glands. The eccrine (pronounced: **eh**-krun) glands are found everywhere in our bodies, although they're mostly in the forehead, palms, and soles of the feet. By producing sweat, these glands help regulate body temperature, and waste products are excreted through them.

The other type of sweat-producing gland, the apocrine glands, develop at puberty and are concentrated in the armpits and pubic region. The sweat from the apocrine glands is thicker than that produced by the eccrine glands. Although this sweat doesn't smell, when it mixes with bacteria on the skin's surface, it can cause body odor. A normal, healthy adult secretes about 1 pint (about half a liter) of sweat daily, but this may be increased by physical activity, fever, or a hot environment.

What Is the Hair and What Does It Do?

The hair on our heads isn't just there for looks. It keeps us warm by preserving heat (we lose about 90% of our body heat through our heads). The hair in our nose, ears, and around our eyes protects these sensitive areas of the body from dust and other small particles. Eyebrows and eyelashes protect our eyes by decreasing the amount of light and particles that go into them. The fine hair that covers our bodies provides warmth and protects our skin. Hair also cushions the body against injury.

Human hair consists of the hair shaft, which projects from the skin's surface, and the root, a soft thickened bulb at the base of the hair embedded in the skin. The root ends in the hair bulb. The hair bulb sits in a sac-like pit in the skin called the follicle, from which the hair grows.

At the bottom of the follicle is the papilla, where hair growth actually takes place. The papilla contains an artery that nourishes the root of the hair. As cells multiply and produce keratin to harden the structure, they're pushed up the follicle and through the skin's surface as a shaft of hair. Each hair has three layers: the medulla at the center, which is soft; the cortex, which surrounds the medulla and is the main part of the hair; and the cuticle, the hard outer layer that protects the shaft.

Hair grows by forming new cells at the base of the root. These cells multiply to form a rod of tissue in the skin. The rods of cells move upward through the skin as new cells form beneath them. As they move up, they're cut off from their supply of nourishment and start to form a hard protein called keratin in a process called keratinization (pronounced: ker-uh-tuh-nuh-**zay**-shun). As this process occurs, the hair cells die. The dead cells and keratin form the shaft of the hair.

Each hair grows about 1/4 inch (about 6 millimeters) every month and keeps on growing for up to 6 years. The hair then falls out and another grows in its place. The length of a person's hair depends on the length of the growing phase of the follicle. Follicles are active for 2 to 6 years; they rest for about 3 months after that. A person becomes bald if the scalp follicles die and no longer produce new hair. Thick hair grows out of large follicles; narrow follicles produce thin hair.

The color of a person's hair is determined by the amount and distribution of melanin in the cortex of each hair (the same melanin that's found in the epidermis). Hair also contains a yellow-red pigment; people who have blonde or red hair have only a small amount of melanin in their hair. Hair becomes gray when people age because pigment no longer forms.

What Are the Nails and What Do They Do?

Nails grow out of deep folds in the skin of the fingers and toes. As epidermal cells below the nail root move up to the surface of the skin, they increase in number, and those closest to the nail root become flattened and pressed tightly together. Each cell is transformed into a thin plate; these plates are piled in layers to form the nail. As with hair, nails are formed by keratinization. When the nail cells accumulate, the nail is pushed forward.

The skin below the nail is called the matrix. The larger part of the nail, the nail plate, looks pink because of the network of tiny blood vessels in the underlying dermis. The whitish crescent-shaped area at the base of the nail is called the lunula.

Fingernails grow about three or four times as quickly as toenails. Like hair, nails grow more rapidly in summer than in winter. If a nail is torn off, it will regrow if the matrix isn't severely injured. White spots on the nail are sometimes due to temporary changes in growth rate.

What Can Go Wrong with the Skin, Hair, and Nails?

Some of the things that can affect the skin, nails, and hair are described below.

Dermatitis

Medical experts use the term dermatitis (pronounced: dur-muh-**tye**-tus) to refer to any inflammation (swelling, itching, and redness) of the skin. There are many types of dermatitis, including:

- **Atopic dermatitis (eczema).** It's a common, hereditary dermatitis that causes an itchy rash primarily on the face, trunk, arms, and legs. It commonly develops in infancy, but can also appear in early childhood. It may be associated with allergic diseases such as asthma.
- **Contact dermatitis** occurs when the skin comes into contact with an irritating substance. The best-known cause of contact dermatitis is poison ivy, but there are many others, including chemicals found in laundry detergent, cosmetics, and perfumes, and metals like the nickel plating on a belt buckle.
- **Seborrheic dermatitis**, an oily rash on the scalp, face, chest, and groin area, is caused by an overproduction of sebum from the sebaceous glands. This condition is common in young infants and adolescents.

Bacterial Skin Infections

- **Impetigo.** Impetigo (pronounced: im-puh-**tee**-go) is a bacterial infection that results in a honey-colored, crusty rash, usually on the face near the mouth and nose.

- **Cellulitis.** Cellulitis (pronounced: sell-yuh-**lye**-tus) is an infection of the skin and subcutaneous tissue that typically occurs when bacteria are introduced through a puncture, bite, or other break in the skin. The area with cellulitis is usually warm, tender, and has some redness.
- **Streptococcal and staphylococcal infections.** These two kinds of bacteria are the main causes of cellulitis and impetigo. Certain types of these bacteria are also responsible for distinctive rashes on the skin, including the rashes associated with scarlet fever and toxic shock syndrome.

Fungal Infections of the Skin and Nails

- **Candidal dermatitis.** A warm, moist environment, such as that found in the folds of the skin in the diaper area of infants, is perfect for growth of the yeast *Candida*. Yeast infections of the skin in older children, teens, and adults are uncommon.
- **Tinea infection (ringworm).** Ringworm, which isn't a worm at all, is a fungus infection that can affect the skin, nails, or scalp. Tinea (pronounced: **tih**-nee-uh) fungi can infect the skin and related tissues of the body. The medical name for ringworm of the scalp is tinea capitis; ringworm of the body is called tinea corporis; and ringworm of the nails is called tinea unguium. With tinea corporis, the fungi can cause scaly, ring-like lesions anywhere on the body.
- **Tinca pedis (athlete's foot).** This infection of the feet is caused by the same types of fungi that cause ringworm. Athlete's foot is commonly found in adolescents and is more likely to occur during warm weather.

Other Skin Problems

- **Parasitic infestations.** Parasites (usually tiny insects or worms) can feed on or burrow into the skin, often resulting in an itchy rash. Scabies and lice are examples of parasitic infestations. Both are contagious—meaning they can be easily caught from other people.
- **Viral infections.** Many viruses cause characteristic rashes on the skin, including varicella (pronounced: var-ih-**seh**-luh), the virus that causes chickenpox and shingles; herpes simplex,

which causes cold sores; papillomavirus (pronounced: pap-ih-**loh**-muh-vye-rus), the virus that causes warts; and a host of others.

- **Acne** (acne vulgaris). Acne is the single most common skin condition in teens. Some degree of acne is seen in 85% of adolescents, and nearly all teens have the occasional pimple, blackhead, or whitehead.

- **Skin cancer.** Skin cancer is rare in children and teens, but good sun protection habits established during these years can help prevent melanoma (pronounced: meh-luh-**no**-ma, a serious form of skin cancer that can spread to other parts of the body) later in life, especially among fair-skinned people who sunburn easily.

In addition to these diseases and conditions, the skin can be injured in a number of ways. Minor scrapes, cuts, and bruises heal quickly on their own, but other injuries—severe cuts and burns, for example—require medical treatment.

Disorders of the Scalp and Hair

- **Tinea capitis**, a type of ringworm, is a fungal infection that forms a scaly, ring-like lesion in the scalp. It's contagious and common among school-age children.

- **Alopecia** (pronounced: ah-luh-**pee**-sha) is an area of hair loss. Ringworm is a common cause of temporary alopecia in children. Alopecia can also be caused by tight braiding that pulls on the hair roots (this condition is called tension alopecia). Alopecia areata (where a person's hair falls out in round or oval patches on the scalp) is a rarer condition that can affect children and teens.

Chapter 2

What Happens When Skin Ages?

Aging Process

One or more benign lesions are present on the skin of virtually all individuals older than 65, and the incidence of skin cancer increases dramatically with age. Like all the body's tissues, the skin undergoes many changes in the course of the normal aging process:

- The cells divide more slowly, and the inner layer of skin (the dermis) starts to thin. Fat cells beneath the dermis begin to atrophy (diminish). In addition, the ability of the skin to repair itself diminishes with age, so wounds are slower to heal. The thinning skin becomes vulnerable to injuries and damage.
- The underlying network of elastin and collagen fibers, which provides scaffolding for the surface skin layers, loosens and unravels. Skin then loses its elasticity. When pressed, it no longer springs back to its initial position but instead sags and forms furrows.
- The sweat- and oil-secreting glands atrophy, depriving the skin of their protective water-lipid emulsions. The skin's ability to retain moisture then diminishes and it becomes dry and scaly.

Various blemishes and precancerous and cancerous lesions appear that are not only unsightly, but potentially serious and are also prevalent.

The skin is also more fragile and may bruise or tear easily and take longer to heal.

The Skin

The skin has three layers and consists of different cell types:

- The outer layer of the skin, the epidermis, is only about 20 cells deep, roughly as thick as a sheet of paper. It is composed of skin cells called keratinocytes. The top part of the epidermis, called the stratum corneum, or horny layer, is composed of dead keratinocytes that are constantly shed. The living keratinocytes underneath are referred to as squamous cells. The lowest part of the epidermis consists of basal cells. These are constantly reproducing from new keratinocytes.
- Below this layer lies the dermis, ranging in thickness from one to four millimeters (about 1/32 to 1/8 inch). The dermis contains tiny blood and lymph vessels, which increase in number deeper in the skin. The skin is the largest organ of the body. The skin and its derivatives (hair, nails, sweat and oil glands) make up the integumentary system. One of the main functions of the skin is protection. It protects the body from external factors such as bacteria, chemicals, and temperature. The skin contains secretions that can kill bacteria and the pigment melanin provides a chemical pigment defense against ultraviolet light that can damage skin cells. Another important function of the skin is body temperature regulation. When the skin is exposed to a cold temperature, the blood vessels in the dermis constrict. This allows the blood, which is warm, to bypass the skin. The skin then becomes the temperature of the cold it is exposed to. Body heat is conserved since the blood vessels are not diverting heat to the skin anymore. Among its many functions the skin is an incredible organ always protecting the body from external agents.
- Cells called melanocytes are found in the transitional layer between the epidermis and dermis. These skin cells produce a brown-black skin pigment called melanin, which helps to protect against the damaging rays of the sun and to determine skin coloring. As a person ages, melanocytes often proliferate, forming concentrated clusters that appear on the surface as small, dark, flat or dome-shaped spots, which are usually harmless moles or liver spots.

Ultraviolet Radiation, Sunlight, and Photoaging

The role of the sun cannot be overestimated as the most important cause of prematurely aging skin (called photoaging) and skin cancers. Overall, exposure to ultraviolet (referred to as UVA or UVB) radiation emanating from sunlight accounts for about 90% of the symptoms of premature skin aging, and most of these effects occur by age 20:

- Even small amounts of UV radiation trigger the process leading to skin wrinkles.
- Long-term repetitive and cumulative exposure to sunlight appears to be responsible for the vast majority of undesirable consequences of aging skin, including basal cell and squamous cell carcinomas.
- Melanoma is more likely to be caused by intense exposure to sunlight in early life.

UVA and UVB Radiation

When sunlight penetrates the top layers of the skin, ultraviolet (referred to as UVA or UVB) radiation bombards the genetic material, the DNA, inside the skin cells and damages it. Both UVB and UVA contribute to skin cancers and less serious skin blemishes, although the mechanisms are not yet fully clear.

- UVB is the primary agent in sunburning and primarily affects the outer skin layers. UVB is most intense at midday when sunlight is brightest. Slightly over 70% of the yearly UVB dose is received during the summer and only 28% is received during the remainder of the year.
- UVA penetrates more deeply and efficiently, however. UVA's intensity also tends to be less variable both during the day and throughout the year than UVB's. For example, only about half of the yearly UVA dose is received during the summer months and the balance is spread over the rest of the year. UVA is also not filtered through window glass (as is UVB).

Damaging Effects of UV Radiation

Both UVA and UVB rays cause damage, including genetic injury, wrinkles, lower immunity against infection, aging skin disorders, and cancer, although the mechanisms are not yet fully clear. The following are some ways in which cancer may develop and some defensive actions that the skin uses to defend itself against DNA damage.

- **Oxidation and Antioxidants.** The effects of UV radiation are implicated in the production of oxidants, also called free radicals. These are unstable molecules produced by normal chemical processes in the body that, in excess, can damage the body's cells and even alter their genetic material, contributing to the aging process and sometimes to cancer. The large surface area of the skin makes this organ a prime target for oxidants.
- **Defective DNA Repair and Protective Enzymes.** Some melanomas and other skin cancers are caused by a breakdown in the mechanisms that help repair DNA damage. This can occur from various causes, including an inherited condition called xeroderma pigmentosum (XP). A number of enzymes in the skin help protect against this damage. One repair enzyme called T4 endonuclease 5 (T4N5) is, in fact, being investigated in lotions to protect against skin cancers.
- **Breakdown of Immune Protection.** Specific immune factors protect the skin, including white blood cells called T lymphocytes and specialized skin cells called Langerhans cells. Such immune factors attack developing cancer cells at the very earliest stages. Unfortunately, certain substances in the skin, of note a chemical called urocanic acid, suppress such immune factors when exposed to sunlight, setting the stage for skin cancers.
- **Defective Cell Death (Apoptosis).** Apoptosis is the last defense of the immune system. It is a natural process of cell-suicide, which occurs when cells are very severely damaged. Apoptosis in the skin kills off cells harmed by UVA so that they do not turn cancerous. (The peeling after sunburn is the result of these dead skin cells.) In some cases, however, genetic mutations or other factors derail apoptosis. If this occurs, the cells can become immortal and continue to proliferate, resulting in skin cancers.

Other Factors Involved in Skin Aging

In addition to sunlight, other factors may hasten the skin-aging process.

Cigarette Smoke: Smoking produces oxygen-free radicals, which are known to accelerate wrinkles and aging skin disorders and increase the risk for nonmelanoma skin cancers. Studies also suggest that smoking and subsequent oxidation produce higher levels of metalloproteinases, which are enzymes associated with wrinkles.

Air Pollution: Ozone, a common air pollutant, may be a particular problem for the skin. One study reported that it might deplete the amount of vitamin E in the skin; this vitamin is an important antioxidant.

Who Is Most Likely to Have Skin Disorders As They Age?

Age and Risk

Exposure to Sun in Childhood: It is estimated that 50% to 80% of skin damage occurs in childhood and adolescence from intermittent, intense sun exposure that causes severe sunburns. In spite of this now well-known effect, many people still believe that a tan in children signifies health. And, even many parents who are concerned about sun exposure still rely too much on sunscreen and not enough on protective clothing.

The Elderly: Nearly half of people between the ages of 65 and 75 years old have at least one significant skin problem. And the majority of people over 75 have at least one skin disorder and many have three or four. Everyone experiences skin changes as they age, but a long life is not the sole determinant of aging skin. Family history, genetics, and behavioral choices all have a profound impact on the onset of aging-skin symptoms.

Activities Leading to Overexposure to Sunlight or Ultraviolet Radiation

Of all the risk factors for aging skin, exposure to UV radiation from sunlight is by far the most serious. Indeed, the vast majority of undesirable consequences of aging skin, including basal cell and squamous cell carcinomas, occur in individuals who are repetitively exposed to the sun. (Melanoma is more likely to be caused by intense exposure to sunlight in early life.) People at risk include the following:

- People who are outdoors for long periods of time either for work or leisure.

- People who regularly attend tanning salons or use tanning beds. A 2002 study indicated that regular use significantly increases the risk for nonmelanoma skin cancers. Fair women under age 50 were at particular risk.
- People who are treated with PUVA [psoralen (P) and ultraviolet light, type A (UVA)] for psoriasis or other skin problems. This procedure uses ultraviolet radiation. Unfortunately, researchers are finding that the increased cancer risks of PUVA may manifest 15 or more years after therapy. Psoriasis, in fact, may increase the risk for squamous cell carcinoma regardless of treatment.

Skin Types and Ethnic Groups

People with light skin, blue, gray, or green eyes, red or blond hair, and lots of freckles are at highest risk than people with other skin types for developing skin cancers, including melanoma. The risk increases for those who are easily sunburned and rarely tan, particularly if they live close to the equator where sunlight is most intense. One study noted that Caucasians, particularly men, who have fewer dark pigment (melanin) cells as measured in the upper inner arm were more likely to develop melanoma and other skin cancers. Darker ethnic groups or those with swarthy complexions are not immune, however.

Smokers

Cigarette smokers are more prone to skin cancers, including squamous cell carcinoma and giant basal cell carcinomas. And heavy smokers are almost five times as likely to have wrinkled facial skin than nonsmokers.

Radiation Therapy

Individuals who have received radiation therapy (such as radiation treatments for leukemia, goiters, ankylosing spondylitis) are at higher risk of developing basal cell carcinomas and squamous cell carcinomas.

What Dietary or Other Lifestyle Measures May Prevent Aging Skin Disorders?

Needless to say, the best long-term prevention for overly wrinkled skin is a healthy lifestyle including the following:

- **Eat Healthily.** A diet with plenty of whole grains, fresh fruits and vegetables, and the use of healthy oils (such as olive oil) may protect against oxidative stress in the skin. In fact, a 2001 study reported that people over 70 years old had fewer wrinkles if they ate such foods. Diet played a role in improving skin regardless of whether the people in the study smoked or lived in sunny countries. Benefits from these foods may be due to high levels of antioxidants found in them. One study indicated that reducing intake of saturated (animal fats) might significantly reduce the risk of actinic keratosis, a common aging skin disorder that can also be a precursor to skin cancer. Certain fatty acids, however, such as those found in monounsaturated fats (e.g., olive and canola oils) or fish oils, may help protect the skin against sun-related diseases.
- **Exercise.** Daily exercise keeps blood flowing, which brings oxygen to the skin, an important ingredient for healthy skin.
- **Reduce Stress.** Reducing stress and tension may have benefits on the skin.
- **Quit Smoking.** Smoking not only increases wrinkles, but smokers have a risk for squamous cell cancers that is 50% higher than nonsmokers' risk. Smokers should quit to prevent many health problems, not just unhealthy skin. The many methods of quitting smoking include counseling and support groups, nicotine patches, gums and sprays, and incremental reduction.

Antioxidant Products: General Information

Antioxidants are substances that act as scavengers of oxygen-free radicals, the unstable particles that can damage cells and are implicated in sun damage and even skin cancers. Antioxidants in the skin are depleted when exposed to sunlight and must be replaced.

- **Topical Products.** Antioxidant topical products (such ointments, creams, and lotions) may help reduce the risk of wrinkles and protect against sun damage. Unlike sunscreens, they accumulate in the skin and are not washed away, so the protection may last. The antioxidants marketed for skin protection include vitamins A, C, E, selenium, coenzyme Q10 (CoQ10), and alpha-lipoic acid. Many are proving to be very beneficial for the skin.
- **Oral Vitamins and Supplements.** Some research has been conducted on the effects on wrinkles using oral antioxidant supplements. One small study found that taking a combination of

vitamins oral C and E supplements may help reduce sunburn reactions, although the protection is much less than from sunscreens. Taking the vitamins singly did not have any effect. In fact, a 2002 study reported that oral vitamin C had no effect on sunburn reaction. Of concern, in the same study some natural antioxidants in the body were reduced in people who took the vitamin.

Vitamin A: Vitamin A is important for skin health and UV radiation produces deficiencies in the skin. Topical products containing natural forms of vitamin A (retinol, retinaldehyde) or vitamin A derivatives called retinoids (tretinoin, tazarotene) have proven to be beneficial for skin damaged by the sun and also by natural aging.

- *Tretinoin (Retin-A).* Tretinoin (known commercially as Retin-A) is the only topical agent approved for treating photoaging and is available in prescription form (Avita, Renova, Differin). This agent produces a rosy glow and reduces fine and large wrinkles, liver spots, and surface roughness. It also may help prevent more serious effects of ultraviolet radiation. Tretinoin may be applied to face, neck, chest, hands, and forearm and should be applied at least twice a week. Noticeable improvement takes from two to six months. Because Retin-A increases a person's sensitivity to the sun, a thin coat is best administered at bedtime. A sunblock should be worn during the day, and overexposure to the sun should be avoided. Almost all patients experience redness, scaling, burning, and itching after two or three days that can last up to three months. In women who experience irritation, a daytime moisturizer or low-dose corticosteroid cream, such as 1% hydrocortisone, may help. There is some concern that overuse of high-dose tretinoin may cause excessive skin thinness over time. Studies now suggest that low concentrations (as low as .02%) of tretinoin can produce significant improvements in wrinkles and skin color, with less irritation than at higher doses.
- *Retinol.* Retinol, a natural form of vitamin A, could not, until recently, be used in skin products because it was unstable and easily broken down by UV radiation. Stable preparations are now sold over the counter. In the right concentrations, retinol may be as effective as tretinoin and studies indicate that it has fewer side effects. An animal study suggests that adding antioxidant creams (such as those containing vitamins C or E) may offer added protection against degradation of retinol, but not tretinoin. The FDA warns that over-the-counter retinol skin products are unregulated;

the amount of active ingredients is unknown, and some preparations, in fact, may contain almost no retinol.

- *Tazarotene.* Tazarotene (Tazorac, Zorac, Avage) is a retinoid used for acne and psoriasis. It has now been approved for treating wrinkles, skin discoloration, and blemishes due to photoaging. One short-term study suggested that it may be as effective as tretinoin and even slightly better at high doses. At such high doses, however, it can cause very severe irritation. Redness and peeling may be reduced by administering tretinoin first to get the skin acclimated. More research is needed to determine if it produces any long-lasting significant benefits.

Warning: Any vitamin A derivative should be avoided by pregnant women and those who may become pregnant. For example, oral tretinoin causes birth defects and women should avoid even topical Retin-A when pregnant or trying to conceive.

Vitamin C: Vitamin C, or ascorbic acid, is a very potent antioxidant and most studies on the effects of antioxidants on the skin have used this vitamin. In laboratory studies, large amounts reduced skin swelling and protected immune factors from sunlight. It may even promote collagen production. Vitamin C by itself is unstable, but products that solve the delivery problem are now available (e.g., Cellex-C, Avon's Anew Formula C Treatment Capsules, Physician Elite, and others). Studies using these formations in 2002 (one using Cellex-C) reported reduction in wrinkles and appeared to improve skin thickness. In one of the studies, wrinkle improvement with a time-released vitamin C product was as effective as with topical retinoids and some laser treatments. Of concern, according to one 2002 study, ascorbyl palmitate, a vitamin C derivative found in many skin products, may actually increase skin damage from UV rays. More research is needed, since other studies have found this chemical to be protective.

Other Antioxidants: Other antioxidants are also being investigated for their value in skin protection. Even with these antioxidants, however, most available brands contain very low concentrations. In addition, they are also not well absorbed and they have a short-term effect. New delivery techniques, however, may prove to offset some of these problems.

- *Vitamin E.* Studies suggest that topical vitamin E, particularly alpha tocopherol (a form of vitamin E) cream decreased skin roughness, length of facial lines, and wrinkle depth. Studies on mice have also reported reductions in UV-induced skin cancer with its use.

- *Selenium* in the form of L-selenomethionine has protected against sun damage and even delayed skin cancer in animal studies. It is not known if such benefits apply to people.
- One 1999 study found that topical application of the antioxidant *Coenzyme Q10* (CoQ10) improved the skin's resistance to the oxidative stress of UV radiation, and when applied long-term, could reduce crow's feet.
- Both *green and black tea* may provide some protection against skin cancers and photoaging. A 2001 study using extracts of topical green tea suggested that it might protect against ultraviolet damage. Of interest was a study in which caffeine and caffeinated green and black tea had some preventive activity on skin tumors in mice. Decaffeinated tea, however, provided no benefits. Thus, while antioxidants in tea may be helpful, caffeine may also be important. In a 2002 study, researchers applied topical caffeine to mice that were exposed to UVB for 20 weeks. At the end of the study there was a small reduction of skin cancer activity.
- The substance *silymarin*, found in the milk thistle family (which includes artichokes), may inhibit UVB-promoted cancers in animals.
- *Aloe, ginger, lemon oil, grape seed extract, and coral extracts* contain antioxidants and are promoted as being healthy for the skin, although evidence of their effects on wrinkles is weak.

What Are Some Common Benign Aging Skin Disorders and What Are Their Treatments?

Wrinkles

In addition to avoiding the sun, hundreds of other methods and cosmetic products are available to retard the progress of wrinkles. Some may actually work to a degree.

Severe Itching (Pruritus) and Preventing Dry Skin

About 30% to 40% of people over age 70 suffer from severe itching (pruritus), which can occur generally or in specific areas, such as bald spots in men.

Causes: Itching can be caused by various conditions, including but not limited to the following:

- *Excessive dryness.* Dry skin is the cause of most cases of itching in older people. In some cases, it can become severe enough to cause general inflammation and even fissures in the skin. It most commonly develops on the legs in the winter.
- *Scabies.* These are tiny parasites typically located under the armpits, in the webs of fingers and toes, or around the ankles. It causes small red pimples, red patches, and scaling. In this case, the itch is usually worse at night.
- *Medications.* A number of drugs can cause itching and rash, particularly in response to sunlight. Stopping the drug resolves both the itch and rash. Common drugs that can cause this reaction include calcium channel blockers and thiazides (which are used for high blood pressure), common pain relievers known as NSAIDs (such as ibuprofen, naproxen, and aspirin and antibiotics).
- *Eczema.*
- *Symptoms of Serious Illness.* In rare cases, itching may be symptomatic of an underlying serious disease, so any persistent itching without an obvious cause should be reported to a physician. Such diseases include systemic lupus erythematosus (lupus), dermatomyositis, lymphomas, iron deficiency, liver and kidney disease, diabetes, and thyroid abnormalities.

Treating Dry Skin: The following measures may be helpful:

- Moisturizing the skin is the most important first step. Patients should avoid hot baths and most soaps. They should take short lukewarm showers and apply oils or moisturizing lotions while the skin is still damp. Moisturizers containing aluminum lactate (AmLactin, Lac-Hydrin) are best, although they can have some side effects, including stinging, and may interact with certain drugs.
- Colloidal preparations added to a lukewarm bath may be helpful. These are available in drugstores (e.g., Aveeno) or can be made at home by preparing a paste of two cups of Linit starch, cornstarch, or oatmeal plus four cups of water. The combination should be boiled then added to a tub half-filled with water. It is

important to stress that these preparations may make the tub slippery.

- For specific itchy areas, over-the-counter lotions may be helpful that contain calamine, menthol, and phenol or combinations of all these ingredients (Sarna, Calamine Lotion, Schamberg's Lotion, Rhuli cream).
- Cold compresses may provide temporary relief.
- Over-the-counter antihistamines, such as Benadryl, that are administered in the evening can help with generalized itching. (It should be noted that Benadryl will cause significant sedation if it is used during the day.)
- Treatment from the physician may include topical corticosteroids (commonly called steroids), anti-itching creams containing the ingredients doxepin or pramoxine, or mild tranquilizers. Some experts do not recommend steroid creams, since in some cases overuse of corticosteroids can cause itchiness, particularly in aged, sun-exposed skin. In some severe cases, phototherapy with UVB radiation is helpful.

Liver Spots

Liver spots (medically referred to as lentigos or sun-induced or pigmented lesions) are flat brown spots on the skin. They are almost universal signs of aging. Occurring most noticeably on the hands and face, these blemishes tend to enlarge and darken over time. The extent and severity of the spots are determined by a combination of skin type, sun exposure, and age. These spots are harmless, but should be distinguished from lentigo maligna, which is an early sign of melanoma.

Liver spots or age spots are a type of skin change that are associated with aging. The increased pigmentation may be brought on by exposure to sun, or other forms of ultraviolet light, or other unknown causes.

Treating Liver Spots: They do not require treatment, although some people are distressed by their appearance. Treatments may include the following:

- Trichloroacetic acid (a chemical peel).
- Tretinoin (Retin-A) alone or in a combination with mequinol (Solagé). Tretinoin is a vitamin A derivative and is also effective in treating wrinkles.

- Gentle freezing with liquid nitrogen (cryotherapy).
- Laser treatment. Specific lasers are effective in eliminating 80% of liver spots in one treatment. (It may be more effective than cryotherapy and have fewer adverse effects.)
- Bleaching creams. These are commonly available but are not as satisfactory as peels, and high concentrations can sometimes cause permanent loss of color.

Chapter 3

Varicose Veins and Spider Veins

What are varicose veins and spider veins?

The heart pumps blood to supply oxygen and nutrients to all parts of the body. Arteries carry blood from the heart toward the body parts, whereas veins carry blood from the body parts back to the heart. As the blood is pumped back to the heart, veins act as one-way valves to prevent the blood from flowing backward. If the one-way valve becomes weak, some of the blood can leak back into the vein, collect there, and then become congested or clogged. This congestion will cause the vein to abnormally enlarge. These enlarged veins can be either varicose veins or spider veins.

Varicose veins are very swollen and raised above the surface of the skin. They are dark purple or blue in color, and can look like cords or very twisted and bulging. They are found most often on the backs of the calves or on the inside of the leg, anywhere from the groin to the ankle. During pregnancy, varicose veins called hemorrhoids can form in the vagina or around the anus.

Spider veins are similar to varicose veins, but they are smaller, are often red or blue in color, and are closer to the surface of the skin than varicose veins. They can look like a tree branch or spiderweb with their short jagged lines. Spider veins can be found on both the legs and the face. They can cover either a very small or very large area of skin.

Excerpted from the article by the National Women's Health Information Center, December 2000. Available online at http://www.4woman.gov; accessed February 2005.

How common are abnormal leg veins?

As many as 60% of all American women and men suffer from some form of vein disorder, but women are more affected—up to 50% overall. It also is estimated that 41% of all women will suffer from abnormal leg veins by the time they are in their fifties.

What causes varicose and spider veins?

No one knows the exact cause of spider and varicose veins, but there are several factors that cause a person to be more likely to develop them. Heredity, or being born with weak vein valves, is the greatest factor. Hormones also play a role. The hormonal changes that occur during puberty, pregnancy, and menopause, as well as taking estrogen, progesterone, and birth control pills can cause a woman to develop varicose veins or spider veins. During pregnancy, besides the increases in hormone levels, there also is a great increase in the volume of blood in the body that can cause veins to enlarge. The enlarged uterus also puts more pressure on the veins. (Within 3 months after delivery, varicose veins usually improve. However, more abnormal veins are likely to develop and remain after additional pregnancies.)

Other factors that weaken vein valves and that may cause varicose or spider veins include aging, obesity, leg injury, and prolonged standing, such as for long hours on the job. Spider veins on the cheeks or nose of a fair-skinned person may occur from sun exposure.

How are varicose and spider veins treated?

Besides a physical examination, your doctor can take x-rays or ultrasound pictures of the vein to assess the cause and severity of the problem. You may want to speak with a doctor who specializes in vein diseases (phlebology). You should discuss which treatment options are best for your condition and lifestyle. It is important to remember that not all cases of varicose veins are the same. Doctors may differ in the ways they treat you. Some available treatments or surgeries include:

Sclerotherapy: Of all available treatments, this one is most commonly used for both spider veins and varicose veins. It involves injecting a solution into the vein that causes the lining of the vein walls to swell, stick together, and eventually seal shut. The flow of blood is stopped and the vein turns into scar tissue. In a few weeks, the vein should fade. Although the same vein may need to be injected with the solution more than once, sclerotherapy is very effective if done correctly. The American Academy of Dermatology states that most patients can expect a 50% to 90% improvement. Also, a new and improved type of sclerotherapy called microsclerotherapy uses improved solutions and injection techniques that increase the success rate for removal of spider veins. Sclerotherapy does not require anesthesia, and can be done in the doctor's office.

Some side effects may only occur at the site of the injection, such as stinging or painful cramps; red raised patches of skin, small skin ulcers, and bruises. Spots, brown lines, or groups of fine red blood vessels could appear around the vein being treated. These usually disappear. The treated vein could become inflamed or develop lumps of coagulated or congested blood. These are not dangerous. Applying heat and taking aspirin or antibiotics can relieve inflammation. Lumps of coagulated blood can be drained. Health insurance coverage varies. If the treatment is done for cosmetic reasons only, it may not be covered.

Electrodesiccation: This treatment is similar to sclerotherapy except the veins are sealed off with an electrical current instead of the injection of solution. This treatment may leave scars.

Laser surgery: Until recently, laser treatments mostly were used for treating spider veins on the face. Varicose veins in the legs did not respond consistently to this treatment, and some doctors doubted whether laser treatment actually worked, and it was not covered by most health insurance plans. Now, however, new technology in laser treatments can effectively treat varicose veins in the legs.

Laser surgery works by sending very strong bursts of light onto the vein that makes the vein slowly fade and disappear. Lasers are very direct and accurate, and only damage the area being treated. All skin types and colors can be safely treated with lasers. The American Academy of Dermatology believes that the new laser technology is more effective with fewer side effects. Laser surgery is more comfortable for patients because there are no needles or incisions. When the laser hits the skin, the patient only feels a small pinch, and the skin is soothed by cooling both before and after the laser is applied. There may be some redness or swelling of the skin right after the treatment, but this disappears within a few days. The skin also may be discolored, but this will disappear within one to two weeks. Treatments last 15 to 20 minutes, and depending on the severity of the veins, two to five treatments are generally needed to remove varicose veins in the legs. Patients can return to normal activity right after treatment.

There are several types of lasers that can be used to treat varicose veins and spider veins on the legs and face. Although your doctor will decide which type is best to treat your condition, some of the lasers used to treat veins include yellow light lasers, green light lasers, and other intense pulsed light systems. Again, health insurance coverage varies. If the treatment is done for cosmetic reasons only, it may not be covered.

Closure Technique: The U.S. Food and Drug Administration (FDA) in March 1999 approved this procedure for use in the United States. Although it is not as widely used as sclerotherapy, some doctors feel it may become the standard for treating varicose veins. It is not very invasive and can be done in a doctor's office. This method involves placing a special catheter or a very small tube into the vein. Once inside, the catheter sends radiofrequency energy to cause the vein wall to shrink and seal shut. Healthier veins surrounding the closed vein can then restore the normal flow of blood. As this happens, symptoms from the varicose vein decrease. The only side effect is slight bruising.

Surgery: Surgery is used mostly to treat very large varicose veins. Available surgical options include:

- *Surgical Ligation and Stripping*—With this treatment, the veins are tied shut and completely removed from the leg. Removing the veins will not affect the circulation of blood in the leg because veins deeper in the leg take care of the larger volumes of blood. The varicose veins mostly removed through surgery are superficial or surface veins, and collect blood only from the skin. This surgery requires either local or general anesthesia and must be done in an operating room on an outpatient basis.

  Serious side effects or complications with this surgery are uncommon. However, with general anesthesia, there always is a risk of cardiac and respiratory complications. Similar to the risks of sclerotherapy, bleeding and congestion of blood can be a problem, but the collected blood usually settles on its own and does not require any further treating. Wound infection, inflammation, swelling, and redness also can occur. This surgery also can leave permanent scars. A very common complication is the damage of nerve tissue around the treated vein. Small sensory nerve branches are difficult to avoid when veins are removed. This damage can cause numbness in small areas of skin, burning, or a change in sensation around the surgical scar. The most serious, but rare, complication of surgery is the creation of a deep vein blood clot that may travel to the lungs and heart. To be safe, many surgeons give injections of heparin, a drug that reduces blood coagulation, for one to two days before the surgery. However, heparin also can increase the normal amount of bleeding and bruising after the operation.

- *Ambulatory Phlebectomy*—With this surgery, a special light source marks the location of the vein. Tiny incisions are made in the vein, and then with surgical hooks, the vein is pulled out of the leg. This surgery requires local or regional anesthesia. The vein usually is removed in one treatment. Side effects and complications are similar to those of ligation and stripping. The most common side effect is slight bruising. Compared to traditional surgery, ambulatory phlebectomy allows the removal of very large varicose veins while leaving only very small scars. Patients can return to normal activity the day after treatment.

Chapter 4

Stretch Marks during Adolescence

Stretch marks are a normal part of puberty for most girls and guys. When a person grows or gains weight really quickly (like during puberty), that person may get fine lines on the body called stretch marks. Stretch marks happen when the tissue under the skin is pulled by rapid growth or stretching. Although the skin is usually fairly elastic, when it's overstretched, the normal production of collagen (the major protein that makes up the connective tissue in your skin) is disrupted. As a result, scars called stretch marks may form.

If you're noticing stretch marks on your body, you're not alone—most girls and women have stretch marks (in girls, they tend to show up on places like the breasts, thighs, hips, and butt, and many women get them during pregnancy). And although stretch marks are more common in girls, guys can get them, too.

Bodybuilders are more prone to getting stretch marks because of the rapid body changes that bodybuilding can produce. People who are obese often have stretch marks. Stretch marks are also more likely to occur if a person uses steroid-containing creams or ointments (such as hydrocortisone) on their skin for more than a few weeks, or if a person has to take high doses of corticosteroids by mouth for months or longer.

"Stretch Marks," provided by KidsHealth, one of the largest resources online for medically reviewed health information written for parents, kids, and teens. For more articles like this one, visit www.KidsHealth.org, or www.TeensHealth.org. Reviewed by Patrice Hyde, M.D., April 2004.

At first, stretch marks may show up as reddish or purplish lines that may appear indented and have a different texture from the surrounding skin. Fortunately, stretch marks often turn lighter (whitish or flesh-colored) and almost disappear over time. But the fact that stretch marks usually fade and become less noticeable over time can be little consolation if you plan to spend most of your summer in a bathing suit.

There are some things that you can do to make stretch marks less noticeable.

Some people find that sunless tanning treatments (both over-the-counter lotions and sprays and in-salon types of treatments) can help cover up stretch marks. This doesn't work for regular tanning or tanning beds, though, because stretch marks themselves are less likely to tan. (And as everyone knows, the sun and tanning beds do more harm than good when it comes to the long-term health of your skin). You can also buy body makeup that, when matched to the tone of your skin, makes stretch marks all but invisible. Although some manufacturers make these cover-up products water-resistant, makeup may not be the best solution if you'll be spending a lot of time in the water.

Speaking of pool or beach time, the good news is that current fashion favors many styles of bathing suits that also just happen to hide stretch marks. "Boy short" style suits (popular with many athletes because they don't ride up when a person moves) work well for hiding stretch marks on the buttocks and upper thighs. And because many swimmers prefer high-neck bathing suits, which can hide stretch marks in the chest area, there are usually lots of styles to choose from.

Although there are tons of creams and other skin products on the market that claim to eliminate stretch marks, the truth is that most of these products are ineffective and often costly. You can't make stretch marks go away entirely without the help of a dermatologist (a doctor who specializes in treating skin problems) or plastic surgeon. These doctors may use one of many types of treatments, from actual surgery to techniques such as microdermabrasion and laser treatment, that reduce the appearance of stretch marks. These techniques are expensive and are not usually recommended for people in their teen years because they are not finished growing and their stretch marks will probably diminish over time anyway.

Chapter 5

Skin Changes during Pregnancy

Now that you are pregnant your skin may begin to change right before your very eyes. Your skin can change from a sudden new glow on your face to pinkish, reddish streaks on your stomach. Not every pregnant woman will experience all the same skin changes. Below is a list of skin changes that are common during pregnancy.

Stretch Marks

What is this? Stretch marks are one of the most famous and talked about skin changes that can occur during pregnancy. Almost 90% of pregnant woman will experience stretch marks. Stretch marks appear as pinkish or reddish streaks running down your abdomen and/or breasts.

What can I do? Exercising and applying lotions that contain vitamin E and alpha hydroxy acids have been said to help in the prevention of stretch marks. These remedies have not been medically proven to have a direct effect on stretch marks but it never hurts to try. If you find that nothing is working for you, take comfort in knowing that these streaks will fade to silvery faint lines after delivery.

Reprinted with permission from the American Pregnancy Association, http://www.americanpregnancy.org,

Mask of Pregnancy

What is this? Mask of pregnancy is also referred to as melasma and chloasma. Melasma causes dark splotchy spots to appear on your face. These spots most commonly appear on your forehead and cheeks and are a result of increased pigmentation. When you become pregnant your body produces more hormones, which causes an increase in your pigmentation. Nearly 50% of pregnant women show some signs of the mask of pregnancy.

What can I do? To prevent mask of pregnancy from happening to you, you should wear a good sunscreen that is at least SPF 15 whenever you plan on being outside. You can also wear your favorite ball cap to protect you face from the sun. Your skin is extra sensitive, and the sun increases your chances of these dark spots showing up on your face.

Pregnancy Glow

What is this? When you are pregnant your body produces 50% more blood, resulting in more blood circulation through your body. This increase in blood circulation causes your face to be brighter. Your body is also producing a fair amount of hormones that cause your oil glands to work in over drive, leaving your face shiny. Both of these things can result in the pregnancy glow you have heard of.

What can I do? If your skin becomes too oily you can use an oil-free cleanser to clean your face. Other than that, do nothing but smile!

Pimple Breakouts and Acne

What is this? If you have a problem with acne already, your acne may become more irritated during pregnancy or it may just clear up. The extra hormones in your body cause your oil glands to secrete more oil, which can cause breakouts.

What can I do? You should keep a strict cleansing routine. You can start with a simple over-the-counter face soap. It is a good idea to use fragrance free soap to avoid nausea. Cleanse your face every night and every morning. Washing your face more than this can cause your skin to be dry. Next use an astringent to remove any remaining oil. Stay away from any acne-medicated astringents; they may contain acne medicine that may not be recommended for pregnant women.

Finally, follow this procedure with an oil-free moisturizer. If you find that you are having problems with acne consult with your doctor on acne treatment during pregnancy.

Varicose Veins

What are these? Varicose veins are bulky bluish veins that usually appear on the legs during pregnancy. This happens because your body is compensating for the extra blood flow that is going to your baby. Varicose veins can be uncomfortable and sometimes painful. Unfortunately if you have a family history of varicose veins, you may be prone to get them during your pregnancy. The good news is that you can take measures now to prevent or decrease the symptoms.

What can I do? To prevent or decrease symptoms, you should:

- Avoid standing for long periods of time.
- Walk as much as possible, to help the blood return to your heart.
- Always prop your feet up on a stool when sitting.
- Avoid sitting for long periods of time.
- Wear support stockings.
- Get enough vitamin C (this helps keeps your veins healthy and elastic).
- Sit with your legs higher than your head for at least half an hour a day.
- Avoid excessive weight gain.

Spider Veins

What are these? Spider veins, also known as spider nevi, are minute reddish tiny blood vessels that branch outward. These spider veins are also caused by the increase in blood circulation. They will usually appear on the face, neck, upper chest, and arms. Spider veins do not hurt and usually disappear shortly after delivery. Spider veins appear more often in Caucasian women than in African American women.

What can I do? Increasing your vitamin C intake and not crossing your legs can help minimize spider veins. Spider veins may also be hereditary in which case there is nothing you can do to prevent them. Fortunately, these will most likely fade shortly after delivery. Laser treatment can also be done to help remove any spider veins that have not faded away.

Dry Itchy Abdomen

What is this? As your beautiful belly grows, your skin stretches and tightens. This causes very uncomfortable dryness and itching. If you begin to experience severe itching late in your pregnancy, possibly accompanied by nausea, vomiting, loss of appetite, fatigue, and possibly jaundice, you should contact your doctor. This could be a sign of cholestasis, which is related to the function of the liver. Your doctor may take blood tests to verify if you are experiencing cholestasis. Cholestasis occurs in about one in every 50 pregnancies and is not a problem after pregnancy.

If the itching is intense and spreads to your arms and legs it could be pruritic urticarial papules and plagues (PUPP). PUPP occurs in about one in every 150 pregnancies. PUPP is itchy, reddish, raised patches on the skin that will go away after delivery.

What can I do? To help alleviate your dry itchy abdomen, you should keep your abdomen moisturized. You can also use anti-itch cream such as calamine lotion to help provide more relief. Cholestasis can be treated with medications. To help alleviate PUPP your doctor can prescribe oral medicine and anti-itch creams. Try taking a nice oatmeal bath to help relieve some of the discomfort.

Linea Nigra

What is this? Linea nigra is the dark line that runs from your navel to your pubic bone. This is a white line that may have always been there, but you may have never noticed. Linea nigra is possibly caused by hormonal imbalance and appears around the fourth or fifth month of pregnancy.

What can I do? There is nothing you can do to prevent this from happening, but after your pregnancy this line will fade.

Skin Tags

What are these? Skin tags are very small, loose growths of skin that usually appear under your arms or breasts.

What can I do? After pregnancy you skin tags may disappear. If they do not disappear, there are ways to remove them.

Darkening of Freckles, Moles, and Other Areas of Your Skin

What is this? Increased hormones cause changes in your skin pigmentation. You will notice that areas with dark pigmentation, such as freckles, moles, nipples, areolas, and labia, can become even darker.

What can I do? There is nothing you can do to prevent this from happening. If you notice that a mole of freckle changes in appearance or shape you should contact your doctor. These darker areas can remain darkened after pregnancy. The change in pigmentation can be noticeable, but not drastic.

Chapter 6

Age-Related Changes in Skin, Hair, and Nails

Chapter Contents

Section 6.1

Age-Related Skin Changes

"Turning Back the Hands of Time: Dermatologists Treat the Five Ways the Face Ages" is reprinted with permission from the American Academy of Dermatology.

You may look in the mirror and notice a wrinkle here or there that you would like to be a little less obvious. Or you may note the overall changes to your face as you age and want a more youthful appearance. No matter what your needs, dermatologists can provide treatment options to revitalize the appearance of the skin.

Melvin Elson, M.D., of Nashville, Tenn., discussed the five types of aging that occur on the face and how dermatologic treatments can improve the skin's texture and return its youthful glow.

"Dermatologists evaluate a patient with aging facial skin for many different factors, including how well the face is aging overall; is there obvious damage to the skin's surface; what does this damage look like; and how deep does it go," stated Dr. Elson. "Once we have a picture of what has occurred on the face over time, dermatologists can identify the steps necessary to reverse the damage—whether that be through a single treatment or a combination of several treatments."

Dr. Elson has identified five independent factors that act together to affect the appearance of the aging face.

Intrinsic Aging

Intrinsic aging is the natural process of aging that begins late in life and is characterized by a loss of substance to the skin and the underlying fat resulting in a gaunt, thin look with hollowed cheeks and eye sockets. The treatment options for this type of aging are aimed at replacement of the lost tissue, such as solid implants, which are surgically placed under the skin, or fat transfer, where fat and tissue from other parts of the patients' body are used to fill in deeper wrinkles and contour the "hills and valleys" associated with aging.

Sleep Lines

Much as a napkin gets a crease when it is folded in a drawer too long, sleep lines etch the surface of the skin and occur from putting the face into the same position on the pillow every night. "Even though these lines may seem to diminish or disappear once a patient is no longer lying in bed, if the patient assumes the same sleeping posture every evening, these lines will return creating more damage," said Dr. Elson. Due to different sleep patterns, women tend to see these types of lines on their chin and cheeks, while men notice them on their foreheads.

Since changing sleep positions is challenging for some patients, dermatologists recommend the use of botulinum rejuvenation to hold the skin taut. Botulinum rejuvenation is an increasingly popular cosmetic procedure where dermatologists carefully inject a low dose of botulinum toxin into a patient's facial muscles, causing temporary relaxation of the injected muscles. The procedure is non-invasive, features practically no recovery time, and can safely and effectively reduce the appearance of facial lines, crow's feet, and wrinkles when performed by a qualified physician.

Expression Lines

Every smile, frown, and laugh affects the face, especially the collagen fibers beneath it. Expression lines are commonly referred to as "laugh lines" and are most noticeable around the large muscles of the eyes and the mouth. While most people do not find these types of lines funny, there is no way to change the way the face reacts to emotion.

One of a dermatologist's most effective treatments for softening or removing these lines is the use of botulinum rejuvenation. Another treatment option is soft-tissue augmentation and a dermatologist can assist patients in selecting from the variety of Food and Drug Administration-approved wrinkle fillers, which produce immediate, yet temporary, results to improve the appearance of lines.

Gravity

No one is immune to the effects of gravity on their body. For the face, this means that as soon as we stand, everything moves downwards—the eyelids fall, the jowls form, the nose tip points downward, the upper lip disappears while the lower lip pouts and even the ears get longer. These facial changes related to gravity become more pronounced as we age.

"No amount of facial exercises or 'good genes' can offset the pull of gravity," stated Dr. Elson. "Dermatologic treatments for the everyday effects of gravity remain surgical, such as a blepharoplasty, a surgical procedure to correct the 'droopy' look of eyelids. Because surgical procedures are invasive and require extensive downtime, it's important to discuss with your dermatologist the option that is right for your lifestyle."

Photodamage

More than 80 percent of the damage on an aging face is from photodamage, which occurs from overexposure to the elements, including the sun and the wind. Individuals with fair skin, light eyes, and a history of long-term sun exposure are more susceptible to photodamage, which is represented by blotchy pigmentation, wrinkling, and scaling.

Dermatologists have a variety of innovative techniques which can improve the appearance of photodamaged skin, including laser resurfacing, a treatment option where heat or light pulses from a laser are used to rejuvenate the skin's tone and texture and minimize fine lines. Depending on the type of laser used, moderate to advanced fine lines and deeper wrinkles can be treated with very little downtime.

An alternative to lasers are chemical peels, which remove levels of the skin to stimulate rapid rejuvenation. The strength of chemical peels can vary from very superficial to deep, and this strength determines the benefit to the skin and the downtime following this procedure. "Aging skin is a fact of life, but patients today need to know that dermatologists can offer them more options than ever before," said Dr. Elson. "It is important that anyone considering a cosmetic procedure for the treatment of the aging face consult with a dermatologist to discuss their expectations and select the best treatment available."

Section 6.2

Age-Related Hair and Nail Changes

Hair Color Changes

Hair color change is probably one of the most obvious signs of aging. Hair color is caused by a pigment (melanin) that is produced by the hair follicle. With aging, the follicle produces less melanin.

Graying often begins in the 30s, although this varies widely. Graying usually begins at the temples and extends to the top of the scalp. Hair becomes progressively lighter, eventually turning white.

By the time they are in their 40s, about 40% of all people have some gray scalp hair. Body and facial hair also turn gray, but usually later than scalp hair. The hair in the armpit, chest, and pubic area may gray less or not at all.

Graying is genetically determined. Gray hair tends to occur earlier in Caucasians and later in Asian races. Nutritional supplements, vitamins, and other products will not stop or decrease the rate of graying.

Hair Thickness Changes

Hair is a protein strand that grows through an opening (follicle) in the skin. A single hair has a normal life cycle of about 4 or 5 years. That hair then falls out and is replaced with a new hair.

How much hair you have on your body and head is determined by your genetic make up. However, almost everyone experiences some hair loss with aging. The rate of hair growth slows.

The hair strands become smaller (and have less pigment), so the thick coarse hair of a young adult eventually becomes thin, fine, light-colored hair.

Many of the hair follicles stop producing new hairs. Both men and women lose hair as they age. About 25% of men begin to show some signs of baldness by the time they are 30 years old, and about two thirds are either bald or have a balding pattern by age 60.

Men develop a typical pattern of baldness associated with the male hormone testosterone (male-pattern baldness). Hair is lost first from the front and top of the scalp.

Women also show a typical pattern of hair loss as they age (female-pattern baldness). The hair becomes less dense all over and the scalp may become visible.

Body and facial hair are also lost. Although the number of hairs is less, individual hairs may become coarser. Women may notice a loss of body hair but may find that they have coarse facial hair, especially on the chin and around the lips.

Men may find the hair of their eyebrows, ears, and nose becoming longer and coarser.

Nail Changes

The nails also change with aging. They grow slower and become dull and brittle. The color may change from translucent to yellowed and opaque.

Nails, especially toenails, may become hard and thick and ingrown toenails may be more common. The tips of the fingernails may fragment.

Sometimes, longitudinal (lengthwise) ridges will develop in the fingernails and toenails. This can be a normal aging change. However, some nail changes can be caused by infections, nutritional problems, trauma, and other problems.

It is a good idea to check with your health care provider if your nails develop pits, ridges, lines, changed shape, or other changes.

Part Two

Acne, Rosacea, and Sweat Gland Disorders

Chapter 7

Questions and Answers about Acne

This chapter contains general information about acne. It describes what acne is and how it develops, the causes of acne, and the treatment options for various forms of acne. Information is also provided on caring for the skin. If you have further questions after reading this chapter, you may wish to discuss them with your doctor.

What Is Acne?

Acne is a disorder resulting from the action of hormones on the skin's oil glands (sebaceous glands), which leads to plugged pores and outbreaks of lesions commonly called pimples or zits. Acne lesions usually occur on the face, neck, back, chest, and shoulders. Nearly 17 million people in the United States have acne, making it the most common skin disease. Although acne is not a serious health threat, severe acne can lead to disfiguring, permanent scarring, which can be upsetting to people who are affected by the disorder.

How Does Acne Develop?

Doctors describe acne as a disease of the pilosebaceous units (PSUs). Found over most of the body, PSUs consist of a sebaceous gland connected to a canal, called a follicle, that contains a fine hair. These units are most numerous on the face, upper back, and chest. The sebaceous

---

National Institute of Arthritis and Musculoskeletal and Skin Diseases, October 2001. Available online at http://www.niams.nih.gov; accessed March 29, 2005.

glands make an oily substance called sebum that normally empties onto the skin surface through the opening of the follicle, commonly called a pore. Cells called keratinocytes line the follicle.

The hair, sebum, and keratinocytes that fill the narrow follicle may produce a plug, which is an early sign of acne. The plug prevents sebum from reaching the surface of the skin through a pore. The mixture of oil and cells allows bacteria *Propionibacterium acnes* (*P. acnes*) that normally live on the skin to grow in the plugged follicles. These bacteria produce chemicals and enzymes and attract white blood cells that cause inflammation. (Inflammation is a characteristic reaction of tissues to disease or injury and is marked by four signs: swelling, redness, heat, and pain.) When the wall of the plugged follicle breaks down, it spills everything into the nearby skin—sebum, shed skin cells, and bacteria—leading to lesions or pimples.

People with acne frequently have a variety of lesions. The basic acne lesion, called the comedo, is simply an enlarged and plugged hair follicle. If the plugged follicle, or comedo, stays beneath the skin, it is called a closed comedo and produces a white bump called a whitehead. A comedo that reaches the surface of the skin and opens up is called a blackhead because it looks black on the skin's surface. This black discoloration is not due to dirt. Both whiteheads and blackheads may stay in the skin for a long time.

Other troublesome acne lesions can develop, including the following:

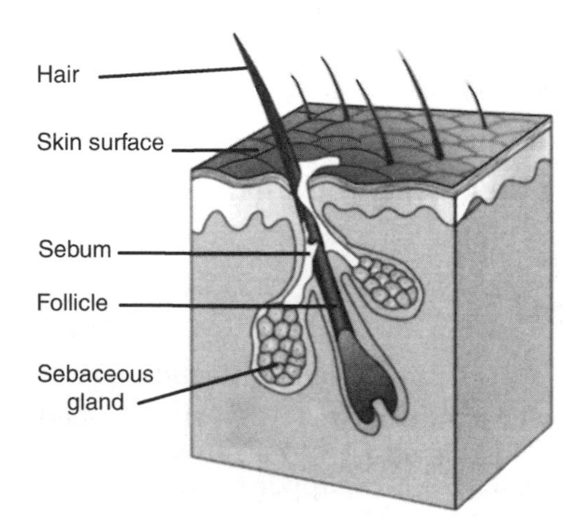

Figure 7.1. *Normal Pilosebaceous Unit*

- Papules—inflamed lesions that usually appear as small, pink bumps on the skin and can be tender to the touch
- Pustules (pimples)—papules topped by pus-filled lesions that may be red at the base
- Nodules—large, painful, solid lesions that are lodged deep within the skin
- Cysts—deep, painful, pus-filled lesions that can cause scarring

What Causes Acne?

The exact cause of acne is unknown, but doctors believe it results from several related factors. One important factor is an increase in hormones called androgens (male sex hormones). These increase in both boys and girls during puberty and cause the sebaceous glands

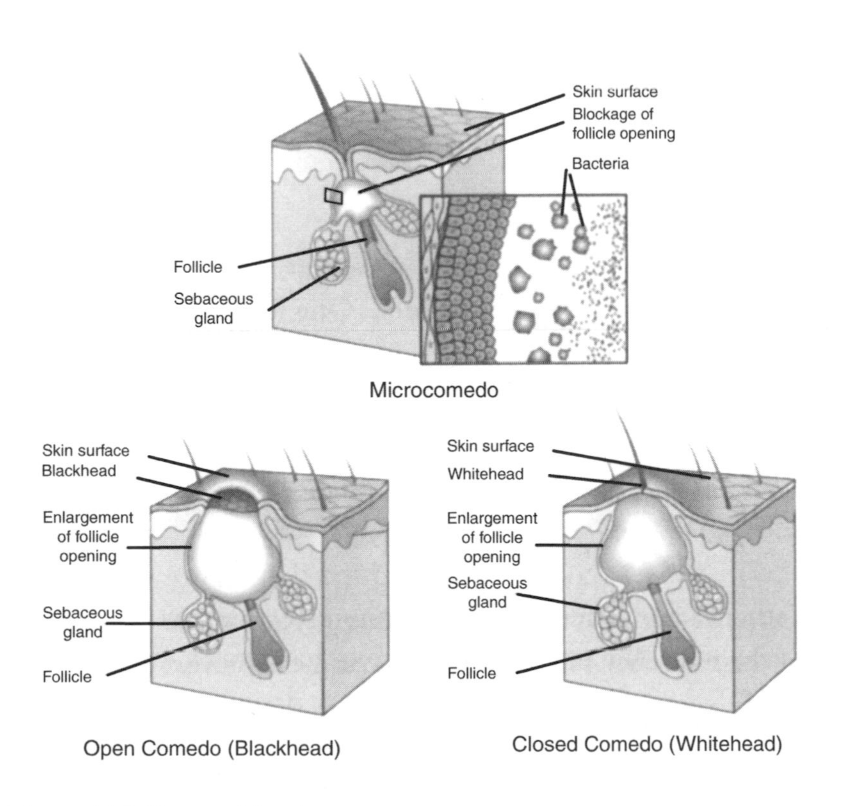

Figure 7.2. *Types of Lesions*

to enlarge and make more sebum. Hormonal changes related to pregnancy or starting or stopping birth control pills can also cause acne.

Another factor is heredity or genetics. Researchers believe that the tendency to develop acne can be inherited from parents. For example, studies have shown that many school-age boys with acne have a family history of the disorder. Certain drugs, including androgens and lithium, are known to cause acne. Greasy cosmetics may alter the cells of the follicles and make them stick together, producing a plug.

Factors That Can Make Acne Worse

Factors that can cause an acne flare include the following:

- Changing hormone levels in adolescent girls and adult women 2 to 7 days before their menstrual period starts
- Friction caused by leaning on or rubbing the skin
- Pressure from bike helmets, backpacks, or tight collars
- Environmental irritants, such as pollution and high humidity
- Squeezing or picking at blemishes
- Hard scrubbing of the skin

Myths about the Causes of Acne

There are many myths about what causes acne. Chocolate and greasy foods are often blamed, but foods seem to have little effect on the development and course of acne in most people. Another common myth is that dirty skin causes acne; however, blackheads and other acne lesions are not caused by dirt. Finally, stress does not cause acne.

Who Gets Acne?

People of all races and ages get acne. It is most common in adolescents and young adults. Nearly 85 percent of people between the ages of 12 and 24 develop the disorder. For most people, acne tends to go away by the time they reach their thirties; however, some people in their forties and fifties continue to have this skin problem.

How Is Acne Treated?

Acne is often treated by dermatologists (doctors who specialize in skin problems). These doctors treat all kinds of acne, particularly severe cases. Doctors who are general or family practitioners, pediatricians, or internists may treat patients with milder cases of acne.

The goals of treatment are to heal existing lesions, stop new lesions from forming, prevent scarring, and minimize the psychological stress and embarrassment caused by this disease. Drug treatment is aimed at reducing several problems that play a part in causing acne: abnormal clumping of cells in the follicles, increased oil production, bacteria, and inflammation. Depending on the extent of the person's acne, the doctor will recommend one of several over-the-counter (OTC) medicines or prescription medicines that are topical (applied to the skin) or systemic (taken by mouth). The doctor may suggest using more than one topical medicine or combining oral and topical medicines.

Treatment for Blackheads, Whiteheads, and Mild Inflammatory Acne

Doctors usually recommend an OTC or prescription topical medication for people with mild signs of acne. Topical medicine is applied directly to the acne lesions or to the entire area of affected skin.

Benzoyl peroxide, resorcinol, salicylic acid, and sulfur are the most common topical OTC medicines used to treat acne. Each works a little differently. Benzoyl peroxide is best at killing *P. acnes* and may reduce oil production. Resorcinol, salicylic acid, and sulfur help break down blackheads and whiteheads. Salicylic acid also helps cut down the shedding of cells lining the follicles of the oil glands. Topical OTC medications are available in many forms, such as gel, lotion, cream, soap, or pad.

In some patients, OTC acne medicines may cause side effects such as skin irritation, burning, or redness. Some people find that the side effects lessen or go away with continued use of the medicine. Severe or prolonged side effects should be reported to the doctor.

OTC topical medicines are somewhat effective in treating acne when used regularly. Patients must keep in mind that it can take 8 weeks or more before they notice their skin looks and feels better.

Treatment for Moderate to Severe Inflammatory Acne

Patients with moderate to severe inflammatory acne may be treated with prescription topical or oral medicines, alone or in combination.

Prescription Topical Medicines

Several types of prescription topical medicines are used to treat acne, including antibiotics, benzoyl peroxide, tretinoin, adapalene, and azelaic acid. Antibiotics and azelaic acid help stop or slow the growth of bacteria and reduce inflammation. Tretinoin, a type of drug called a retinoid that contains an altered form of vitamin A, is an effective topical medicine for stopping the development of new comedones. It works by unplugging existing comedones, thereby allowing other topical medicines, such as antibiotics, to enter the follicles. The doctor may also prescribe newer retinoids or retinoid-like drugs, such as tazarotene or adapalene, that help decrease comedo formation.

Like OTC topical medicines, prescription topical medicines come as creams, lotions, solutions, or gels. The doctor will consider the patient's skin type when prescribing a product. Creams and lotions provide moisture and tend to be good for people with sensitive skin. Gels and solutions are generally alcohol-based and tend to dry the skin. Therefore, patients with very oily skin or those who live in hot, humid climates may prefer them. The doctor will tell the patient how to apply the medicine and how often to use it.

Some people develop side effects from using prescription topical medicines. Initially, the skin may look worse before improving. Common side effects include stinging, burning, redness, peeling, scaling, or discoloration of the skin. With some medicines, like retinoids, these side effects usually decrease or go away after the medicine is used for a period of time. Patients should report prolonged or severe side effects to their doctor. Between 4 and 8 weeks will most likely pass before patients see their skin improve.

Prescription Oral Medicines

For patients with moderate to severe acne, the doctor often prescribes oral antibiotics (taken by mouth). Oral antibiotics are thought to help control acne by curbing the growth of bacteria and reducing inflammation. Prescription oral and topical medicines may be combined. For example, benzoyl peroxide may be combined with clindamycin, erythromycin, or sulfur. Other common antibiotics used to treat acne are tetracycline, minocycline, and doxycycline. Some people have side effects when taking these antibiotics, such as an increased tendency to sunburn, upset stomach, dizziness or lightheadedness, and changes in skin color. Tetracycline is not given to pregnant women, nor is it given to children under 8 years of age because it might discolor developing teeth. Tetracycline and minocycline may also decrease the effectiveness of birth control pills. Therefore, a backup or another form of birth control may be needed. Prolonged treatment with oral antibiotics may be necessary to achieve the desired results.

Treatment for Severe Nodular or Cystic Acne

People with nodules or cysts should be treated by a dermatologist. For patients with severe inflammatory acne that does not improve with medicines such as those described above, a doctor may prescribe isotretinoin (Accutane), a retinoid. [Note: Brand names included in this chapter are provided as examples only, and their inclusion does not mean that these products are endorsed by the National Institutes of Health or any other Government agency. Also, if a particular brand name is not mentioned, this does not mean or imply that the product is unsatisfactory.] Isotretinoin is an oral drug that is usually taken once or twice a day with food for 15 to 20 weeks. It markedly reduces the size of the oil glands so that much less oil is produced. As a result, the growth of bacteria is decreased.

Advantages of Isotretinoin (Accutane)

Isotretinoin is a very effective medicine that can help prevent scarring. After 15 to 20 weeks of treatment with isotretinoin, acne completely or almost completely goes away in up to 90 percent of patients. In those patients where acne recurs after a course of isotretinoin, the doctor may institute another course of the same treatment or prescribe other medicines.

Disadvantages of Isotretinoin (Accutane)

Isotretinoin can cause birth defects in the developing fetus of a pregnant woman. It is important that women of childbearing age are not pregnant and do not get pregnant while taking this medicine. Women must use two separate effective forms of birth control at the same time for 1 month before treatment begins, during the entire course of treatment, and for 1 full month after stopping the drug. They should ask their doctor when it is safe to get pregnant after they have stopped taking Accutane.

Some people with acne become depressed by the changes in the appearance of their skin. Changes in mental health may be intensified during treatment or soon after completing a course of medicines like Accutane. A doctor should be consulted if a person feels unusually sad or has other symptoms of depression, such as loss of appetite or trouble concentrating.

Other possible side effects include dry eyes, mouth, lips, nose, or skin; itching; nosebleeds; muscle aches; sensitivity to the sun; and, sometimes, poor night vision. More serious side effects include changes in the blood, such as an increase in triglycerides and cholesterol, or a change in liver function. To make sure Accutane is stopped if side effects occur, the doctor monitors blood studies that are done before treatment is started and periodically during treatment. Side effects usually go away after the medicine is stopped.

Treatments for Hormonally Influenced Acne in Women

Clues that help the doctor determine whether acne in an adult woman is due to an excess of androgen hormones are hirsutism (excessive growth of hair in unusual places), premenstrual acne flares, irregular menstrual cycles, and elevated blood levels of certain androgens. The doctor may prescribe one of several drugs to treat women with this type of acne. Low-dose estrogen birth control pills help suppress the androgen produced by the ovaries. Low-dose corticosteroid drugs, such as prednisone or dexamethasone, may suppress the androgen produced by the adrenal glands. Finally, the doctor may prescribe an antiandrogen drug, such as spironolactone (Aldactone). This medicine reduces excessive oil production. Side effects of antiandrogen drugs may include irregular menstruation, tender breasts, headache, and fatigue.

Other Treatments for Acne

Doctors may use other types of procedures in addition to drug therapy to treat patients with acne. For example, the doctor may remove the patient's comedones during office visits. Sometimes the doctor will inject cortisone directly into lesions to help reduce the size and pain of inflamed cysts and nodules.

Early treatment is the best way to prevent acne scars. Once scarring has occurred, the doctor may suggest a medical or surgical procedure to help reduce the scars. A superficial laser may be used to treat irregular scars. Another kind of laser allows energy to go deeper into the skin and tighten the underlying tissue and plump out depressed scars. Dermabrasion (or microdermabrasion), which is a form of "sanding down" scars, is sometimes combined with the subsurface laser treatment. Another treatment option for deep scars caused by cystic acne is the transfer of fat from one part of the body to the face.

How Should People with Acne Care for Their Skin?

Clean Skin Gently

Most doctors recommend that people with acne gently wash their skin with a mild cleanser, once in the morning and once in the evening and after heavy exercise. Some people with acne may try to stop outbreaks and oil production by scrubbing their skin and using strong detergent soaps and rough scrub pads. However, scrubbing will not improve acne; in fact, it can make the problem worse. Patients should ask their doctor or another health professional for advice on the best type of cleanser to use. Patients should wash their face from under the jaw to the hairline. It is important that patients thoroughly rinse their skin after washing it. Astringents are not recommended unless the skin is very oily, and then they should be used only on oily spots. Doctors also recommend that patients regularly shampoo their hair. Those with oily hair may want to shampoo it every day.

Avoid Frequent Handling of the Skin

People who squeeze, pinch, or pick their blemishes risk developing scars or dark blotches. People should avoid rubbing and touching their skin lesions.

Shave Carefully

Men who shave and who have acne can test both electric and safety razors to see which is more comfortable. Men who use a safety razor should use a sharp blade and soften their beard thoroughly with soap and water before applying shaving cream. Nicking blemishes can be avoided by shaving lightly and only when necessary.

Avoid a Sunburn or Suntan

Many of the medicines used to treat acne can make a person more prone to sunburn. A sunburn that reddens the skin or suntan that darkens the skin may make blemishes less visible and make the skin feel drier. However, these benefits are only temporary, and there are known risks of excessive sun exposure, such as more rapid skin aging and a risk of developing skin cancer.

Choose Cosmetics Carefully

People being treated for acne often need to change some of the cosmetics they use. All cosmetics, such as foundation, blush, eye shadow, and moisturizers, should be oil free. Patients may find it difficult to apply foundation evenly during the first few weeks of treatment because the skin may be red or scaly, particularly with the use of topical tretinoin or benzoyl peroxide. Oily hair products may eventually spread over the forehead, causing closed comedones. Products that are labeled as noncomedogenic (do not promote the formation of closed pores) should be used; in some people, however, even these products may cause acne.

What Research Is Being Done on Acne?

Medical researchers are working on new drugs to treat acne, particularly topical antibiotics to replace some of those in current use. As with many other types of bacterial infections, doctors are finding that, over time, the bacteria that are associated with acne are becoming resistant to treatment with certain antibiotics. Research is also being conducted by industry on the potential side effects of isotretinoin and the long-term use of medicines used for treating acne.

Scientists are working on other means of treating acne. For example, researchers are studying the biology of sebaceous cells and testing a laser in laboratory animals to treat acne by disrupting sebaceous glands. Scientists are also studying the treatment of androgenic disorders, including acne, in men by inhibiting an enzyme that changes testosterone to a more potent androgen.

Chapter 8

Accutane: The Benefits and Risks of a Breakthrough Acne Drug

Acne plagued Julie Harper throughout high school and college. She depended on makeup and wore her hair down over the side of her face. She gave up chocolate and french fries, only to find that neither made a difference. And she went through medicine after medicine, from over-the-counter creams to oral antibiotics.

These were not occasional pimples that vanish after a couple of days. This acne covered her face and left scars on her neck. "I had tried everything and felt frustrated all the time," says Harper, now a physician and assistant professor of dermatology at the University of Alabama-Birmingham—a career she chose due in large part to her struggle with acne.

Harper finally found a successful treatment nine years ago at the age of 22. She took a drug called isotretinoin (trade name Accutane) and watched her skin improve in just a couple of months. By the third month, her acne had disappeared. She says with clearer skin came more self-confidence and higher self-esteem.

Considered the biggest breakthrough in acne drug treatment over the last 20 years, Accutane is the only drug that has the potential to clear severe acne permanently after one course of treatment. One course, which is typically five months, results in prolonged remission of acne in up to 85 percent of patients. A member of a class of drugs

---

"The Power of Accutane: The Benefits and Risks of a Breakthrough Acne Drug," U.S. Food and Drug Administration, *FDA Consumer,* March 2001. By Michelle Meadows. Available online at http://www.fda.gov; accessed March 2005.

known as retinoids, Accutane is highly effective. But it doesn't work for everyone, and some patients need more than one course of treatment. Dr. Harper took a second course of Accutane one year after the first and has been free of severe acne ever since, now only occasionally using a topical medication.

No other acne medicine works as well for severe acne. Patients generally have to keep using other medications because they only suppress acne temporarily. But as powerful as Accutane can be in improving patients' lives, its adverse effects can be just as powerful. The drug is known to cause miscarriage and severe birth defects. Patients taking Accutane may develop potentially serious problems affecting a number of organs, including the liver, intestines, eyes, ears, and skeletal system. And some patients taking Accutane have developed serious psychiatric problems, including depression. More rarely, patients have developed suicidal behavior and killed themselves.

Because it is a high-risk drug, Accutane should be reserved for cases of "severe recalcitrant nodular acne," according to the product's labeling. This type of acne is resistant to standard acne treatment, including oral antibiotics, and is characterized by many nodules or cysts—inflammatory lesions filled with pus and lodged deep within the skin. These lesions can cause pain, permanent scarring, and negative psychological effects.

"Sometimes people tend to dismiss the impact of acne because it's not life-threatening, says Kathy O'Connell, M.D., PhD, a medical reviewer for Accutane in FDA's division of dermatologic and dental drug products, Center for Drug Evaluation and Research (CDER). "But patients with severe acne know all too well the very real suffering caused by this disfiguring disease."

FDA approved Accutane in 1982, and since then, about 5 million people in the United States and 12 million worldwide have been treated with it, according to its manufacturer, Hoffmann-La Roche of Nutley, N.J. The number of patients taking the drug has increased, and half are females, most of whom are in their childbearing years (age 15 to 44). Because of concern about the drug's risks, FDA continues to evaluate Accutane and work with the manufacturer to maximize safe use of the drug.

Warning about Pregnancy Risks

When FDA approved Accutane, the drug was known to be teratogenic—able to cause birth defects. It was designated as Category X, meaning that it must be avoided under all circumstances during pregnancy. Nursing mothers also should not use Accutane.

Though not every fetus exposed to Accutane becomes deformed, the risk of birth defects among pregnant women is extremely high. These defects include hydrocephaly (enlargement of the fluid-filled spaces of the brain) and microcephaly (small head), heart defects, facial deformities such as cleft lip and missing ears, and mental retardation.

Reports in the literature suggest that about 25 to 35 percent of babies will suffer a malformation after exposure, and that doesn't account for other defects, such as learning disabilities, that aren't detectable at birth. Miscarriages and premature births have also been reported.

Though FDA approved labeling in 1982 that warned Accutane should not be used in pregnant women, reports of severe birth defects associated with the drug began to arrive in June 1983. Over the following years, a series of labeling changes and letters to pharmacists and prescribers of the drug stressed pregnancy warnings and sought to increase awareness about reported malformations.

Then, after an FDA review of pregnancy exposures to Accutane, Roche launched the Pregnancy Prevention Program (PPP) in late 1988 to further educate women using Accutane and their physicians about the dangers. The goal was to ensure that prescriptions would only be given to women with severe recalcitrant nodular acne who could comply with contraceptive requirements.

Roche sent PPP kits to physicians and encouraged them to review pregnancy prevention materials with patients before starting the drug. Materials included a contraceptive booklet, checklists to help assess whether patients could adhere to the drug's requirements, and consent forms that patients sign to acknowledge their understanding of the risk of birth defects. Roche also set up a toll-free line, made contraceptive information available in 13 languages, and offered to pay for contraceptive counseling and pregnancy testing by a specialist.

To further reinforce pregnancy prevention, Roche began packaging Accutane in blister packs that include red and black warnings, along with a drawing of a malformed baby and the "Avoid Pregnancy" symbol.

Even though Accutane's labeling recommended use of two reliable forms of contraception, there have been reports of pregnancies occurring in patients who used hormonal contraception, including pills, injectables, and implantables, while taking Accutane. Accutane's labeling was updated in the summer of 2000. One change emphasized the need for two reliable forms of contraception for at least one month before taking Accutane, during treatment, and for one month after discontinuing Accutane, even when one of the forms of contraception is hormonal.

Evaluating Compliance

Yolonda Lawrence of Santa Monica, Calif., says there was no way she could miss the point about pregnancy prevention before she used Accutane for severe adult-onset acne in 1998. "I got a pamphlet, I signed papers, the doctor told me over and over, and the pictures of what can happen were very clear—babies with no ears" and other deformities, she says.

But reports of Accutane-exposed pregnancies continue, and that's enough to make FDA concerned, says Peter Honig, M.D., director of FDA's office of post-marketing drug risk assessment (OPDRA) in CDER.

Shortly after the Pregnancy Prevention Program began, Roche sponsored a survey of women taking Accutane to assess compliance with the program, and the company encouraged doctors to enroll patients. Run by the Slone Epidemiology Unit at Boston University's School of Public Health, the survey set out to track pregnancy rates and outcomes, patients' awareness of risks, and patient and physician behavior.

Of the 500,000 women enrolled in the Slone survey from 1989 to 1998, there have been 958 pregnancies, 834 of which were terminations (either elective, spontaneous or due to ectopic pregnancies), 110 that resulted in live births, and 14 patients that had unknown outcomes. Of the 60 infants with available medical records, eight had congenital abnormalities. Since Accutane's approval, Roche has received close to 2,000 reports of Accutane-exposed pregnancies, 70 percent of which occurred after the PPP began.

According to FDA, exactly how well the PPP has worked is unclear. Experts say the PPP is a significant program that has prevented many pregnancies and is the first of its kind initiated by a pharmaceutical company. Roche has made extraordinary efforts to educate patients that they must not become pregnant while taking Accutane, says a Roche spokesperson.

At a September 2000 meeting of FDA's Dermatologic and Ophthalmic Drugs Advisory Committee, a Roche representative reported that from the company's perspective, pregnancy rates have declined. Amarilys Vega, M.D., an FDA medical officer, agreed. However, because

use of the product has increased over the years, the actual number of pregnancies occurring while taking Accutane has not declined. One limitation is that the survey is voluntary and only captures about 30 to 40 percent of all patients on Accutane. So there's no way to know exactly how many pregnancy exposures there have been, according to FDA experts. Of serious concern is that women who enroll in the survey may be more likely to comply with the contraceptive requirements than those who don't enroll in the survey. This leaves open critical questions about how representative the PPP group is and about unreported pregnancies among women who don't enroll in the PPP.

Most patients in the Slone survey have reported that they understood Accutane may cause birth defects. And according to Roche, the percentage of female patients who reported they were pregnant when they began Accutane dropped from 30 percent of pregnancies reported in 1989 to 11 percent of pregnancies reported for the period of 1991 to 1997. But substantial noncompliance with the PPP continues to be reported.

For example, a 1997 report on the survey shows that 25 percent of women in the program did not report having a pregnancy test before starting Accutane, and 33 percent did not report postponing the start of Accutane until a pregnancy test result was known. It is estimated that 40 percent of women taking Accutane are sexually active.

The only patients exempt from Accutane's contraceptive requirements are men, and women who have had a hysterectomy or who say they will abstain from sex during treatment. But the challenge is that going from sexually inactive to active can happen overnight.

Possible Psychiatric Link

Many patients say they feel better about themselves after receiving successful treatment for acne. Evelyn Germanakos, of Los Angeles, Calif., struggled with acne as an adult, and says she felt like her old self after Accutane cleared up lumpy blemishes in 1997. "I had gotten to the point where I didn't even want to go outside or be with people, let alone look in the mirror," she says. But while Accutane may help lift psychosocial distress such as embarrassment, evidence suggests that it may actually cause serious psychiatric disorders in some people.

Though the drug's label previously listed depression as a possible reaction, FDA strengthened the label warning in 1998 after reviewing cases with serious outcomes reported in the years after the drug was approved. The new labeling states that Accutane may cause depression and psychosis, and that in rare cases it may cause suicidal ideation (thoughts of suicide), suicide attempts, and suicide.

The label also advises providers that simply discontinuing the drug may not remedy any psychiatric problems and that further evaluation may be necessary. "In some cases, stopping Accutane alone may not be enough to relieve the mood changes," says Jonathan Wilkin, M.D., director of CDER's division of dermatologic and dental drug products. "Psychiatric treatment may also be needed."

The relationship between Accutane and depression remains unproven, but some patients have reported that their depression subsided when they stopped the medication and came back when they resumed taking it. And some who have reported problems with depression while taking Accutane had no previous psychiatric history. FDA considers the number of reports of serious depression associated with Accutane high compared to other drugs in its database.

From 1982 to May 2000, FDA received reports of 37 U.S. Accutane patients who committed suicide, 24 while on the drug and 13 after stopping the drug. In addition to suicides, FDA received reports of 110 U.S. Accutane users hospitalized for depression, suicidal ideation, and suicide attempt during the same time period. As of May 2000, FDA had received reports of 284 Accutane users with non-hospitalized depression.

Several factors make it hard to definitively link depression with Accutane. Depression is a common problem, and some patients may be suffering from it before starting Accutane therapy. Additionally, some patients who reported depression with Accutane had previous courses of the drug without depression. Even so, it is recommended that doctors act as if Accutane could have psychiatric effects until there is more information, says FDA's Wilkin.

The Future of Accutane

Roche does not want to have any Accutane-exposed pregnancies, a company spokesperson says, and plans to continue educational efforts. This year Roche launched a targeted Pregnancy Prevention Program that focuses on women who are at highest risk of becoming pregnant while taking Accutane.

Experts agree that pregnancy prevention education should remain a key part of risk management for Accutane use. But more labeling changes and letters are not likely to make a significant difference, according to FDA's Honig. "During all the time the drug has been on the market and after all of those labeling changes, there are still pregnancies," he says. "It is not expected that another labeling change or 'Dear Doctor' letter will change behavior at this point." Psychiatric adverse events have also continued after labeling changes.

FDA's Dermatologic and Ophthalmic Drugs Advisory Committee met in September 2000 to discuss options for Accutane, and to evaluate whether a framework for safer use of the drug can be developed. One change since then is that all Accutane prescriptions now come with a new Medication Guide that contains warnings about pregnancy and psychiatric issues, plus other important warnings and precautions regarding potentially serious or life-threatening effects.

FDA has also proposed a mandatory registration of patients taking Accutane, prescribers, and pharmacists. "The main reason is to ensure that pregnancy testing is done before the drug is prescribed," says Julie Beitz, M.D., of FDA's office of post-marketing drug risk assessment. The goal would be to have doctors document negative pregnancy tests and to have pharmacies dispense the drug only to women who have had negative pregnancy tests. The program to track Accutane patients is expected to be in place by summer 2001.

The registry for prescribers may involve a continuing education course that doctors would have to take to be able to prescribe Accutane. According to Hoffmann-La Roche, about 85 percent of Accutane prescriptions come from dermatologists and 15 percent come from primary care physicians. The course would be open to all medical doctors. And all Accutane patients would have to sign a mandatory consent form that would address both pregnancy and psychiatric issues, Beitz says.

The American Academy of Dermatology and the Dermatologic Nurses Association were among those who testified at the September 2000 committee meeting in opposition to a mandatory registration, saying that it would be a disservice to patients, making it harder for them to obtain the drug. Others, including the March of Dimes and the Public Citizen's Health Research Group, testified that they want to see stricter measures for Accutane.

FDA's experts say it's a balancing act. The value of Accutane is clear, but when it comes to even one report of death—whether it's suicide, miscarriage, or some other cause—FDA must make choices that will best protect the public's health.

Chapter 9

Rosacea

What is rosacea?

Rosacea is a chronic (long-term) disease that affects the skin and sometimes the eyes. The disorder is characterized by redness, pimples, and, in advanced stages, thickened skin. Rosacea usually affects the face; other parts of the upper body are only rarely involved.

Who gets rosacea?

Approximately 14 million people in the United States have rosacea. It most often affects adults between the ages of 30 and 60. Rosacea is more common in women (particularly during menopause) than men. Although rosacea can develop in people of any skin color, it tends to occur most frequently and is most apparent in people with fair skin.

What does rosacea look like?

There are several symptoms and conditions associated with rosacea. These include frequent flushing, vascular rosacea, inflammatory rosacea, and several other conditions involving the skin, eyes, and nose.

Frequent flushing of the center of the face—which may include the forehead, nose, cheeks, and chin—occurs in the earliest stage of rosacea.

Excerpted from "Questions and Answers About Rosacea," National Institute of Arthritis and Musculoskeletal and Skin Diseases, June 2002. Available online at http://www.niams.nih.gov; accessed March 2005.

The flushing often is accompanied by a burning sensation, particularly when creams or cosmetics are applied to the face. Sometimes the face is swollen slightly.

A condition called vascular rosacea causes persistent flushing and redness. Blood vessels under the skin of the face may dilate (enlarge), showing through the skin as small red lines. This is called telangiectasia. The affected skin may be swollen slightly and feel warm.

A condition called inflammatory rosacea causes persistent redness and papules (pink bumps) and pustules (bumps containing pus) on the skin. Eye inflammation and sensitivity as well as telangiectasia also may occur.

In the most advanced stage of rosacea, the skin becomes a deep shade of red and inflammation of the eye is more apparent. Numerous telangiectases are often present, and nodules in the skin may become painful. A condition called rhinophyma also may develop in some men; it is rare in women. Rhinophyma is characterized by an enlarged, bulbous, and red nose resulting from enlargement of the sebaceous (oil-producing) glands beneath the surface of the skin on the nose. People who have rosacea also may develop a thickening of the skin on the forehead, chin, cheeks, or other areas.

How is the eye affected?

In addition to skin problems, up to 50 percent of people who have rosacea have eye problems caused by the condition. Typical symptoms include redness, dryness, itching, burning, tearing, and the sensation of having sand in the eye. The eyelids may become inflamed and swollen. Some people say their eyes are sensitive to light and their vision is blurred or otherwise impaired.

What causes rosacea?

Doctors do not know the exact cause of rosacea but believe that some people may inherit a tendency to develop the disorder. People who blush frequently may be more likely to develop rosacea. Some researchers believe that rosacea is a disorder where blood vessels dilate too easily, resulting in flushing and redness.

Factors that cause rosacea to flare up in one person may have no effect on another person. Although the following factors have not been well-researched, some people claim that one or more of them have aggravated their rosacea: heat (including hot baths), strenuous exercise, sunlight, wind, very cold temperatures, hot or spicy foods and drinks, alcohol consumption, menopause, emotional stress, and long-term use of topical steroids on the face. Patients affected by pustules may assume they are caused by bacteria, but researchers have not established a link between rosacea and bacteria or other organisms on the skin, in the hair follicles, or elsewhere in the body.

Can rosacea be cured?

Although there is no cure for rosacea, it can be treated and controlled. A dermatologist (a medical doctor who specializes in diseases of the skin) usually treats rosacea. The goals of treatment are to control the condition and improve the appearance of the patient's skin. It may take several weeks or months of treatment before a person notices an improvement of the skin.

Some doctors will prescribe a topical antibiotic, such as metronidazole, which is applied directly to the affected skin. For people with more severe cases, doctors often prescribe an oral (taken by mouth) antibiotic. Tetracycline, minocycline, erythromycin, and doxycycline are the most common antibiotics used to treat rosacea. The papules and pustules symptomatic of rosacea may respond quickly to treatment, but the redness and flushing are less likely to improve.

Some people who have rosacea become depressed by the changes in the appearance of their skin. Information provided by the National Rosacea Society indicates that people who have rosacea often experience low self-esteem, feel embarrassed by their appearance, and claim their social and professional interactions with others are adversely affected. A doctor should be consulted if a person feels unusually sad or has other symptoms of depression, such as loss of appetite or trouble concentrating.

Doctors usually treat the eye problems of rosacea with oral antibiotics, particularly tetracycline or doxycycline. People who develop infections of the eyelids must practice frequent eyelid hygiene. The doctor may recommend scrubbing the eyelids gently with diluted baby shampoo or an over-the-counter eyelid cleaner and applying warm (but not hot) compresses several times a day. When eyes are severely affected, doctors may prescribe steroid eyedrops.

Electrosurgery and laser surgery are treatment options if red lines caused by dilated blood vessels appear in the skin or if rhinophyma develops. For some patients, laser surgery may improve the skin's appearance with little scarring or damage. For patients with rhinophyma, surgical removal of the excess tissue to reduce the size of the nose usually will improve the patient's appearance.

Chapter 10

All about Sweat Gland Disorders

Chapter Contents

Section 10.1

Hyperhidrosis

"Hyperhidrosis: Frequently Asked Questions," by Mark D. Iannettoni, M.B.A., M.D., Harold M. Burkhart, M.D., and Timothy L. Vannatta, M.D., University of Iowa Hospitals and Clinics, Iowa City, Iowa 52242, © May 2004. Copyright protected material used with permission of the authors and the University of Iowa's Virtual Hospital, www.vh.org.

What Is It?

Hyperhidrosis is an involuntary sweating response generated by the sympathetic nervous system. The body uses sweating as a means to regulate our own body temperature in response to changes in generated body heat or environment. Besides the environmental changes, which can make us sweat, hormonal or emotional stimuli can cause sweating. There are two types of sweat glands that are primarily responsible for sweating and temperature regulation. There are 4 to 5 million exocrine glands in the body and approximately one third of them are in the palms. The feedback system that regulates sweating is located in the sympathetic chain and runs along the posterior chest parallel to vertebral column.

What Are the Symptoms?

The symptoms of hyperhidrosis represent excessive sweating, which may or may not be related to temperature, emotional response, or activity. The incidence of this disease is approximately 0.5 to 1% of the population. It is important to determine whether hyperhidrosis is primary or secondary. Primary hyperhidrosis refers to sweating that is excessive with no known cause and unrelated to any other medical condition. This may be in response to emotional stimuli such as public speaking or situations that make one apprehensive or anxious. Secondary hyperhidrosis is sweating that occurs due to underlying conditions or diseases such as hyperthyroidism or medications. Another cause of secondary hyperhidrosis can be diabetes, which results in a dysfunction of the autonomic nervous system.

Hyperhidrosis can occur at multiple sites including the hands, the feet, the axilla, and less likely, in the groin and buttocks.

What Are the Concerns?

Hyperhidrosis can result in emotional and social embarrassment and in children can result in developmental delay in social skills because of concerns of ridicule or avoidance of personal relationships. This disease tends to become most prevalent in the years during puberty and remain stable after that age. Although hyperhidrosis is not a dangerous disease, it can significantly affect a person's ability to interact with other people and result in situational avoidance and emotional development delay.

What Are the Treatment Options?

There are two basic treatment options: medical therapy or surgical therapy.

Medicine

Topical remedies reduce the amount of sweating but must be applied two to four times per day. Most patients prior to surgery will have tried this remedy. The lotions can cause chapping and cracking of the hands and has a wide range of effectiveness.

Oral medications such as anti-cholinergic drugs are groups of medicines, which inhibit the autonomic nervous systems from firing and results in the inability to sweat. There are significant side effects that occur with these medications, such as dry mouth, dry eyes, and GI dysfunction, and for these reasons have not gained significant popularity.

Iontophoresis is a technique, which uses ionic transfer to interrupt the sympathetic chain but must be used daily for many hours and can be somewhat uncomfortable. The result is transient. Patients frequently find this an unacceptable method of treatment.

Surgery

Thoracic sympathectomy has been performed for many years to treat many different diseases. This procedure was used to increase blood flow to the hand in patients who have reflux sympathetic dystrophy. This disease causes intense vasoconstriction, which is also under the control of the sympathetic nervous system and can result in tissue loss of the fingers. Originally this operation was performed by making a large incision in the chest called a thoracotomy with approximately a 3% risk of long-term pain syndromes. In order to save the fingers, this was an acceptable complication.

When we are talking about simply relieving excessive sweating on the hands and both sides are required to be operated on, this was an unacceptable complication and a relatively large operation for a small problem. Another approach was to perform an axillary thoracotomy, although much more cosmetically appealing and less invasive, it was not without significant risk, such as postoperative pain syndrome, and a significant recovery time.

In the early 1990s, thoracoscopic surgery was developed and resulted in major advances for minimally invasive techniques performed on the chest. This is similar to other endoscopic surgical techniques such as laparoscopic surgery used in general surgery or arthroscopic surgery used in orthopedic surgery. In 1993, we started performing thoracoscopic sympathectomies, which required a 2- to 3-day hospital stay and one side was operated on at a time. In 1994, because of better anesthetic and surgical techniques, bilateral sympathectomies were performed, however, the patient was still admitted for 2 to 3 days. In 1997, with the development of new instrumentation and more experience, patients were able to have a bilateral thoracoscopic sympathectomy and these patients were now being operated upon on an outpatient basis.

Section 10.2

Dyshidrosis

Dyshidrosis is a common disorder affecting the hands and feet. The exact cause is not known, but it possibly comes from some abnormal function in the sweating mechanism. The condition may be mild with only a little peeling or very severe with big blisters and cracks which are so uncomfortable that the patient cannot work.

Acute and Chronic Stages

The first (acute) stage shows tiny blisters deep in the skin, associated with itching and burning sensations. The later and more chronic stage shows more peeling, cracking or crusting. Some patients will have mostly one stage, and some patients will have mostly the other. Sometimes both stages occur at the same time.

Dyshidrosis does not have any quick cure. It often runs a chronic course, but sometimes it does go away for long periods. Many times flare-ups occur after a period of nervous tension, worry or other emotional conflict, just as tension may aggravate ulcer symptoms in patients with ulcer disease.

Treatment

Treatment varies with the stage of the disease. In the acute, blistering stage, cool compresses or soaks with Burow's solution (one packet or tablet dissolved in one pint of water) used for 15 to 30 minutes 2 to 4 times a day may help to dry up the blisters. Following the soaks, these areas should be dried and the medicated cream or gel applied.

In the chronic stage, cortisone creams or ointments help to reduce inflammation and itching and speed recovery. In severe cases cortisone tablets or injections may be used for limited periods.

Sometimes the affected areas may become secondarily infected with bacteria at the site of cracks or broken blisters. If this happens, your doctor will use appropriate additional treatment.

Although at present dyshidrosis is not curable, satisfactory control can usually be obtained by the treatments outlined. Most people sooner or later have less and less trouble—as time goes on the disorder subsides. Do not lose hope!

Section 10.3

Hidradenitis Suppurativa

Hidradenitis is a chronic disease of the apocrine glands (a form of sweat gland found on certain parts of the body). For unknown reasons, people with hidradenitis develop plugging or clogging of their apocrine glands. It causes chronic scarring and pus formation of the underarms (axilla) and groin/inner thigh areas.

In women it can also occur under the breasts. It is similar to acne, which is also a disease of the sebaceous glands. Hidradenitis is more common in people who have had acne. It may be an unusual type of adult acne.

This condition is slightly more common in women and African Americans. Hidradenitis usually starts as one or more red, tender, swellings in the groin or armpits. Over a period of hours to days the lesions enlarge and often open to the skin surface, draining clear to yellow fluid. The involved area then heals with scarring. The condition usually continues for years with periods of flare and remission.

Bacterial infection produces the pain and odor. Hidradenitis is made worse by being overweight, however this condition is not caused by obesity and weight loss will improve but not cure hidradenitis. Hidradenitis may become worse under stress. Hidradenitis is not caused by poor hygiene.

Initial treatments are usually oral antibiotics (minocycline, tetracycline, erythromycin, Augmentin, others) and topical antibiotics (clindamycin or erythromycin). Intralesional injections into the affected places reduce swelling and tenderness within days. Anti-inflammatory pills (Celebrex, Advil, Naprosyn, Aleve, and others) are helpful in addition to the antibiotics, especially if it is a severe case. Some women respond to high estrogen birth control pills (Demulen 1/50, Ortho Novum 1/50) and spironolactone pills.

Tight-fitting clothing and shaving the areas are to be strictly avoided. Dirt does not cause hidradenitis. The involved areas should be cleaned daily using an antibacterial soap, as this will reduce any odor associated with this condition. Retin-A cream, a prescription, helps some people. Accutane, a drug for severe acne, offers modest help for moderately bad cases. There is medical control, but not a cure for hidradenitis.

Surgery is the most effective treatment for hidradenitis. Aggressive surgery will cure an area of severe, chronic hidradenitis but it has to remove scarred tissue or even large areas of skin. Skin grafts may be needed. Incision (lancing) and draining will reliably help smaller affected areas. Because surgery scars and may have complications, medical treatments are usually tried first.

Part Three

Rashes, Skin Signs of Systemic Diseases, and Allergic Skin Conditions

Chapter 11

General Information about Skin Rashes

Definition

Rashes involve changes in the color or texture of your skin.

Considerations

Often, the cause of a rash can be determined from its visible characteristics and other symptoms.

Common Causes

A simple rash is called dermatitis, meaning inflammation of the skin. Contact dermatitis is caused by things your skin touches, such as:

- Dyes and other chemicals in clothing
- Chemicals in elastic, latex, and rubber products
- Cosmetics, soaps, and detergents
- Poison ivy, oak, or sumac

Seborrheic dermatitis is a rash that appears in patches of redness and scaling around the eyebrows, eyelids, mouth, nose, the trunk, and behind the ears. If it happens on your scalp, it is called dandruff in adults and cradle cap in infants.

Age, stress, fatigue, weather extremes, oily skin, infrequent shampooing, and alcohol-based lotions aggravate this harmless but bothersome condition.

Other common causes of a rash include:

- Eczema (atopic dermatitis)—tends to happen in people with allergies or asthma. The rash is generally red, itchy, and scaly.
- Psoriasis—tends to occur as red, scaly, itchy patches over joints and along the scalp. Fingernails may be affected.
- Impetigo—common in children, this infection is from bacteria that live in the top layers of the skin. Appears as red sores that turn into blisters, ooze, then crust over.
- Shingles—a painful blistered skin condition caused by the same virus as chickenpox. The virus can lie dormant in your body for many years and re-emerge as shingles.
- Childhood illnesses like chicken pox, measles, roseola, rubella, hand-foot-mouth disease, fifth disease, and scarlet fever.
- Medications and insect bites or stings.

Many medical conditions can cause a rash as well. For example:

- Lupus erythematosus
- Rheumatoid arthritis, especially the juvenile type
- Kawasaki disease

Home Care

Most simple rashes will improve with gentle skin care and avoiding irritating substances. Follow these general guidelines:

- Avoid scrubbing your skin.
- Use as little soap as possible. Use gentle cleansers instead.
- Avoid applying cosmetic lotions or ointments directly on the rash.
- Use warm (not hot) water for cleaning. Pat dry, don't rub.
- Eliminate any newly added cosmetics or lotions.
- Leave the affected area exposed to the air as much as possible.
- Try calamine medicated lotion for poison ivy, oak, or sumac as well as other types of contact dermatitis.

Hydrocortisone cream (1%) is available without a prescription and may soothe many rashes. If you have eczema, apply moisturizers over your skin. Try oatmeal bath products, available at drugstores, to relieve symptoms of eczema, psoriasis, or shingles.

For psoriasis, you may need a prescription. You could also talk to your doctor about ultraviolet (UV) light therapy. It is safest to have such treatment under medical supervision. However, not all clinics or hospitals offer light therapy. Home units are available, but the cost is not always covered by insurance. If you do purchase a home unit, look for a device that delivers narrow band UVB light.

For seborrheic dermatitis, try applying small amounts of antidandruff shampoo to patches of this scaly rash on your skin, especially near hairy areas like your eyebrows. Leave on for 10 minutes and then carefully rinse off. If the shampoo feels irritating or your skin becomes redder, STOP use.

For impetigo, an antibacterial cream or oral antibiotic is generally prescribed.

Call Your Health Care Provider If

Call 911 if:

- You are short of breath, your throat is tight, or your face is swollen.
- Your child has a purple rash that looks like a bruise.

Call your health care provider if:

- You have joint pain, fever, or a sore throat.
- You have streaks of redness, swelling, or very tender areas. These may indicate an infection.
- You are taking a new medication. **Do not** change or stop any of your medications without talking to your doctor.
- You may have a tick bite.
- Home treatment is ineffective, or your symptoms get worse.

What to Expect at Your Health Care Provider's Office

Your doctor will perform a physical examination. He or she will ask questions about your medical conditions, medications, health problems that run in your family, and recent illnesses or exposures. Questions may include:

- When did the rash begin?
- What parts of your body are affected?
- Does anything make the rash better? Worse?
- Have you used any new soaps, detergents, lotions, or cosmetics recently?
- Have you been in any wooded areas recently?
- Have you had any change in your medications?
- Have you noticed a tick or insect bite?
- Have you eaten anything unusual of late?
- Do you have any other symptoms like itching or scaling?
- What are your underlying medical problems? Do you have, for example, asthma or allergies?

Diagnostic tests may include:

- Skin biopsy
- Skin scrapings
- Blood tests

Depending on the cause of your rash, treatments may include medicated creams or lotions, medications taken by mouth, or skin surgery.

Many primary care doctors are comfortable dealing with common rashes, but for more complicated skin disorders, a referral to a dermatologist may be necessary.

Prevention

- Identify and then stay away from products that irritate your skin. If allergies are suspected, your doctor may want to consider skin testing.
- Receive appropriate vaccines for childhood illnesses, like the varicella vaccine for chicken pox and MMR immunization (a combination vaccine that protects against measles, mumps, and rubella).

- Get strep throat treated right away to prevent scarlet fever.
- Wash your hands frequently to prevent spreading viruses like roseola, hand-foot-mouth disease, and fifth disease.
- Learn relaxation methods like yoga, meditation, or tai chi. Stress aggravates many rashes, including eczema, psoriasis, and seborrheic dermatitis.

Chapter 12

Allergy Testing and the Skin

How are allergies diagnosed?

First, your doctor will ask you questions about your health and symptoms. Make sure to tell your doctor if anyone in your family has allergies. If family members have allergies, your chances of having allergies increase. Your doctor uses the following information to make a diagnosis of allergy:

- Physical exam
- History of your symptoms and family history
- Allergy tests (not always needed)

Allergy tests can be done to help identify if you are allergic and what you are allergic to. Once allergies are identified specific avoidance and treatment measures can be recommended. There are several types of allergy testing.

What types of allergy testing can be done?

Prick Skin Testing: A reliable test for allergies is the prick skin test. A small amount of each thing you may be allergic to (allergen) is placed on the skin, often the back. The skin is then pricked. If you

---

are allergic to an allergen, you will get a bump and redness where the skin is pricked. After a short time, each skin test reaction is measured for swelling and redness. If there is a large enough skin reaction, it means that you may be allergic to the allergen placed at that site. The information from your prick skin test results and your history of symptoms will help your doctor to determine if you have an allergy.

Antihistamines can affect the skin test results. Your doctor may tell you to stop these medications for days to weeks before the testing is done. Other medicines can also affect the results and may need to be avoided. Ask your health care provider what medicines to avoid before your prick skin tests are done.

Intradermal Skin Testing: Another form of skin testing for allergy is by intradermal skin testing. This method is not as reliable as prick skin testing. It is most often used when prick skin testing is negative and there is a strong suspicion of allergy from the history. A small amount of each thing you may be allergic to (allergen) is placed under the skin with a needle, usually on the arm. If you are allergic to an allergen, you will get a bump and redness where the needle has gone under the skin. After a short time, each skin test reaction is measured for swelling and redness. If there is a large enough skin reaction, it means that you may be allergic to the allergen placed at that site. The information from these test results and your history of symptoms will help your doctor to determine if you have an allergy.

Antihistamines and other medicines can also affect these skin test results. Ask your health care provider what medicines to avoid before your skin tests are done.

Blood Testing: A blood test is another kind of test that can be done to help find out if you have allergies. There is some evidence that blood tests are not as sensitive as prick skin tests in determining allergies. However, a blood test may be done if you have skin problems or there is concern that someone will have a severe reaction to a skin test. This is very rare. There are many types of blood tests that can be used to detect allergies. The most common one is called RAST [radioallergosorbent] testing.

Patch Skin Testing: Patch skin testing may be used to find out if a rash is from direct contact with an allergen. Small amounts of allergens are placed on the skin, often the back. The skin is covered with a watertight bandage for several days. After several days the patch is removed and the skin reactions are measured to find out if you may have a contact allergy.

Food Challenge: If you have a positive skin test to foods, your doctor may consider a food challenge. In some cases, this test is the only way to make a diagnosis of food allergy. Increasing doses of the suspected food are given and you are checked for symptoms. The food challenge may be double blind. This means the patient or person giving the test does not know the food being challenged. The doctor prescribing the challenge knows the food. Food challenges are done in a medical setting where emergency care is available. This test is rarely done if there is a history of a life-threatening reaction to a food.

Unproven Methods: There are many other tests to diagnose allergies. Many have not been scientifically proven to be effective and accurate. Talk with your doctor or a board-certified allergist about the best way to determine your allergies.

Should you see an allergy expert?

Many people with allergies see a family doctor for allergy care. You may choose to visit a doctor who is an expert in allergies. These doctors are called board-certified allergists. Here are a few reasons to see an allergy expert:

- Your symptoms make daily activities hard.
- Your symptoms are getting worse.
- You are concerned about side effects of medicine.
- Your regular doctor refers you to an expert for tests.

Allergy tests can be done to help identify if you are allergic and what you are allergic to. Once allergies are identified specific avoidance and treatment measures can be recommended. Talk with you doctor if you think you may have allergies.

Chapter 13

Overview of Common Allergic Skin Conditions: Hives and Angioedema

What is urticaria?

Urticaria, also known as hives, is an outbreak of swollen, pale red bumps or patches (wheals) on the skin that appear suddenly as a result of the body's adverse reaction to certain allergens or for unknown reasons. Hives usually cause itching but may also burn or sting. They can appear anywhere on the body including the face, lips, tongue, throat, or ears. Hives vary in size (from a pencil eraser to a dinner plate) and may join together to form larger areas known as plaques. They can last for hours or up to 3 to 4 days before fading.

What is angioedema?

Angioedema is tissue swelling similar to urticaria, but the swelling occurs beneath the skin instead of on the surface. Angioedema is characterized by deep swelling around the eyes and lips and sometimes of the genitals, hands, and feet. Angioedema generally lasts longer than urticaria, but the swelling usually goes away in less than 24 hours.

"Urticaria and Angioedema," © 2005 The Cleveland Clinic Foundation, 9500 Euclid Avenue, Cleveland, OH 44195, www.clevelandclinic.org. Additional information is available from the Cleveland Clinic Health Information Center, 216-444-3771, toll-free 800-223-2273 extension 43771, or at http://www.clevelandclinic.org/health.

Occasionally, severe, prolonged tissue swelling can be disfiguring. Rarely, angioedema of the throat, tongue, or the lungs can block the airways, causing difficulty breathing and become life threatening.

What causes hives and angioedema?

Hives and angioedema form when blood plasma leaks out of small blood vessels in the skin because a chemical called histamine is released. Histamine is released from mast cells along the blood vessels in the skin. Allergic reactions, chemicals in foods, insect stings, sunlight exposure, or medications can cause histamine release. Sometimes it's impossible to find out why hives have formed.

What are the different types of urticaria and angioedema?

Acute urticaria: Hives lasting less than six weeks. The most common causes are foods, medications, latex, or infections. Insect bites and internal disease may also be responsible. The most common foods that cause hives are nuts, chocolate, fish, tomatoes, eggs, fresh berries, and milk. Fresh foods cause hives more often than cooked foods. Food additives and preservatives may also be the cause. Medications that can cause hives and angioedema include aspirin and other nonsteroidal anti-inflammatory medications such as ibuprofen, high blood pressure medications (ACE inhibitors), or painkillers such as codeine.

Chronic urticaria and angioedema: Hives lasting more than six weeks. The cause of this type of hives is usually more difficult to identify than that of acute urticaria. In patients with chronic urticaria, the cause is found in only a small number of patients and is unknown for more than 80 percent of patients. Chronic urticaria and angioedema can effect other internal organs (such as the lungs and gastrointestinal tract), and can cause symptoms of shortness of breath, vomiting, and diarrhea.

Physical urticaria: Hives caused by direct physical stimulation of the skin such as cold, heat, sun exposure, vibration, pressure, sweating, exercise, and others. The hives usually occur at the site of direct stimulation and rarely, appear on other skin areas. Most of the hives appear within one hour after exposure.

Dermatographism: Hives that form after firmly stroking or scratching the skin. These hives can also occur along with other forms of urticaria. This type of hives is considered a normal variant of the skin.

How are hives and angioedema diagnosed?

Your doctor will need to ask many questions in an attempt to find the possible cause. Since there are no specific tests for hives or the associated swelling of angioedema, testing will depend on your medical history and a thorough examination by your dermatologist. Skin tests may be performed to determine the substance that you are allergic to. Routine blood tests are done to determine if a systemic illness is present.

How are hives and angioedema treated?

The best treatment for hives and associated swelling is to identify and remove the trigger. This is not an easy task. Antihistamines are usually prescribed by your dermatologist to provide relief from symptoms. Antihistamines work best if taken on a regular schedule to prevent hives from forming.

Chronic hives may be treated with antihistamines or combination medications. When antihistamines do not provide relief, oral corticosteroids may be prescribed. For severe hive or angioedema outbreaks, an injection of epinephrine (adrenaline) or a cortisone medication may be needed.

How can hives be managed?

While you're waiting for the hives and swelling to disappear, here are some tips:

- Avoid hot water; use lukewarm water instead.
- Use gentle, mild soap.
- Apply cool compresses or wet cloths to the affected areas.
- Try to work and sleep in a cool room.
- Wear loose-fitting lightweight clothes.

When should I call the doctor?

If hives or angioedema occur with any of the following symptoms, please contact your doctor right away:

- Dizziness
- Wheezing
- Difficulty breathing

- Tightness in the chest
- Swelling of the tongue, lips, or face

Also contact your doctor if your hives have lasted longer than a few days, if they continue to recur over a month or longer, or if you have symptoms of angioedema or anaphylaxis.

Chapter 14

Atopic Dermatitis (Eczema)

Chapter Contents

Section 14.1

All about Atopic Dermatitis

Excerpted from "Atopic Dermatitis" from the National Institute of Arthritis and Musculoskeletal and Skin Diseases (NIAMS), updated April 2003. Available online at http://www.niams.nih.gov; accessed May 10, 2005.

Defining Atopic Dermatitis

Atopic dermatitis is a chronic (long-lasting) disease that affects the skin. It is not contagious; it cannot be passed from one person to another. The word "dermatitis" means inflammation of the skin. "Atopic" refers to a group of diseases where there is often an inherited tendency to develop other allergic conditions, such as asthma and hay fever. In atopic dermatitis, the skin becomes extremely itchy. Scratching leads to redness, swelling, cracking, weeping clear fluid, and finally, crusting and scaling. In most cases, there are periods of time when the disease is worse (called exacerbations or flares) followed by periods when the skin improves or clears up entirely (called remissions). As some children with atopic dermatitis grow older, their skin disease improves or disappears altogether, although their skin often remains dry and easily irritated. In others, atopic dermatitis continues to be a significant problem in adulthood. Although atopic dermatitis may occur at any age, it most often begins in infancy and childhood.

Atopic dermatitis is often referred to as eczema, which is a general term for the several types of inflammation of the skin. Atopic dermatitis is the most common of the many types of eczema. Several have very similar symptoms.

Incidence and Prevalence of Atopic Dermatitis

Atopic dermatitis is very common. It affects males and females and accounts for 10 to 20 percent of all visits to dermatologists (doctors who specialize in the care and treatment of skin diseases). Although atopic dermatitis may occur at any age, it most often begins in infancy and childhood. Scientists estimate that 65 percent of patients develop symptoms in the first year of life, and 90 percent develop symptoms before the age of 5. Onset after age 30 is less common and is often due to exposure of the skin to harsh or wet conditions. Atopic dermatitis is a common cause of workplace disability. People who live in cities and in dry climates appear more likely to develop this condition.

Although it is difficult to identify exactly how many people are affected by atopic dermatitis, an estimated 20 percent of infants and young children experience symptoms of the disease. Roughly 60 percent of these infants continue to have one or more symptoms of atopic dermatitis in adulthood. This means that more than 15 million people in the United States have symptoms of the disease.

Types of Eczema (Dermatitis)

- **Allergic contact eczema (dermatitis):** a red, itchy, weepy reaction where the skin has come into contact with a substance that the immune system recognizes as foreign, such as poison ivy or certain preservatives in creams and lotions
- **Atopic dermatitis:** a chronic skin disease characterized by itchy, inflamed skin
- **Contact eczema:** a localized reaction that includes redness, itching, and burning where the skin has come into contact with an allergen (an allergy-causing substance) or with an irritant such as an acid, a cleaning agent, or other chemical
- **Dyshidrotic eczema:** irritation of the skin on the palms of hands and soles of the feet characterized by clear, deep blisters that itch and burn
- **Neurodermatitis:** scaly patches of the skin on the head, lower legs, wrists, or forearms caused by a localized itch (such as an insect bite) that become intensely irritated when scratched
- **Nummular eczema:** coin-shaped patches of irritated skin—most common on the arms, back, buttocks, and lower legs—that may be crusted, scaling, and extremely itchy
- **Seborrheic eczema:** yellowish, oily, scaly patches of skin on the scalp, face, and occasionally other parts of the body
- **Stasis dermatitis:** a skin irritation on the lower legs, generally related to circulatory problems

Cost of Atopic Dermatitis

In a recent analysis of the health insurance records of 5 million Americans under age 65, medical researchers found that approximately 2.5 percent had atopic dermatitis. Annual insurance payments for medical care of atopic dermatitis ranged from $580 to $1,250 per patient. More than one quarter of each patient's total health care costs were for atopic dermatitis and related conditions. The researchers project that U.S. health insurance companies spend more than $1 billion per year on atopic dermatitis.

Causes of Atopic Dermatitis

The cause of atopic dermatitis is not known, but the disease seems to result from a combination of genetic (hereditary) and environmental factors.

Children are more likely to develop this disorder if one or both parents have had it or have had allergic conditions like asthma or hay fever. Although some people outgrow skin symptoms, approximately three fourths of children with atopic dermatitis go on to develop hay fever or asthma. Environmental factors can bring on symptoms of atopic dermatitis at any time in individuals who have inherited the atopic disease trait.

Atopic dermatitis is also associated with malfunction of the body's immune system: the system that recognizes and helps fight bacteria and viruses that invade the body. Scientists have found that people with atopic dermatitis have a low level of a cytokine (a protein) that is essential to the healthy function of the body's immune system and a high level of other cytokines that lead to allergic reactions. The immune system can become misguided and create inflammation in the skin even in the absence of a major infection. This can be viewed as a form of autoimmunity, where a body reacts against its own tissues.

In the past, doctors thought that atopic dermatitis was caused by an emotional disorder. We now know that emotional factors, such as stress, can make the condition worse, but they do not cause the disease.

Skin Features of Atopic Dermatitis

- **Atopic pleat (Dennie-Morgan fold):** an extra fold of skin that develops under the eye
- **Cheilitis:** inflammation of the skin on and around the lips

- **Hyperlinear palms:** increased number of skin creases on the palms
- **Hyperpigmented eyelids:** eyelids that have become darker in color from inflammation or hay fever
- **Ichthyosis:** dry, rectangular scales on the skin
- **Keratosis pilaris:** small, rough bumps, generally on the face, upper arms, and thighs
- **Lichenification:** thick, leathery skin resulting from constant scratching and rubbing
- **Papules:** small raised bumps that may open when scratched and become crusty and infected
- **Urticaria:** hives (red, raised bumps) that may occur after exposure to an allergen, at the beginning of flares, or after exercise or a hot bath

Symptoms of Atopic Dermatitis

Symptoms (signs) vary from person to person. The most common symptoms are dry, itchy skin and rashes on the face, inside the elbows and behind the knees, and on the hands and feet. Itching is the most important symptom of atopic dermatitis. Scratching and rubbing in response to itching irritates the skin, increases inflammation, and actually increases itchiness. Itching is a particular problem during sleep when conscious control of scratching is lost.

The appearance of the skin that is affected by atopic dermatitis depends on the amount of scratching and the presence of secondary skin infections. The skin may be red and scaly, be thick and leathery, contain small raised bumps, or leak fluid and become crusty and infected. These features can also be found in people who do not have atopic dermatitis or who have other types of skin disorders.

Atopic dermatitis may also affect the skin around the eyes, the eyelids, and the eyebrows and lashes. Scratching and rubbing the eye area can cause the skin to redden and swell. Some people with atopic dermatitis develop an extra fold of skin under their eyes. Patchy loss of eyebrows and eyelashes may also result from scratching or rubbing.

Researchers have noted differences in the skin of people with atopic dermatitis that may contribute to the symptoms of the disease. The outer layer of skin, called the epidermis, is divided into two parts: an inner part containing moist, living cells, and an outer part, known as the horny layer or stratum corneum, containing dry, flattened, dead cells. Under normal conditions the stratum corneum acts as a barrier, keeping the rest of the skin from drying out and protecting other layers of skin from damage caused by irritants and infections. When this barrier is damaged, irritants act more intensely on the skin.

The skin of a person with atopic dermatitis loses moisture from the epidermal layer, allowing the skin to become very dry and reducing its protective abilities. Thus, when combined with the abnormal skin immune system, the person's skin is more likely to become infected by bacteria (for example, Staphylococcus and Streptococcus) or viruses, such as those that cause warts and cold sores.

Stages of Atopic Dermatitis

When atopic dermatitis occurs during infancy and childhood, it affects each child differently in terms of both onset and severity of symptoms. In infants, atopic dermatitis typically begins around 6 to 12 weeks of age. It may first appear around the cheeks and chin as a patchy facial rash, which can progress to red, scaling, oozing skin. The skin may become infected. Once the infant becomes more mobile and begins crawling, exposed areas, such as the inner and outer parts of the arms and legs, may also be affected. An infant with atopic dermatitis may be restless and irritable because of the itching and discomfort of the disease. The skin may improve by 18 months of age, although the infant has a greater than normal risk of developing dry skin or hand eczema later in life.

In childhood, the rash tends to occur behind the knees and inside the elbows; on the sides of the neck; around the mouth; and on the wrists, ankles, and hands. Often, the rash begins with papules that become hard and scaly when scratched. The skin around the lips may be inflamed, and constant licking of the area may lead to small, painful cracks in the skin around the mouth.

In some children, the disease goes into remission for a long time, only to come back at the onset of puberty when hormones, stress, and the use of irritating skin care products or cosmetics may cause the disease to flare.

Although a number of people who developed atopic dermatitis as children also experience symptoms as adults, it is also possible for the disease to show up first in adulthood. The pattern in adults is similar to that seen in children; that is, the disease may be widespread or limited to only a few parts of the body. For example, only the hands or feet may be affected and become dry, itchy, red, and cracked. Sleep patterns and work performance may be affected, and long-term use of medications to treat the atopic dermatitis may cause complications. Adults with atopic dermatitis also have a predisposition toward irritant contact dermatitis, where the skin becomes red and inflamed from contact with detergents, wool, friction from clothing, or other potential irritants. It is more likely to occur in occupations involving frequent hand washing or exposure to chemicals. Some people develop a rash around their nipples. These localized symptoms are difficult to treat. Because adults may also develop cataracts, the doctor may recommend regular eye exams.

Diagnosing Atopic Dermatitis

Each person experiences a unique combination of symptoms, which may vary in severity over time. The doctor will base a diagnosis on the symptoms the patient experiences and may need to see the patient several times to make an accurate diagnosis and to rule out other diseases and conditions that might cause skin irritation. In some cases, the family doctor or pediatrician may refer the patient to a dermatologist (doctor specializing in skin disorders) or allergist (allergy specialist) for further evaluation.

A medical history may help the doctor better understand the nature of a patient's symptoms, when they occur, and their possible causes. The doctor may ask about family history of allergic disease; whether the patient also has diseases such as hay fever or asthma; and about exposure to irritants, sleep disturbances, any foods that seem to be related to skin flares, previous treatments for skin-related symptoms, and use of steroids or other medications. A preliminary diagnosis of atopic dermatitis can be made if the patient has three or more features from each of two categories: major features and minor features.

Currently, there is no single test to diagnose atopic dermatitis. However, there are some tests that can give the doctor an indication of allergic sensitivity.

Pricking the skin with a needle that contains a small amount of a suspected allergen may be helpful in identifying factors that trigger flares of atopic dermatitis. Negative results on skin tests may help rule out the possibility that certain substances cause skin inflammation. Positive skin prick test results are difficult to interpret in people with atopic dermatitis because the skin is very sensitive to many substances, and there can be many positive test sites that are not meaningful to a person's disease at the time. Positive results simply indicate that the individual has IgE (allergic) antibodies to the substance tested. IgE (immunoglobulin E) controls the immune system's allergic response and is often high in atopic dermatitis.

Recently, it was shown that if the quantity of IgE antibodies to a food in the blood is above a certain level, it is diagnostic of a food allergy. If the level of IgE to a specific food does not exceed the level needed for diagnosis but a food allergy is suspected, a person might be asked to record everything eaten and note any reactions. Physician-supervised food challenges (that is, the introduction of a food) following a period of food elimination may be necessary to determine if symptomatic food allergy is present. Identifying the food allergen may be difficult when a person is also being exposed to other possible allergens at the same time or symptoms may be triggered by other factors, such as infection, heat, and humidity.

Factors That Make Atopic Dermatitis Worse

Many factors or conditions can make symptoms of atopic dermatitis worse, further triggering the already overactive immune system, aggravating the itch-scratch cycle, and increasing damage to the skin. These factors can be broken down into two main categories: irritants and allergens.

Irritants are substances that directly affect the skin and, when present in high enough concentrations with long enough contact, cause the skin to become red and itchy or to burn. Specific irritants affect people with atopic dermatitis to different degrees. Over time, many patients and their family members learn to identify the irritants causing the most trouble. For example, frequent wetting and drying of the skin may affect the skin barrier function. Also, wool or synthetic fibers and rough or poorly fitting clothing can rub the skin, trigger inflammation, and cause the itch-scratch cycle to begin. Soaps and detergents may have a drying effect and worsen itching, and some perfumes and cosmetics may irritate the skin. Exposure to certain substances, such as solvents, dust, or sand, may also make the condition worse. Cigarette smoke may irritate the eyelids. Because the effects of irritants vary from one person to another, each person can best determine what substances or circumstances cause the disease to flare.

Allergens are substances from foods, plants, animals, or the air that inflame the skin because the immune system overreacts to the substance. Inflammation occurs even when the person is exposed to small amounts of the substance for a limited time. Although it is known that allergens in the air, such as dust mites, pollens, molds, and dander from animal hair or skin, may worsen the symptoms of atopic dermatitis in some people, scientists aren't certain whether inhaling these allergens or their actual penetration of the skin causes the problems. When people with atopic dermatitis come into contact with an irritant or allergen they are sensitive to, inflammation-producing cells become active. These cells release chemicals that cause itching and redness. As the person responds by scratching and rubbing the skin, further damage occurs.

A number of studies have shown that foods may trigger or worsen atopic dermatitis in some people, particularly infants and children. In general, the worse the atopic dermatitis and the younger the child, the more likely food allergy is present. An allergic reaction to food can cause skin inflammation (generally an itchy red rash), gastrointestinal symptoms (abdominal pain, vomiting, diarrhea), and/or upper respiratory tract symptoms (congestion, sneezing, and wheezing). The most common allergenic (allergy-causing) foods are eggs, milk, peanuts, wheat, soy, and fish. A recent analysis of a large number of studies on allergies and breastfeeding indicated that breastfeeding an infant for at least 4 months may protect the child from developing allergies. However, some studies suggest that mothers with a family history of atopic diseases should avoid eating common allergenic foods during late pregnancy and breastfeeding.

In addition to irritants and allergens, emotional factors, skin infections, and temperature and climate play a role in atopic dermatitis. Although the disease itself is not caused by emotional factors, it can be made worse by stress, anger, and frustration. Interpersonal problems or major life changes, such as divorce, job changes, or the death of a loved one, can also make the disease worse.

Bathing without proper moisturizing afterward is a common factor that triggers a flare of atopic dermatitis. The low humidity of winter or the dry year-round climate of some geographic areas can make the disease worse, as can overheated indoor areas and long or hot baths and showers. Alternately sweating and chilling can trigger a flare in some people. Bacterial infections can also trigger or increase the severity of atopic dermatitis. If a patient experiences a sudden flare of illness, the doctor may check for infection.

Common Irritants

- Wool or synthetic fibers
- Soaps and detergents

- Some perfumes and cosmetics
- Substances such as chlorine, mineral oil, or solvents
- Dust or sand
- Cigarette smoke

Treatment of Atopic Dermatitis

Treatment is more effective when a partnership develops that includes the patient, family members, and doctor. The doctor will suggest a treatment plan based on the patient's age, symptoms, and general health. The patient or family member providing care plays a large role in the success of the treatment plan by carefully following the doctor's instructions and paying attention to what is or is not helpful. Most patients will notice improvement with proper skin care and lifestyle changes. Treatment is more effective when a partnership develops that includes the patient, family members, and doctor.

The doctor has two main goals in treating atopic dermatitis: healing the skin and preventing flares. These may be assisted by developing skin care routines and avoiding substances that lead to skin irritation and trigger the immune system and the itch-scratch cycle. It is important for the patient and family members to note any changes in the skin's condition in response to treatment, and to be persistent in identifying the treatment that seems to work best.

Medications

New medications known as immuno-modulators have been developed that help control inflammation and reduce immune system reactions when applied to the skin. Examples of these medications are tacrolimus ointment (Protopic) and pimecrolimus cream (Elidel). They can be used in patients older than 2 years of age and have few side effects (burning or itching the first few days of application). They not only reduce flares, but also maintain skin texture and reduce the need for long-term use of corticosteroids. [*Note:* Brand names included in this chapter are provided as examples only, and their inclusion does not mean that these products are endorsed by the National Institutes of Health or any other Government agency. Also, if a particular brand name is not mentioned, this does not mean or imply that the product is unsatisfactory.]

Corticosteroid creams and ointments have been used for many years to treat atopic dermatitis and other autoimmune diseases affecting the skin. Sometimes over-the-counter preparations are used, but in many cases the doctor will prescribe a stronger corticosteroid cream or ointment. When prescribing a medication, the doctor will take into account the patient's age, location of the skin to be treated, severity of the symptoms, and type of preparation (cream or ointment) that will be most effective. Sometimes the base used in certain brands of corticosteroid creams and ointments irritates the skin of a particular patient. Side effects of repeated or long-term use of topical corticosteroids can include thinning of the skin, infections, growth suppression (in children), and stretch marks on the skin.

When topical corticosteroids are not effective, the doctor may prescribe a systemic corticosteroid, which is taken by mouth or injected instead of being applied directly to the skin. An example of a commonly prescribed corticosteroid is prednisone. Typically, these medications are used only in resistant cases and only given for short periods of time. The side effects of systemic corticosteroids can include skin damage, thinned or weakened bones, high blood pressure, high blood sugar, infections, and cataracts. It can be dangerous to suddenly stop taking corticosteroids, so it is very important that the doctor and patient work together in changing the corticosteroid dose.

Antibiotics to treat skin infections may be applied directly to the skin in an ointment, but are usually more effective when taken by mouth. If viral or fungal infections are present, the doctor may also prescribe specific medications to treat those infections.

Certain antihistamines that cause drowsiness can reduce nighttime scratching and allow more restful sleep when taken at bedtime. This effect can be particularly helpful for patients whose nighttime scratching makes the disease worse.

In adults, drugs that suppress the immune system, such as cyclosporine, methotrexate, or azathioprine, may be prescribed to treat severe cases of atopic dermatitis that have failed to respond to other forms of therapy. These drugs block the production of some immune cells and curb the action of others. The side effects of drugs like cyclosporine can include high blood pressure, nausea, vomiting, kidney problems, headaches, tingling or numbness, and a possible increased risk of cancer and infections. There is also a risk of relapse after the drug is stopped. Because of their toxic side effects, systemic corticosteroids and immunosuppressive drugs are used only in severe cases and then for as short a period of time as possible. Patients requiring systemic corticosteroids should be referred to dermatologists or allergists specializing in the care of atopic dermatitis to help identify trigger factors and alternative therapies.

In rare cases, when home-based treatments have been unsuccessful, a patient may need a few days in the hospital for intense treatment.

Phototherapy

Use of ultraviolet A or B light waves, alone or combined, can be an effective treatment for mild to moderate dermatitis in older children (over 12 years old) and adults. A combination of ultraviolet light therapy and a drug called psoralen can also be used in cases that are resistant to ultraviolet light alone. Possible long-term side effects of this treatment include premature skin aging and skin cancer. If the doctor thinks that phototherapy may be useful to treat the symptoms of atopic dermatitis, he or she will use the minimum exposure necessary and monitor the skin carefully.

Treating Atopic Dermatitis in Infants and Children

- Give lukewarm baths.
- Apply lubricant immediately following the bath.
- Keep child's fingernails filed short.
- Select soft cotton fabrics when choosing clothing.
- Consider using sedating antihistamines to promote sleep and reduce scratching at night.
- Keep the child cool; avoid situations where overheating occurs.
- Learn to recognize skin infections and seek treatment promptly.
- Attempt to distract the child with activities to keep him or her from scratching.
- Identify and remove irritants and allergens.

Skin Care

Healing the skin and keeping it healthy are important to prevent further damage and enhance quality of life. Developing and sticking with a daily skin care routine is critical to preventing flares.

A lukewarm bath helps to cleanse and moisturize the skin without drying it excessively. Because soaps can be drying to the skin, the doctor may recommend use of a mild bar soap or nonsoap cleanser. Bath oils are not usually helpful.

After bathing, a person should air-dry the skin, or pat it dry gently (avoiding rubbing or brisk drying), and then apply a lubricant to seal in the water that has been absorbed into the skin during bathing. In addition to restoring the skin's moisture, lubrication increases the rate of healing and establishes a barrier against further drying and irritation. Lotions that have a high water or alcohol content evaporate more quickly, and alcohol may cause stinging. Therefore, they generally are not the best choice. Creams and ointments work better at healing the skin.

Another key to protecting and restoring the skin is taking steps to avoid repeated skin infections. Signs of skin infection include tiny pustules (pus-filled bumps), oozing cracks or sores, or crusty yellow blisters. If symptoms of a skin infection develop, the doctor should be consulted and treatment should begin as soon as possible.

Protection from Allergen Exposure

The doctor may suggest reducing exposure to a suspected allergen. For example, the presence of the house dust mite can be limited by encasing mattresses and pillows in special dust-proof covers, frequently washing bedding in hot water, and removing carpeting. However, there is no way to completely rid the environment of airborne allergens.

Changing the diet may not always relieve symptoms of atopic dermatitis. A change may be helpful, however, when the medical history, laboratory studies, and specific symptoms strongly suggest a food allergy. It is up to the patient and his or her family and physician to decide whether the dietary restrictions are appropriate. Unless properly monitored by a physician or dietitian, diets with many restrictions can contribute to serious nutritional problems, especially in children.

Atopic Dermatitis and Quality of Life

Despite the symptoms caused by atopic dermatitis, it is possible for people with the disorder to maintain a good quality of life. The keys to quality of life lie in being well-informed; awareness of symptoms and their possible cause; and developing a partnership involving the patient or caregiving family member, medical doctor, and other health professionals. Good communication is essential.

When a child has atopic dermatitis, the entire family may be affected. It is helpful if families have additional support to help them cope with the stress and frustration associated with the disease. A child may be fussy and difficult and unable to keep from scratching and rubbing the skin. Distracting the child and providing activities that keep the hands busy are helpful but require much effort on the part of the parents or caregivers. Another issue families face is the social and emotional stress associated with changes in appearance caused by atopic dermatitis. The child may face difficulty in school or with social relationships and may need additional support and encouragement from family members.

Adults with atopic dermatitis can enhance their quality of life by caring regularly for their skin and being mindful of the effects of the disease and how to treat them. Adults should develop a skin care regimen as part of their daily routine, which can be adapted as circumstances and skin conditions change. Stress management and relaxation techniques may help decrease the likelihood of flares. Developing a network of support that includes family, friends, health professionals, and support groups or organizations can be beneficial. Chronic anxiety and depression may be relieved by short-term psychological therapy.

Recognizing the situations when scratching is most likely to occur may also help. For example, many patients find that they scratch more when they are idle, and they do better when engaged in activities that keep the hands occupied. Counseling also may be helpful to identify or change career goals if a job involves contact with irritants or involves frequent hand washing, such as kitchen work or auto mechanics.

Atopic Dermatitis and Vaccination against Smallpox

Although scientists are working to develop safer vaccines, persons diagnosed with atopic dermatitis (or eczema) should not receive the current smallpox vaccine. According to the Centers for Disease Control and Prevention (CDC), a U.S. Government organization, persons who have ever been diagnosed with atopic dermatitis, even if the condition is mild or not presently active, are more likely to develop a serious complication if they are exposed to the virus from the smallpox vaccine.

People with atopic dermatitis should exercise caution when coming into close physical contact with a person who has been recently vaccinated, and make certain the vaccinated person has covered the vaccination site or taken other precautions until the scab falls off (about 3 weeks). Those who have had physical contact with a vaccinated person's unhealed vaccination site or to their bedding or other items that might have touched that site should notify their doctor, particularly if they develop a new or unusual rash.

During a smallpox outbreak, these vaccination recommendations may change. Persons with atopic dermatitis who have been exposed to smallpox should consult their doctor about vaccination.

Section 14.2

Safety Concerns of Two Common Atopic Dermatitis Drugs

"FDA Issues Public Health Advisory Informing Health Care Providers of Safety Concerns Associated with the Use of Two Eczema Drugs, Elidel and Protopic," March 10, 2005. Available online at http://www.fda.gov; accessed April 29, 2005.

The Food and Drug Administration (FDA) today advised health care professionals to prescribe Elidel (pimecrolimus) and Protopic (tacrolimus) only as directed and only after other eczema treatments have failed to work because of a potential cancer risk associated with their use. In addition, FDA is adding a black box warning to the health professional label for the two products and developing a Medication Guide for patients.

Today's actions follow the recommendations made by the FDA's Pediatric Advisory Committee during its February 15, 2005 meeting. At this meeting, findings of cancer in three different animal species were reviewed. The data showed that the risk of cancer increased as the amount of the drug given increased. The data also included a small number of reports of cancers in children and adults treated with Elidel or Protopic.

The manufacturers of the products have agreed to conduct research to determine whether there is an actual risk of cancer in humans, and, if so, its extent.

Both products are applied to the skin to control eczema by suppressing the immune system. FDA's Public Health Advisory specifically advises physicians to weigh the risks and benefits of these drugs in adults and children and consider the following:

- Elidel and Protopic are approved for short-term and intermittent treatment of atopic dermatitis (eczema) in patients unresponsive to, or intolerant of other treatments.
- Elidel and Protopic are not approved for use in children younger than 2 years old. The long-term effect of Elidel and Protopic on the developing immune system in infants and children is not known. In clinical trials, infants and children younger than 2 years of age treated with Elidel had a higher rate of upper respiratory infections than those treated with placebo cream.
- Elidel and Protopic should be used only for short periods of time, not continuously. The long-term safety of these products is unknown.
- Children and adults with a weakened or compromised immune system should not use Elidel or Protopic.
- Use the minimum amount of Elidel and Protopic needed to control the patient's symptoms. The animal data suggest that the risk of cancer increases with increased exposure to Elidel or Protopic.

Protopic was approved in 2000 and Elidel in 2001 to treat eczema.

Chapter 15

Contact Dermatitis

Definition

Contact dermatitis is an inflammation of the skin caused by direct contact with an irritating substance.

Causes, Incidence, and Risk Factors

Contact dermatitis is an inflammation of the skin caused by direct contact with an irritating or allergy-causing substance (irritant or allergen) and varies in the same individual over time. A history of any type of allergies increases the risk for this condition.

Irritant dermatitis, the most common type of contact dermatitis, involves inflammation resulting from contact with acids, alkaline materials such as soaps and detergents, solvents, or other chemicals. The reaction usually resembles a burn.

The second most common type of contact dermatitis is caused by exposure to a material to which the person has become hypersensitive or allergic. The skin inflammation varies from mild irritation and redness to open sores, depending on the type of irritant, the body part affected, and the sensitivity of the individual.

Overtreatment dermatitis is a form of contact dermatitis that occurs when treatment for another skin disorder causes irritation.

Common allergens associated with contact dermatitis include:

- Poison ivy, poison oak, poison sumac
- Other plants
- Nickel or other metals
- Medications
  - Antibiotics, especially those applied to the surface of the skin (topical)
  - Topical anesthetics
  - Other medications
- Rubber
- Cosmetics
- Fabrics and clothing
- Detergents
- Solvents
- Adhesives
- Fragrances, perfumes
- Other chemicals and substances

Contact dermatitis may involve a reaction to a substance that the person is exposed to or uses repeatedly. Although there may be no initial reaction, repeated use (for example, nail polish remover, preservatives in contact lens solutions, or repeated contact with metals in earring posts and the metal backs of watches) can cause eventual sensitization and reaction to the product.

Some products cause a reaction only when they contact the skin and are exposed to sunlight (photosensitivity). These include shaving lotions, sunscreens, sulfa ointments, some perfumes, coal tar products, and oil from the skin of a lime. A few airborne allergens, such as ragweed or insecticide spray, can cause contact dermatitis.

Symptoms

- Itching (pruritus) of the skin in exposed areas
- Skin redness or inflammation in the exposed area
- Tenderness of the skin in the exposed area
- Localized swelling of the skin
- Warmth of the exposed area (may occur)

- Skin lesion or rash at the site of exposure
  - Lesions of any type: redness, rash, papules (pimple-like), vesicles, and bullae (blisters)
  - May involve oozing, draining, or crusting
  - May become scaly, raw, or thickened

Signs and Tests

The diagnosis is primarily based on the skin appearance and a history of exposure to an irritant or an allergen.

According to the American Academy of Allergy, Asthma, and Immunology, "Patch testing is the gold standard for contact allergen identification." Allergy testing with skin patches may isolate the suspected allergen that is causing the reaction.

Patch testing is used for patients who have chronic, recurring contact dermatitis. It requires three office visits and must be done by a clinician with detailed experience in the procedures and interpretation of results. Patients should bring suspected materials with them, especially if they have already tested those materials on a small area of their skin and noticed a reaction.

Other tests may be used to rule out other possible causes, including skin lesion biopsy or culture of the skin lesion.

Treatment

Initial treatment includes thorough washing with lots of water to remove any trace of the irritant that may remain on the skin. Further exposure to known irritants or allergens should be avoided.

In some cases, the best treatment is to do nothing to the area.

Topical corticosteroid medications may reduce inflammation. Carefully adhere to instructions when using topical steroids because overuse of these medications, even low-strength over-the-counter topical steroids, may cause a troublesome skin condition. In severe cases, systemic corticosteroids may be needed to reduce inflammation. These are usually tapered gradually over about 12 days to prevent recurrence of the rash.

Wet dressings and soothing, antipruritic (anti-itch), or drying lotions may be recommended to reduce other symptoms.

Expectations (Prognosis)

Contact dermatitis usually clears up without complications within 2 or 3 weeks but may recur if the causal agent cannot be identified or avoided. Change of occupation or occupational habits may be necessary if the disorder is caused by occupational exposure.

Complications

Secondary bacterial skin infections may occur.

Calling Your Health Care Provider

Call your health care provider if symptoms indicate contact dermatitis and it is severe or there is no improvement after treatment.

Prevention

Avoid contact with known allergens. Use protective gloves or other barriers if contact with substances is likely or unavoidable. Wash skin surfaces thoroughly after contact with substances. Avoid overtreating skin disorders.

Chapter 16

Dermatitis Herpetiformis

Dermatitis herpetiformis (DH) is a chronic disease of the skin marked by groups of watery, itchy blisters that may resemble pimples or blisters. The ingestion of gluten (from wheat, rye, and barley) triggers an immune system response that deposits a substance, IgA (Immunoglobulin A), under the top layer of skin. IgA is present in affected as well as unaffected skin. DH is a hereditary autoimmune gluten intolerance disease linked with celiac disease. If you have DH, you always have gluten intolerance. With DH, the primary lesion is on the skin, whereas with celiac disease the lesions are in the small intestine. The degree of damage to the small intestine is often less severe or more patchy than those with celiac disease. Both diseases are permanent and symptoms and damage will occur after consuming gluten.

Symptoms

The IgA deposits under the skin result in eruptions of red raised patches of skin, similar to the beginning of a pimple, that can develop into small watery blisters. The itching and burning of the eruptions are severe and the urge to scratch them is intense. Scratching will further irritate the eruptions. Eruptions commonly occur on pressure points, such as around the elbows, the front of the knees, the buttocks, back, face, and scalp but can appear anywhere on the body. Eruptions are usually bilateral—occurring on both sides of the body. Sixty percent of those diagnosed are men and the most common age at diagnosis is 15 to 40 years old. Although it is uncommon to diagnose young children with DH, we are seeing more cases of early childhood DH.

Diagnosis

Your dermatologist will take a small biopsy of the unaffected skin very close to an eruption or eruption site. The presence of IgA deposits confirms a diagnosis of DH. Sometimes the dermatologist may also want you to have blood work for celiac disease and see a gastroenterologist.

Treatment

Just as with celiac disease, strictly following a gluten-free diet for life is the only complete treatment. It may take two or more years on a gluten-free diet for the IgA deposits under the skin to clear. Your doctors may prescribe medications for immediate relief from the itching and burning eruptions. The most common medication used is Dapsone. This medication has serious side effects and requires regular monitoring by your physician. When taken to relieve the symptoms of DH, Dapsone should be taken in the smallest effective doses for as short a time as possible. Medications for DH should not be used during pregnancy.

If you use medications to relieve the itching caused from DH, but do not follow a gluten-free diet, you run the risk of also developing the intestinal problem celiac disease and other complications.

Questions to Ask Your Doctor:

- Should I take medication for this disease?
- How long will I need to take this medicine and how will I know when to stop taking it?
- What are the side effects of the medicine?
- How often do I need to get my blood drawn to monitor this medicine's effect on my body?
- What else can trigger DH?

Prognosis

The prognosis of dermatitis herpetiformis is excellent, if you stay on the gluten-free diet. The severity and frequency of eruptions will decrease as you continue with the diet. Iodine can trigger eruptions in some people. However, iodine is an essential nutrient and should not be removed from the diet without a physician's supervision.

Related Disorders

Thyroid disease is most commonly associated with DH. Other autoimmune disorders that people with CD are at greater risk to develop include Addison disease, autoimmune chronic active hepatitis, alopecia areata, Graves disease, insulin-dependent diabetes mellitus (type 1), myasthenia gravis, scleroderma, Sjögren syndrome, systemic lupus erythematosus, and thyroid disease. This is not a complete list. Thyroid diseases and diabetes are the two most commonly associated diseases. It is not uncommon to have other skin conditions as well.

Chapter 17

Mastocytosis

The Disorder

Mastocytosis is a disorder in both children and adults. It is caused by the presence of too many mast cells in your body. You can find mast cells in skin, linings of the stomach and intestine, and connective tissue (such as cartilage or tendons). Mast cells play an important role in helping your immune system defend these tissues from disease. Mast cells attract other key players of the immune defense system to areas of your body where they are needed by releasing chemical "alarms" such as histamine and cytokines.

Mast cells seem to have other roles as well. Found to gather around wounds, they may play a part in wound healing. For example, the typical itching you feel around a healing scab may be caused by histamine released by mast cells. Researchers also think mast cells may have a role in the growth of blood vessels. No one with too few or no mast cells has ever been found. This fact indicates to some scientists that having too few mast cells may be incompatible with life.

The presence of too many mast cells, or mastocytosis, can occur in two forms—cutaneous and systemic. The most common cutaneous (skin) form is also called urticaria pigmentosa, which occurs when mast cells infiltrate the skin. Systemic mastocytosis is caused by mast

---

From the National Institute of Allergy and Infectious Disease (NIAID), January 2005. Available online at http://www.niaid.nih.gov; accessed May 15, 2005.

cells accumulating in the tissues and can affect organs such as the liver, spleen, bone marrow, and small intestine.

Researchers first described urticaria pigmentosa in 1869. Systemic mastocytosis was first reported in the scientific literature in 1933. The true incidence of either type of mastocytosis remains unknown, but mastocytosis generally is considered to be an "orphan disease." (Orphan diseases affect approximately 200,000 or fewer people in the United States.)

Symptoms

Chemicals released by mast cells cause changes in your body's functioning that lead to typical allergic responses such as flushing, itching, abdominal cramping, and even shock. When too many mast cells are in your body, the additional chemicals can cause:

- Musculoskeletal pain
- Abdominal discomfort
- Nausea and vomiting
- Ulcers
- Diarrhea
- Skin lesions

It can also cause episodes of hypotension (very low blood pressure and faintness) or anaphylaxis (shock).

Diagnosis

Your doctor can diagnose urticaria pigmentosa by the appearance of your skin and confirm it by finding an abnormally high number of mast cells on a skin biopsy. The diagnosis of systemic mastocytosis is made when an increased number of abnormal mast cells is found during an examination of your bone marrow.

Other tests that are important in evaluating a suspected case of mastocytosis include a search for specific genetic mutations that health experts associate with this disease.

Treatment

Doctors use several medicines to treat mastocytosis symptoms, including antihistamines (to prevent the effect of mast cell histamine) and anticholinergics (to relieve intestinal cramping). A number of medicines treat specific symptoms of mastocytosis.

- Antihistamines frequently treat itching and other skin complaints.
- Antihistamines that work specifically against ulcers and proton pump inhibitors relieve ulcer-like symptoms.
- Two types of antihistamines treat severe flushing and low blood pressure before symptoms appear and epinephrine after symptoms begin.
- Topical steroids temporarily reduce skin lesions that are cosmetically disturbing.
- Steroids treat malabsorption, or impaired ability to take in nutrients.

In cases in which mastocytosis is malignant, cancerous, or associated with a blood disorder, steroids and/or chemotherapy may be necessary.

Research

The National Institute of Allergy and Infectious Diseases (NIAID) scientists have studied and treated patients with mastocytosis for more than two decades at the National Institutes of Health (NIH) Clinical Center.

Some of the most important research advances for this rare disorder include improved diagnosis of mast cell disease, identification of growth factors that are responsible for increased mast cell production, and improved treatment. For example, researchers have developed drugs that help block the action of chemicals released from mast cells. Researchers are evaluating other drugs that slow down mast cell production.

Scientists also are focusing on identifying disease-associated gene mutations. Several such mutations have been identified at NIH in a receptor for a mast cell growth factor. Understanding such mutations helps researchers to understand the causes of mastocytosis, improve diagnosis, and lead to better treatment methods.

Chapter 18

Dermatomyositis

What is dermatomyositis? What are the signs and symptoms?

Dermatomyositis (DM) affects people of any age or sex, but is found in more women than men. DM is thought to be an autoimmune disease, meaning the body's immune system, which normally fights infections and viruses, does not stop fighting once the infection or virus is gone. The immune system then attacks the body's own normal, healthy tissue through inflammation, or swelling.

DM is the easiest type of myositis to diagnose because of the skin rash. The DM rash looks patchy, dusky, and reddish or purple. It is found on the eyelids, cheeks, nose, back, upper chest, elbows, knees, and knuckles. Some people also have hardened bumps under the skin, called calcinosis. The rash is often seen before muscle weakness is felt. The skin rash and weak muscles are caused by inflammation, or swelling, in the blood vessels under the skin and in the muscles, also called vasculitis.

Muscle weakness usually happens over a period of days, weeks, or months. Patients who have the skin rash but feel no muscle weakness have amyopathic DM, or DM sine myositis. The weakness begins with muscles that are closest to and within the trunk of the body. Neck, hip, back, and shoulder muscles are examples. Some DM patients have muscle pain and difficulty swallowing, or dysphagia.

What tests will the doctor run to decide if I have dermatomyositis?

Your doctor may first ask you questions about your health in general, including your health history. The doctor will want to know when you first saw signs of the skin rash or muscle weakness. He or she will then look at your skin and muscles for signs of DM.

Finally, the doctor may ask the hospital's lab to run one or more of the following tests:

- Blood tests for muscle enzymes (including CPK and aldolase tests)
- Muscle biopsy
- Magnetic resonance imaging (MRI)
- Electromyogram (EMG)

There may be other tests to rule out another type of disease or condition. If you have questions about any test, be sure to talk with your doctor or lab technician.

How is it treated?

Many patients do well with oral prednisone. This is a steroid medicine that stops your body from attacking the muscle by slowing down your immune system. If prednisone does not work for you, there are other treatments, including methotrexate; hydroxychloroquine, also known as Plaquenil; and cyclosporine. Some DM patients respond to intravenous immunoglobulin, a medicine given through a needle for a few hours each time.

Your doctor might also want you to do special exercises or a rehabilitation program. Someone will show you how to do the exercises and help you, to make sure that you are doing them right.

Talk with your doctor about DM. If you have DM, it is important to start treatment as soon as possible. Patients that are diagnosed and treated quickly have better results.

What is happening to my skin?

To diagnose dermatomyositis, or DM, doctors look for a number of changes in the skin. The most obvious changes are an itchy or burning red-purple rash; swelling in the fingers; and shawl sign, or a red-purple rash along the collar area of the back of the neck. Other changes include swelling with no redness, calcinosis, and mechanic's hands (thickened, scaly, and cracked skin on the palm side of the fingers and hands).

Going from head to toe, the following is a list of possible skin changes in DM patients:

- Scalp itching, burning, and redness with some hair thinning possible—the hair most often grows back when the rash is treated;
- Heliotrope rash, or rash around the eyes that has the coloring of the reddish-purple heliotrope flower;
- Red-purple rash on the open collar area of the lower neck and upper chest;
- Shawl sign, or red-purple rash over the back of the neck, upper back, and shoulder areas, covering the same area that a shawl would cover;
- Gottron's sign, or red-purple rash over the elbows, knees, and or knuckles (the rash of lupus patients tends to avoid the knuckles and instead shows up on the hair-bearing skin between the knuckles);
- Gottron's papules, or red-purple bumps over the knuckles that may be pressed down in the bump's center;
- Small but visible blood vessels in the skin at the base of the fingernails;
- Ragged, irregular, and cracked cuticles (skin at the base and sides of fingernails);
- Red-purple patches of skin on the body (usually the back and buttocks);
- Holster sign, or red-purple rash over the outer hip area.

A combination of these changes makes it easier and quicker to reach a correct diagnosis. Remember that every DM patient is different, so you may have redness, itching, or scaly skin on just about any part of your body.

The early skin changes of DM are less evident in individuals with more darkly pigmented skin, which can result in a delay in diagnosis of the skin changes of DM.

What is done to treat the skin symptoms?

It can be hard to treat the rash because it's not just a rash. The skin rash and weak muscles are caused by inflammation or swelling in the blood vessels under the skin and in the muscles, also called vasculitis. The blood vessels under your skin are damaged, usually starting with the smaller blood vessels in your body. This is why your fingers and feet may show signs of the rash first. Using a cream or ointment on the skin may not be enough to treat the rash. Your doctor may have you take other medicines, including prednisone; methotrexate; hydroxychloroquine, also known as Plaquenil; or cyclosporine.

An important part of any treatment is prevention. Stop the rash from becoming worse by changing your habits, if necessary. If you are going to be in the sun or wind, be sure to moisturize your skin. Also use sunscreen and sun protective clothing, even on cloudy days. Use a milder soap that won't dry out your skin. Choose soaps that don't have alcohol in them.

What is calcinosis, and how is it treated?

Calcinosis occurs more often in childhood dermatomyositis (JM, or juvenile myositis) than in dermatomyositis that begins in adults (DM). These are hard, sometimes painful lumps of calcium under the skin that appear on the fingers, hands, elbows, and knees. Painful sores can appear if these lumps break the skin.

Calcinosis is usually not one of the first signs or symptoms of JM but occurs later in the illness.

People sometimes expect the calcinosis to get better right away when they begin taking medicines for it, but it may take four months or more to see some healing. Healing means the calcium lumps already there stop growing and new calcium deposits don't show up. The lumps already there may not go away.

Most information is based on what doctors see in their patients, not on controlled studies. When JM patients are treated with higher doses of prednisone after just being diagnosed, they are less likely to form these calcium deposits in the first place. Some doctors carefully treat the disease that likely causes these lumps of calcium.

This may include the following treatments:

- Plaquenil, also called hydroxychloroquine
- intravenous immunoglobulin, or IVIG
- cyclosporine, also called Neoral
- methotrexate.

Check with your doctor about taking vitamin supplements, particularly vitamins C and E, to help the pain and infections that may be caused by calcinosis.

Chapter 19

Diaper Rash

What is diaper rash?

Diaper rash is any rash that affects your child's diaper area. It is a common condition in infants.

What causes it?

- Too much moisture in the diaper area.
- Chafing or rubbing.
- Yeast or bacterial infection.
- Skin stays in contact with urine or feces for a long period.
- Allergic reaction to the material a diaper is made of.
- Allergic reaction to products that come into contact with the skin.

Who can get it?

- Many babies between the ages of 4 months and 15 months get diaper rash.
- It is most common between the ages of 8 to 10 months.

- It is more common in babies who have many stools, especially if the diaper is not changed overnight.
- It is more common in babies who have started to eat solid foods.
- It is more common in babies who are taking antibiotics.
- It is more common in babies who are nursing from mothers who are taking antibiotics.
- Babies with a sensitive skin condition, such as eczema, are more likely to get diaper rash.

What are the signs and symptoms?

- The skin might be red.
- The rash is usually on the stomach, genitals, and inside the skin folds of the thighs and bottom.
- The rash may be warmer than other skin.
- Your baby may seem uncomfortable, especially when you are changing her diaper or washing her diaper area.
- More severe cases may have painful, open sores.

Is it contagious?

Diaper rash is usually not contagious.

How is it treated?

- It may be helpful to remove the diaper and let your baby's skin be open to the air. Set your baby on a few cloth diapers or on a blanket over a plastic sheet. Use the time to play.
- If you use disposable baby wipes and your baby has a rash, you may need to switch to another brand or stop use all together. Plain water is best.
- Some products can irritate young skin. If you use harsh detergent, bleach, or fabric softener, you may need to change brands or stop using the product.
- Use a thick ointment such as Desitin or Balmex on your baby's bottom. It helps protect the skin. Apply after each changing. Ask your doctor first.

- Avoid using adult products on your baby's skin.
- You may want to try using a different brand of diapers if you think they are irritating your baby's skin.
- Avoid using talcum powder. If inhaled, it could irritate your baby's lungs.
- Avoid using cornstarch. It may help bacteria grow in your baby's diaper area.
- The best treatment is prevention. See the suggestions below.

How long does it last?

- Mild cases may clear up in 3 to 4 days without any treatment.
- Some cases take several days to improve, even with treatment.
- The rash can last for weeks.

Can it be prevented?

- Keep the diaper area dry and clean. Change your baby's diaper often. Babies usually have 6 to 8 wet diapers every 24 hours.
- Avoid using disposable baby wipes. They can irritate or dry out the skin. Wash your baby with each change using water instead. Use a water bottle, wet washcloth, or soak a cotton ball in water. Pat the skin to clean it. Do not rub.
- Avoid using harsh soap. Gentle soap is best. Using soap once a day is enough. Gently pat the diaper area dry after washing it. Do not rub it or use a hair-dryer.
- Avoid dressing your child in plastic pants. They do not let the diaper area get enough air.
- Avoid using tight-fitting diapers that could rub against the skin.
- Use mild detergents to wash diapers.
- Avoid using fabric softeners or antistatic sheets when washing diapers.

When should I call the doctor?

- Call your doctor if your baby has a diaper rash that does not go away after 1 or 2 days.

- Call the doctor if your baby has a rash with blisters or bumps.
- Call if the rash is crusty, oozing pus, or bleeding.
- Call the doctor if your baby has a fever with her rash.
- Call the doctor if your baby has a rash and also has many liquid stools or urine that has a very strong smell. These symptoms could be signs of dehydration.
- Call the doctor if there is still a rash after treatment.
- Call your doctor to ask which ointment is best to use on your baby's skin.
- Call the doctor if you have questions or concerns about your child's treatment or condition.

Chapter 20

Seborrheic Dermatitis: Dandruff and Cradle Cap

Definition

Seborrheic dermatitis is a skin condition characterized by loose, greasy or dry, white to yellowish scales, with or without associated reddened skin. Cradle cap is the term used when seborrheic dermatitis affects the scalp of infants.

Causes, Incidence, and Risk Factors

Seborrheic dermatitis may involve the skin of the scalp, eyebrows, eyelids, nasolabial creases, lips, behind the ears, in the external ear, and the skin of the trunk, particularly over the sternum and along skin folds. The cause is unknown.

Seborrheic dermatitis appears to run in families. Stress, fatigue, weather extremes, oily skin, infrequent shampoos or skin cleaning, use of lotions that contain alcohol, skin disorders (such as acne), or obesity may increase the risk.

Neurologic conditions, including Parkinson's disease, head injury, and stroke, can also be associated with seborrheic dermatitis. Human immunodeficiency virus (HIV) is also associated with increased cases of seborrheic dermatitis.

Cradle cap appears as thick, crusty, yellow or brown scales over the child's scalp. Similar scales may also be found on the eyelids, ear,

---

around the nose, and in the groin. Cradle cap may be seen in newborns and small children up to the age of 3 years, and is a harmless, temporary condition.

Cradle cap is not contagious, nor is it caused by poor hygiene. It is not an allergy, and it is not dangerous. Cradle cap may or may not itch. If it itches, excessive scratching of the area may cause additional inflammation, and breaks in skin may cause mild infections or bleeding.

Symptoms

- Skin lesions
- Plaques over large area
- Greasy, oily areas of skin
- Skin scales—white and flaking, or yellowish, oily, and adherent—dandruff
- Plaques may include the scalp, eyebrows, nose, forehead, or ears
- Itching—may become more itchy if infected
- Mild redness
- Hair loss may also be associated with this disease

Signs and Tests

The diagnosis is based on the appearance and location of the skin lesions.

Treatment

You can treat flaking and dryness with over-the-counter dandruff or medicated shampoos. Shampoo the hair vigorously and frequently (preferably daily). Loosen scales with the fingers, scrub for at least 5 minutes, and rinse thoroughly.

Active ingredients in these shampoos include salicylic acid, coal tar, zinc, resorcin, or selenium.

Shampoos or lotions containing selenium, ketoconazole, or corticosteroids may be prescribed for severe cases. To apply shampoos, part the hair into small sections, apply to a small area at a time, and massage into the skin. If on face or chest, apply medicated lotion twice per day.

Seborrheic dermatitis may improve in the summer, especially after outdoor activities.

For infants with cradle cap:

1. Massage your baby's scalp gently with your fingers or a soft brush to loosen the scales and improve scalp circulation.
2. Give your child daily, gentle shampoos with a mild soap while scales are present. After scales have disappeared, you may reduce shampoos to twice weekly.
3. Be sure to rinse off all soap.
4. Brush your child's hair with a clean, soft brush after each shampoo and several times during the day.
5. If scales do not easily loosen and wash off, apply some mineral oil to the baby's scalp and wrap warm, wet cloths around his head for up to an hour before shampooing. Then, shampoo as directed above. Remember that your baby loses a lot of heat through his scalp. If you use warm, wet cloths with the mineral oil, check frequently to be sure that the cloths have not become cold. Cold, wet cloths could drastically reduce your baby's temperature.
6. If the scales continue to be a problem or concern, or if your child seems uncomfortable or scratches his scalp, contact your physician. He may prescribe a cream or lotion to apply to your baby's scalp several times a day.

Expectations (Prognosis)

Seborrheic dermatitis is a chronic condition, controllable with treatment. It often has extended inactive periods followed by flare-ups.

Complications

- Psychological distress, low self-esteem, embarrassment
- Secondary bacterial or fungal infections

Calling Your Health Care Provider

Call for an appointment with your health care provider if seborrheic dermatitis symptoms do not respond to self-care or over-the-counter treatments.

Also call if patches of seborrheic dermatitis drain fluid or pus, form crusts, or become very red or painful.

Prevention

The tendency to develop seborrheic dermatitis may be inherited. The severity can be lessened by controlling the risk factors and by careful attention to skin care.

Chapter 21

Rashes Related to Drug Allergies

Definition

Drug allergies are a group of symptoms caused by an allergic reaction to a drug (medication).

Causes, Incidence, and Risk Factors

In general, adverse reactions to drugs are not uncommon, and almost any drug can cause an adverse reaction. Reactions range from irritating or mild side effects (such as nausea and vomiting), to allergic response including life-threatening anaphylaxis. Some drug reactions are idiosyncratic (unusual effects of the medication). For example, aspirin can cause nonallergic hives (no antibodies formed), or it may trigger asthma. Only a small proportion of these reactions are allergic in nature. Many individuals may confuse an uncomfortable but not serious side effect of a medicine, such as nausea, with a drug allergy, which can be life threatening.

"True" drug allergies occur when there is an allergic reaction to a medication. This is caused by hypersensitivity of the immune system, leading to a misdirected response against a substance that does not cause a response in most people. The body becomes sensitized (the immune system is triggered) by the first exposure to the medication. The second or subsequent exposure causes an immune response, including the production of antibodies and release of histamine.

Most drug allergies cause minor skin rashes and hives. However, other symptoms occasionally develop and life-threatening acute allergic reaction involving the whole body (anaphylaxis) can occur. Serum sickness is a delayed type of drug allergy that occurs a week or more after exposure to a medication or vaccine.

Penicillin and related antibiotics are the most common cause of drug allergies. Other common allergy-causing drugs include sulfa drugs, barbiturates, anticonvulsants, insulin preparations (particularly animal sources of insulin), local anesthetics such as Novocain, and iodine (found in many x-ray contrast dyes).

Symptoms

- hives (common)
- skin rash (common)
- itching of the skin or eyes (common)
- wheezing
- swelling of the lips, tongue, and/or face
- anaphylaxis, or severe allergic reaction (see below)

Symptoms of anaphylaxis include:

- difficulty breathing with wheeze or hoarse voice
- hives over different parts of the body
- fainting and light-headedness
- dizziness
- confusion
- rapid pulse
- sensation of feeling the heart beat (palpitations)
- nausea and vomiting
- diarrhea
- abdominal pain or cramping

Signs and Tests

An examination of the skin and face may show hives, rash, or angioedema (swelling of the lips, face, and/or tongue). Decreased blood pressure, wheezing, and other signs may indicate an anaphylactic reaction.

Skin testing may confirm allergy to penicillin-type medications. Testing may be ineffective (or in some cases, dangerous) for other medications. A history of allergic-type reaction after use of a medication is often considered adequately diagnostic for drug allergy. (No further testing is required to demonstrate the allergy.) The same applies to other substances that are not considered drugs but are used in hospitals, such as s-ray contrast dyes.

Treatment

The treatment goal is relief of symptoms and prevent consequences of a severe reaction, if present.

Antihistamines usually relieve mild symptoms (rash, hives, itching). Topical (applied to a localized area of the skin) corticosteroids may also be recommended. Bronchodilators such as albuterol may be prescribed to reduce asthma-like symptoms (moderate wheezing or cough). Epinephrine by injection may be necessary to treat anaphylaxis.

The offending medication should be avoided. Health care providers (including dentists, hospital personnel, etc.) should be advised of drug allergies before treating the allergic patient. Identifying jewelry or cards (such as Medic-Alert or others) may be advised.

Occasionally a penicillin allergy responds to desensitization (immunotherapy) in which increasing doses (each dose of the drug is slightly larger than the previous dose) are given to improve tolerance of the drug. This should only be done by a physician.

Expectations (Prognosis)

Most drug allergies respond readily to treatment. A few cases cause severe asthma, anaphylaxis, or death.

Complications

- discomfort
- asthma
- anaphylaxis (life threatening)

Calling Your Health Care Provider

Call your health care provider if you are taking a medication and develop symptoms indicating drug allergy.

Go to the emergency room or call the local emergency number (such as 911) if you have difficulty breathing or develop other symptoms of severe asthma or anaphylaxis (see above); these are emergency conditions!

Prevention

There is no known way to prevent development of a drug allergy. In people who have a known drug allergy, avoiding the medication is the best means to prevent an allergic reaction. In some cases, a physician may recommend pre-treatment.

The medication may be given safely after pre-treatment with corticosteroids (such as prednisone) and antihistamines (such as diphenhydramine).

Chapter 22

Rashes Related to Water Exposure

Chapter Contents

Section 22.1

Hot Tub Rash

"Hot Tub Rash: *Pseudomonas* Dermatitis/Folliculitis," Centers for Disease Control and Prevention, February 26, 2003. Available online at http://www.cdc.gov; accessed May 10, 2005.

What is hot tub rash?

Hot tub rash or dermatitis is an infection of the skin. The skin may become itchy and progress to a bumpy red rash that may become tender.

There may also be pus-filled blisters that are usually found surrounding hair follicles. Because a swimsuit can keep contaminated water in longer contact with the skin, the rash may be worse under a person's swimsuit.

What causes hot tub rash?

Hot tub rash infections are often caused by the germ *Pseudomonas aeruginosa*. This germ is common in the environment (such as in water and soil) and is microscopic so that it can't be seen with the naked eye. Most rashes clear up in a few days without medical treatment. However, if your rash persists, consult your health care provider.

How is hot tub rash spread?

Hot tub rash is spread by direct skin contact with contaminated water. The rash usually occurs within a few days of swimming in poorly maintained hot tubs or spas but can also be spread by swimming in a contaminated pool or lake.

How can I protect myself from hot tub rash?

Be aware that hot tubs and spas have warmer water than pools, so chlorine or other disinfectants break down faster. This leaves hot tubs and spas at risk for the spread of RWIs (recreational water illnesses). Therefore, ask your pool manager about the disinfectant and pH testing program at your hot tub or pool.

Ensuring frequent testing, control of disinfectant (usually chlorine or bromine) levels, and pH control are likely to prevent the spread of dermatitis.

Section 22.2

Swimmer's Rash: Cercarial Dermatitis

"Swimmer's Itch," Wisconsin Department of Health and Family Services, June 2001. Available online at http://dhfs.wisconsin.gov; accessed May 10, 2005.

What is swimmer's itch?

Swimmer's itch is a skin rash caused by a parasite (schistosomes), which ordinarily infects birds, semi-aquatic mammals, and snails.

Common grackles, red-winged blackbirds, ducks, geese, swans, muskrats, and moles have been found to carry the parasite. As part of their developmental life cycle, these parasites are released from infected snails, migrate through the water, and are capable of penetrating the skin of humans. After penetration, these parasites remain in the skin and die but can cause an allergic reaction in some people. The parasite in humans does not mature, reproduce, or cause any permanent infection.

Who gets swimmer's itch?

Only about one third of the people who come in contact with the parasite develop swimmer's itch. People who swim or wade in infested water may experience this itchy rash. All age groups and both sexes can be involved, but children are most often infected due to their habits of swimming or wading in shallow water and playing on the beach as the water evaporates from the skin. Swimmer's itch may be prevalent among bathers in lakes in many parts of the world, including the Great Lakes region of North America and certain coastal beaches.

How is swimmer's itch spread?

An individual may get the infection by swimming or wading in infested water and then allowing water to evaporate off the skin rather than drying the skin with a towel. Person-to-person spread does not occur.

What are the symptoms of swimmer's itch?

Whenever infested water is allowed to evaporate off the skin, an initial tingling sensation may be felt and is associated with the penetration of the parasite into the skin. The irritated spot reaches its maximum size after about 24 hours; the itching may continue for several days. The symptoms should disappear within a week.

How soon do the symptoms begin?

A person's first exposure to infested water may not result in the itchy rash. Repeated exposure increases a person's allergic sensitivity to the parasite and increases the likelihood of rash development. Symptoms may appear within 1 to 2 hours of exposure.

What is the treatment for swimmer's itch?

There is no treatment necessary for swimmer's itch. Some people may get relief from the itching by applying skin lotions or creams to the infected site.

When can you get swimmer's itch?

The first outbreaks usually occur in late May or early June. In some lakes it may last the entire summer.

What can be done to reduce the chances of getting swimmer's itch?

- Toweling off immediately after swimming or wading in infested water can be very helpful in preventing rash development.
- Swim in water away from the shore.
- Avoid swimming in areas where snails have accumulated.
- Don't encourage birds to stay near swimming areas by feeding them.

For more information, contact your local public health department.

Chapter 23

Other Rashes

Chapter Contents

Section 23.1

Perioral Dermatitis

Perioral dermatitis is a facial rash that tends to occur around the mouth. Most often it is red and slightly scaly or bumpy. Any itching or burning is mild. It may spread up around the nose and occasionally the eyes while avoiding the skin adjacent to the lips. It is rarer in men and children. Perioral dermatitis may come and go for months or years.

There may be more than one cause of perioral dermatitis. One of the most common factors is prolonged use of topical steroid creams and inhaled prescription steroid sprays used in the nose and the mouth. Overuse of heavy face creams and moisturizers are another common cause. Other causes include skin irritations, fluorinated toothpastes, and rosacea.

A dermatologist diagnoses perioral dermatitis by examination. No other tests are usually done. The first step in treating perioral dermatitis is to discontinue all topical steroid creams, even non-prescription hydrocortisone. Once the steroid cream is discontinued, the rash appears and feels worse for days to weeks before it starts to improve. Heavy face creams should also be stopped. One must resist the temptation to apply any of these creams to the face when this happens. Think of the face as a cream junkie that needs a "fix"—one needs to go cold turkey.

A mild soap or soap substitute, such as Dove or Cetaphil, should be used for washing. Scrubbing should be avoided. Try stopping fluorinated toothpaste for stubborn cases. Non-fluorinated toothpaste is available at a health food store. The most reliably effective treatment is oral antibiotics. These are taken in decreasing doses for three to twelve weeks. Topical antibacterial creams and lotions may also be used for faster relief. These can be continued for several months in order to prevent recurrences.

Even after successful treatment, perioral dermatitis sometimes comes back later. Usually, the same type of treatment will again be effective. Many cases that come back eventually turn into rosacea. Perioral dermatitis is a common skin problem, but fortunately most people do very well with proper treatment.

Section 23.2

Pityriasis Rosea

From *Gale Encyclopedia of Medicine, 2nd Edition*, by Carol A. Turkington, Volume 4. © 2002 Gale Group. Reprinted by permission of the Gale Group.

Definition

Pityriasis rosea is a mild, noncontagious skin disorder common among children and young adults, and characterized by a single round spot on the body, followed later by a rash of colored spots on the body and upper arms.

Description

Pityriasis rosea is most common in young adults, and appears up to 50% more often in women. Its cause is unknown; however, some scientists believe that the rash is an immune response to some type of infection in the body.

Causes and Symptoms

Doctors do not think that pityriasis rosea is contagious, but the cause is unknown. Some experts suspect the rash, which is most common in spring and fall, may be triggered by a virus, but no infectious agent has ever been found.

It is not sexually transmitted, and does not appear to be contagious from one person to the next.

Sometimes, before the symptoms appear, people experience preliminary sensations including fever, malaise, sore throat, or headache. Symptoms begin with a single, large round spot called a "herald patch" on the body, followed days or weeks later by slightly raised, scaly-edged round or oval pink-copper colored spots on the trunk and upper arms. The spots, which have a wrinkled center and a sharp border, sometimes resemble a Christmas tree. They may be mild to severely itchy, and they can spread to other parts of the body.

Diagnosis

A physician can diagnose the condition with blood tests, skin scrapings, or a biopsy of the lesion.

Treatment

The rash usually clears up on its own, although a physician should rule out other conditions that may cause a similar rash (such as syphilis).

Treatment includes external and internal medications for itching and inflammation. Mild inflammation and itching can be relieved with antihistamine drugs or calamine lotion, zinc oxide, or other mild lubricants or anti-itching creams. Gentle, soothing strokes should be used to apply the ointments, since vigorous rubbing may cause the lesions to spread. More severe itching and inflammation is treated with topical steroids. Moderate exposure to sun or ultraviolet light may help heal the lesions, but patients should avoid being sunburned.

Soap makes the rash more uncomfortable; patients should bathe or shower with plain lukewarm water, and apply a thin coating of bath oil to freshly dried skin afterward.

Prognosis

These spots, which may be itchy, last for between 3 to 12 weeks. Symptoms rarely recur.

Part Four

Pigmentation Disorders, Vascular Skin Changes, and Benign Skin Growths

Chapter 24

Albinism

The word "albinism" refers to a group of inherited conditions. People with albinism have little or no pigment in their eyes, skin, or hair. They have inherited genes that do not make the usual amounts of a pigment called melanin.

One person in 17,000 in the United States has some type of albinism. Albinism affects people from all races. Most children with albinism are born to parents who have normal hair and eye color for their ethnic backgrounds.

Often people do not recognize that they have albinism. A common myth is that by definition people with albinism have red eyes. In fact there are different types of albinism, and the amount of pigment in the eyes varies. Although some individuals with albinism have reddish or violet eyes, most have blue eyes. Some have hazel or brown eyes.

Vision Problems

People with albinism always have problems with vision, and many have low vision. Many are legally blind, but most use their vision for reading, and do not use braille. Some have vision good enough to drive a car.

Vision problems in albinism result from abnormal development of the retina and abnormal patterns of nerve connections between the eye and the brain. It is the presence of these eye problems that defines the

---

"What Is Albinism?" is reprinted with permission from the National Organization for Albinism and Hypopigmentation (NOAH), http://www.albinism.org,

diagnosis of albinism. Therefore the main test for albinism is simply an eye exam.

Types of Albinism

While most people with albinism have very light skin and hair, not all do. Oculocutaneous albinism involves the eyes, hair, and skin. Ocular albinism involves primarily the eyes, while skin and hair may appear similar or slightly lighter than that of other family members.

Over the years researchers have used various systems for classifying oculocutaneous albinism. In general, these systems contrasted types of albinism having almost no pigmentation with types having slight pigmentation. In less pigmented types of albinism, hair and skin are cream-colored, and vision is often in the range of 20/200. In types with slight pigmentation, hair appears more yellow or red-tinged, and vision often corrects to 20/60. Early descriptions of albinism called these main categories of albinism "complete" and "incomplete" albinism. Later researchers used a test that involved plucking a hair root, and seeing if it would make pigment in a test tube. This test separated "ty-neg" (no pigment) from "ty-pos" (some pigment). Further research showed that this test was inconsistent, and added little information to the clinical exam.

Recent research has used analysis of DNA [deoxyribonucleic acid], the chemical which encodes genetic information, to arrive at a more firm classification system for albinism. Type 1 albinism (also called tyrosinase-related albinism) is the type involving almost no pigmentation. Type 1 albinism results from a genetic defect in an enzyme called tyrosinase. This enzyme helps the body to change the amino acid tyrosine into pigment. (An amino acid is a "building block" of protein, and comes from protein in the diet.) Type 2, a type with slight pigmentation, results from a defect in a different gene called the "P" gene.

Researchers have identified several other genes that cause forms of albinism. In one form of albinism, the Hermansky-Pudlak syndrome, there can be problems with bleeding, and with lung and bowel disease as well. Hermansky-Pudlak syndrome is a less common form of albinism, but should be suspected if a child with albinism shows unusual bruising or bleeding.

Genetics of Albinism

For nearly all types of albinism both parents must carry an albinism gene to have a child with albinism. Because the body has two sets of genes, a person may have normal pigmentation but carry the albinism gene. If a person has one gene for normal pigmentation and one gene for albinism, he or she will have enough genetic information to make normal pigment. The albinism gene is "recessive"—it does not result in albinism unless a person has two copies of the gene for albinism and no copy of the gene that makes normal pigment.

When both parents carry the gene, and neither parent has albinism, there is a one in four chance at each pregnancy that the baby will be born with albinism. This type of inheritance is called autosomal recessive inheritance. (The most common type of ocular albinism follows a different pattern of inheritance.)

Each parent of a child with oculocutaneous albinism must carry the gene. Both the father and the mother must carry the gene for albinism. For couples who have not had a child with albinism, there is no simple test to determine whether a person carries a gene for albinism. Researchers have analyzed DNA of people with albinism and found the changes that cause albinism, but these changes are not always in exactly the same place, even for a given type of albinism. Therefore the tests for the gene may be inconclusive.

If parents have had a child with albinism previously, there is a way to test in subsequent pregnancies to see if the fetus has albinism. The test uses amniocentesis (placing a needle into the uterus to draw off fluid). Cells in the fluid are examined to see if they have an albinism gene from each parent.

For specific information and genetics and testing, seek the advice of a qualified genetic counselor. Genetic counselors are usually associated with universities and children's hospitals. The National Society of Genetic Counselors at (610) 872-7608 in Philadelphia maintains a referral list. Those considering prenatal testing should be made aware that people with albinism can adapt well to their disabilities, and lead fulfilling lives.

Vision Rehabilitation

Eye conditions common in albinism include:

- Nystagmus, irregular rapid movement of the eyes back and forth
- Strabismus, muscle imbalance of the eyes ("crossed eyes" or "lazy eye")
- Sensitivity to bright light and glare
- People with albinism may be either farsighted or nearsighted, and often have astigmatism (distortion of a viewed image)

These eye problems result from abnormal development of the eye because of lack of pigment. The retina, the surface inside the eye that receives light, does not develop normally before birth and in infancy. The nerve signals from the retina to the brain do not follow the usual nerve routes.

The iris, the colored area in the center of the eye, does not have enough pigment to screen out stray light coming into the eye. (Light normally enters the eye only through the pupil, the dark opening in the center of the iris, but in albinism light can pass through the iris as well.)

For the most part, treatment of the eye conditions consists of visual rehabilitation. Surgery to correct strabismus may improve the appearance of the eyes. However, since surgery will not correct the misrouting of nerves from the eyes to the brain, surgery will not provide fine binocular vision. In the case of esotropia or "crossed eyes," surgery may help vision by expanding the visual field (the area that the eyes can see while looking at one point).

People with albinism are sensitive to glare, but they do not prefer to be in the dark, and need light to see just like anyone else. Sunglasses or tinted contact lenses help outdoors. Indoors, it is important to place lights for reading or close work over a shoulder rather than in front.

Various optical aids are helpful to people with albinism, and the choice of an optical aid depends on how a person uses his or her eyes in jobs, hobbies, or other usual activities. Some people do well using bifocals which have a strong reading lens, prescription reading glasses, or contact lenses. Others use handheld magnifiers or special small telescopes. Some use bioptics, glasses which have small telescopes mounted on, in, or behind their regular lenses, so that one can look through either the regular lens or the telescope. Newer designs of bioptics use smaller light-weight lenses. Some states allow the use of bioptic telescopes for driving.

Optometrists or ophthalmologists who are experienced in working who have people with low vision can recommend various optical aids. Clinics should provide aids on trial loan, and provide instruction in their use. The American Foundation for the Blind (1-800-AFB-LINE) maintains a directory of low vision clinics.

Medical Problems

In the United States, people with albinism live normal life spans and have the same types of general medical problems as the rest of the population. The lives of people with Hermansky-Pudlak syndrome can be shortened by lung disease or other problems. In tropical countries, those who do not use skin protection may develop life-threatening skin cancers. If they use appropriate skin protection, such as sunscreen lotions rated 20 or higher, and opaque clothing, people with albinism can enjoy outdoor activities even in summer.

People with albinism are at risk of isolation, because the condition is often misunderstood. Social stigmatization can occur, especially within communities of color, where the race or paternity of a person with albinism may be questioned. Families and schools must make an effort not to exclude children with albinism from group activities.

Contact with others with albinism or who have albinism in their families is most helpful. NOAH can provide the names of contacts in many regions of the country.

Chapter 25

McCune-Albright Syndrome

Introduction

The McCune-Albright syndrome is named for the two physicians who described it over 50 years ago. They reported a group of children, most of them girls, with an unusual pattern of associated abnormalities:

- bone disease, with fractures, asymmetry and deformity of the legs, arms, and skull;
- endocrine disease, including early puberty with menstrual bleeding, development of breasts and pubic hair and an increased rate of growth; and
- skin changes, with areas of increased pigment distributed in an asymmetric and irregular pattern.

Today, the term McCune-Albright syndrome is used to describe patients who have some or all of these bone, endocrine, and skin abnormalities. In the years since it was first identified, however, researchers have studied many additional patients, and have learned that the condition has a broad spectrum of severity. Sometimes, children are diagnosed in early infancy with obvious bone disease and markedly increased endocrine secretions from several glands; a very few of these severely affected children have died. At the opposite end

From the National Institute of Child Health and Human Development, 1993. Available online at http://www.nichd.nih.gov; accessed May 12, 2005. Updated and revised by David A. Cooke, M.D., June 2005.

of the spectrum, many children are entirely healthy, and have little or no outward evidence of bone or endocrine involvement. They may enter puberty close to the normal age, and have no unusual skin pigment at all. Because of this marked variability among patients, the components of this complicated syndrome are described separately below.

In recent years, the underlying cause of the diverse problems that affect patients with McCune-Albright syndrome has become understood. Mutations in a gene named *GNAS1* cause a molecular "switch" inside cells to become stuck in the "on" position. This abnormally activated "switch" has effects in different cell types throughout the body, and is especially important in glandular cells as it usually increases their activity. This explains the tendency of patients with McCune-Albright syndrome to develop problems due to overactivity of various endocrine systems.

The great variability of symptoms between patients occurs because only some of the cells in affected patients' bodies carry this gene mutation. The mutation is not present in the sperm or egg; during the first few rounds of cell division after conception, a DNA copying error occurs in one of the resulting cells and that cell's descendants carry the same error. Therefore, patients with McCune-Albright syndrome have a mixture of normal and abnormal cells. The severity of the disease is thought to depend on how high a percentage of the body cells are abnormal.

It has been observed that patients with McCune-Albright syndrome do not pass the disease on to their children. It appears that the mutation that causes the disease is lethal if all of the fetal cells carry it. Therefore, only children conceived from normal cells are able to survive to birth.

Endocrine Abnormalities

Precocious Puberty

When the signs of puberty (development of breasts, testes, pubic and underarm hair, body odor, menstrual bleeding, and increased growth rate) appear before the age of 8 years in a girl or 9½ years in a boy, it is termed precocious puberty. In the most common form of precocious puberty, there is early activation of the regions in the brain, which control the maturation of the gonads (ovaries in a girl and testes in a boy). One brain center, the hypothalamus, secretes a substance called gonadotropin-releasing-hormone, or GnRH. This acts, in turn, on another part of the brain, the pituitary gland, to cause increased secretion of hormones called gonadotropins (luteinizing hormone [LH] and follicle-stimulating hormone [FSH]) that travel through the bloodstream, and act on the ovaries or testes to stimulate secretion of estrogen or testosterone. Endocrinologists determine if a child with precocious puberty has early activation of the hypothalamus and pituitary by measuring the levels of LH and FSH in the blood after an injection of a synthetic preparation of GnRH.

After studying many girls with McCune-Albright syndrome, however, researchers have learned that most do not appear to have early activation of the hypothalamus and pituitary, because the levels of LH and FSH are usually low, or similar to those of prepubertal children. The precocious puberty in McCune-Albright girls is caused by estrogens, which are secreted into the bloodstream by ovarian cysts, which enlarge, and then decrease in size over periods of weeks to days. The cysts can be visualized and measured by ultrasonography, in which sound waves are used to outline the dimensions of the ovaries. The cysts may become quite big, occasionally over 50 cc in volume (about the size of a golf ball). Frequently, menstrual bleeding and breast enlargement accompany the growth of a cyst. In fact, menstrual bleeding under 2 years of age has been the first symptom of McCune-Albright syndrome in 85 percent of patients. Although ovarian cysts and irregular menstrual bleeding may continue into adolescence and adulthood, many adult women with McCune-Albright syndrome are fertile, and can bear normal children.

The precocious puberty in McCune-Albright syndrome has been difficult to treat. After surgical removal of the cyst or of the entire affected ovary, cysts usually recur in the remaining ovary. A progesterone-like hormone called Provera can be given to suppress the menstrual bleeding, but does not appear to slow the rapid rates of growth and bone development, and may have unwanted effects on adrenal functioning. The synthetic forms of GnRH (Deslorelin, Histrelin, and Lupron) that suppress LH and FSH, and are used to treat the common, gonadotropin-dependent form of precocious puberty, are not effective in most girls with McCune-Albright syndrome. An investigational form of treatment, using oral medications that block estrogen synthesis (testolactone) is now being tested in girls with McCune-Albright syndrome, and has been beneficial in many patients. Tamoxifen, a medication with anti-estrogen activity that is used for treating breast cancer appears to be effective for treating precocious puberty in McCune-Albright syndrome. Letrozole, an aromatase inhibitor that interferes with estrogen production, also seems promising.

Thyroid Function

Almost 50 percent of patients with McCune-Albright syndrome have thyroid gland abnormalities; these include generalized enlargement called goiter, and irregular masses called nodules and cysts. Some patients have subtle structural changes detected only by ultrasonography. Pituitary thyroid-stimulating-hormone (TSH) levels are low in these patients, and thyroid hormone levels may be normal or elevated. Therapy with drugs that block thyroid hormone synthesis (Propylthiouracil or Methimazole) can be given if thyroid hormone levels are excessively high.

Growth Hormone

Excessive secretion of pituitary growth hormone has been seen in a few patients with McCune-Albright syndrome. Most of these have been diagnosed as young adults, when they developed the coarsening of facial features, enlargement of hands and feet, and arthritis characteristic of the condition termed acromegaly. Therapy has included surgical removal of the area of the pituitary that is secreting the hormone, and use of new, synthetic analogs of the hormone somatostatin, which suppress growth hormone secretion.

Other Endocrine Abnormalities

Although rare, adrenal enlargement and excessive secretion of the adrenal hormone cortisol is seen in McCune-Albright syndrome. This may cause obesity of the face and trunk, weight gain, skin fragility, and cessation of growth in childhood. These symptoms are called Cushing syndrome. Treatment is removal of the affected adrenal glands, or use of drugs that block cortisol synthesis.

Some children with McCune-Albright syndrome have very low levels of phosphorus in their blood due to excessive losses of phosphate in their urine. This may cause bone changes associated with rickets, and may be treated with oral phosphates and supplemental vitamin D.

Bone Disease—Polyostotic Fibrous Dysplasia

The term polyostotic fibrous dysplasia means "abnormal fibrous tissue growth in many bones." However, the severity of bone disease in McCune-Albright syndrome is quite variable. In affected areas, normal bone is replaced by irregular masses of fibroblast cells. When this occurs in weight-bearing bones, such as the femur (upper leg bone), limping, deformity, and fractures may occur. In many children, the arms and/or legs are of unequal length, even in the absence of actual fracture. Regions of fibrous dysplasia are also very common in the bones that form the skull and upper jaw. If these areas begin to expand, skull and facial asymmetry may result.

Polyostotic fibrous dysplasia can often be seen in a plain X-ray picture of the skeleton. A more sensitive method of finding lesions is a bone scan, in which a small amount of radioactivity (an isotope of technetium) is injected into a vein, taken up by the abnormal tissues, and detected by a scanner.

Some children may be minimally affected, with no asymmetry, deformity or fracture, and lesions detected only by a bone scan. In a few children, lesions are found only in the base of the skull. By repeating bone scans at intervals of 1 to 2 years, it has been shown that the bone disease in some children may become more extensive over time. Unfortunately, severe bone disease can have permanent effects upon physical appearance and mobility.

There is no known hormonal or medical treatment effective in controlling progressive polyostotic fibrous dysplasia. Surgical procedures to correct fracture and deformity include grafting, pinning, and casting. Skull and jaw changes are often corrected surgically, with great improvement in appearance.

Treatment and therapy for this bone disease is usually the most difficult aspect of caring for a child who has severe polyostotic fibrous dysplasia.

Skin Abnormalities

The irregular, flat areas of increased skin pigment in McCune-Albright syndrome are called café-au-lait spots because, in children with light complexions, they are the color of coffee with milk. In dark-skinned individuals, these spots may be difficult to see. Most children have the pigment from birth, and it almost never becomes more extensive. The pattern of the pigment distribution is unique, often starting or ending abruptly at the midline on the abdomen in front or at the spine in back. Some children have no café-au-lait pigment at all; in a few, it is confined to small areas, such as the nape of the neck or crease of the buttocks.

There are seldom any medical problems associated with the areas of café-au-lait pigment. Some adolescent children may want to use makeup to obscure areas of dark pigment on the face.

Recent Research

Because the underlying molecular defect that causes McCune-Albright syndrome is now known, there is considerable research devoted to finding ways to better treat the abnormalities seen in the disease.

Chapter 26

Questions and Answers about Vitiligo

What is vitiligo?

Vitiligo is a pigmentation disorder in which melanocytes (the cells that make pigment) in the skin, the mucous membranes (tissues that line the inside of the mouth and nose and genital and rectal areas), and the retina (inner layer of the eyeball) are destroyed. As a result, white patches of skin appear on different parts of the body. The hair that grows in areas affected by vitiligo usually turns white.

The cause of vitiligo is not known, but doctors and researchers have several different theories. One theory is that people develop antibodies that destroy the melanocytes in their own bodies. Another theory is that melanocytes destroy themselves. Finally, some people have reported that a single event such as sunburn or emotional distress triggered vitiligo; however, these events have not been scientifically proven to cause vitiligo.

Who is affected by vitiligo?

About 1 to 2 percent of the world's population, or 40 to 50 million people, have vitiligo. In the United States, 2 to 5 million people have the disorder. Ninety-five percent of people who have vitiligo develop it before their 40th birthday. The disorder affects all races and both sexes equally.

Excerpted from the article by the National Institute of Arthritis and Musculoskeletal and Skin Diseases (NIAMS), May 2001. Available online at http://www.niams.nih.gov; accessed May 18, 2005.

Vitiligo seems to be more common in people with certain autoimmune diseases (diseases in which a person's immune system reacts against the body's own organs or tissues). These autoimmune diseases include hyperthyroidism (an overactive thyroid gland), adrenocortical insufficiency (the adrenal gland does not produce enough of the hormone called corticosteroid), alopecia areata (patches of baldness), and pernicious anemia (a low level of red blood cells caused by failure of the body to absorb vitamin B12). Scientists do not know the reason for the association between vitiligo and these autoimmune diseases. However, most people with vitiligo have no other autoimmune disease.

Vitiligo may also be hereditary, that is, it can run in families. Children whose parents have the disorder are more likely to develop vitiligo. However, most children will not get vitiligo even if a parent has it, and most people with vitiligo do not have a family history of the disorder.

What are the symptoms of vitiligo?

People who develop vitiligo usually first notice white patches (depigmentation) on their skin. These patches are more common in sun-exposed areas, including the hands, feet, arms, face, and lips. Other common areas for white patches to appear are the armpits and groin and around the mouth, eyes, nostrils, navel, and genitals.

Vitiligo generally appears in one of three patterns. In one pattern (focal pattern), the depigmentation is limited to one or only a few areas. Some people develop depigmented patches on only one side of their bodies (segmental pattern). But for most people who have vitiligo, depigmentation occurs on different parts of the body (generalized pattern). In addition to white patches on the skin, people with vitiligo may have premature graying of the scalp hair, eyelashes, eyebrows, and beard. People with dark skin may notice a loss of color inside their mouths.

What treatment options are available?

The goal of treating vitiligo is to restore the function of the skin and to improve the patient's appearance. Therapy for vitiligo takes a long time—it usually must be continued for 6 to 18 months. The choice of therapy depends on the number of white patches and how widespread they are and on the patient's preference for treatment. Each patient responds differently to therapy, and a particular treatment may not work for everyone. Current treatment options for vitiligo include medical, surgical, and adjunctive therapies (therapies that can be used along with surgical or medical treatments).

Medical Therapies

Topical Steroid Therapy: Steroids may be helpful in repigmenting the skin (returning the color to white patches), particularly if started early in the disease. Corticosteroids are a group of drugs similar to the hormones produced by the adrenal glands (such as cortisone). Doctors often prescribe a mild topical corticosteroid cream for children under 10 years old and a stronger one for adults. Patients must apply the cream to the white patches on their skin for at least 3 months before seeing any results. It is the simplest and safest treatment but not as effective as psoralen photochemotherapy (see below). The doctor will closely monitor the patient for side effects such as skin shrinkage and skin striae (streaks or lines on the skin).

Psoralen Photochemotherapy: Psoralen photochemotherapy (psoralen and ultraviolet A therapy, or PUVA) is probably the most beneficial treatment for vitiligo available in the United States. The goal of PUVA therapy is to repigment the white patches. However, it is time-consuming and care must be taken to avoid side effects, which can sometimes be severe. Psoralens are drugs that contain chemicals that react with ultraviolet light to cause darkening of the skin. The treatment involves taking psoralen by mouth (orally) or applying it to the skin (topically). This is followed by carefully timed exposure to ultraviolet A (UVA) light from a special lamp or to sunlight. Patients usually receive treatments in their doctors' offices so they can be carefully watched for any side effects. Patients must minimize exposure to sunlight at other times.

Topical Psoralen Photochemotherapy: Topical psoralen photochemotherapy often is used for people with a small number of depigmented patches (affecting less than 20 percent of the body). It is also used for children 2 years old and older who have localized patches of vitiligo. Treatments are done in a doctor's office under artificial UVA light once or twice a week. The doctor or nurse applies a thin coat of psoralen to the patient's depigmented patches about 30 minutes before UVA light exposure. The patient is then exposed to an amount of UVA light that turns the affected area pink. The doctor usually increases the dose of UVA light slowly over many weeks. Eventually, the pink areas fade and a more normal skin color appears. After each treatment, the patient washes his or her skin with soap and water and applies a sunscreen before leaving the doctor's office.

There are two major potential side effects of topical PUVA therapy: (1) severe sunburn and blistering and (2) too much repigmentation or darkening of the treated patches or the normal skin surrounding the vitiligo (hyperpigmentation). Patients can minimize their chances of sunburn if they avoid exposure to direct sunlight after each treatment. Hyperpigmentation is usually a temporary problem and eventually disappears when treatment is stopped.

Oral Psoralen Photochemotherapy: Oral PUVA therapy is used for people with more extensive vitiligo (affecting greater than 20 percent of the body) or for people who do not respond to topical PUVA therapy. Oral psoralen is not recommended for children under 10 years of age because of an increased risk of damage to the eyes, such as cataracts. For oral PUVA therapy, the patient takes a prescribed dose of psoralen by mouth about 2 hours before exposure to artificial UVA light or sunlight. The doctor adjusts the dose of light until the skin areas being treated become pink. Treatments are usually given two or three times a week, but never 2 days in a row.

For patients who cannot go to a PUVA facility, the doctor may prescribe psoralen to be used with natural sunlight exposure. The doctor will give the patient careful instructions on carrying out treatment at home and monitor the patient during scheduled checkups.

Known side effects of oral psoralen include sunburn, nausea and vomiting, itching, abnormal hair growth, and hyperpigmentation. Oral psoralen photochemotherapy may increase the risk of skin cancer. To avoid sunburn and reduce the risk of skin cancer, patients undergoing oral PUVA therapy should apply sunscreen and avoid direct sunlight for 24 to 48 hours after each treatment. Patients should also wear protective UVA sunglasses for 18 to 24 hours after each treatment to avoid eye damage, particularly cataracts.

Depigmentation: Depigmentation involves fading the rest of the skin on the body to match the already white areas. For people who have vitiligo on more than 50 percent of their bodies, depigmentation may be the best treatment option. Patients apply the drug monobenzyl ether of hydroquinone (monobenzone or Benoquin) twice a day to pigmented areas until they match the already depigmented areas. Patients must avoid direct skin-to-skin contact with other people for at least 2 hours after applying the drug.

The major side effect of depigmentation therapy is inflammation (redness and swelling) of the skin. Patients may experience itching, dry skin, or abnormal darkening of the membrane that covers the white of the eye. Depigmentation is permanent and cannot be reversed. In addition, a person who undergoes depigmentation will always be abnormally sensitive to sunlight.

Note: Brand names included in this chapter are provided as examples only, and their inclusion does not mean that these products are endorsed by the National Institutes of Health or any other Government agency. Also, if a particular brand name is not mentioned, this does not mean or imply that the product is unsatisfactory.

Surgical Therapies

All surgical therapies must be viewed as experimental because their effectiveness and side effects remain to be fully defined.

Autologous Skin Grafts: In an autologous (use of a person's own tissues) skin graft, the doctor removes skin from one area of a patient's body and attaches it to another area. This type of skin grafting is sometimes used for patients with small patches of vitiligo. The doctor removes sections of the normal, pigmented skin (donor sites) and places them on the depigmented areas (recipient sites). There are several possible complications of autologous skin grafting. Infections may occur at the donor or recipient sites. The recipient and donor sites may develop scarring, a cobblestone appearance, or a spotty pigmentation, or may fail to repigment at all. Treatment with grafting takes time and is costly, and most people find it neither acceptable nor affordable.

Skin Grafts Using Blisters: In this procedure, the doctor creates blisters on the patient's pigmented skin by using heat, suction, or freezing cold. The tops of the blisters are then cut out and transplanted to a depigmented skin area. The risks of blister grafting include the development of a cobblestone appearance, scarring, and lack of repigmentation. However, there is less risk of scarring with this procedure than with other types of grafting.

Micropigmentation (Tattooing): Tattooing implants pigment into the skin with a special surgical instrument. This procedure works best for the lip area, particularly in people with dark skin; however, it is difficult for the doctor to match perfectly the color of the skin of the surrounding area. Tattooing tends to fade over time. In addition, tattooing of the lips may lead to episodes of blister outbreaks caused by the herpes simplex virus.

Autologous Melanocyte Transplants: In this procedure, the doctor takes a sample of the patient's normal pigmented skin and places it in a laboratory dish containing a special cell culture solution to grow melanocytes. When the melanocytes in the culture solution have multiplied, the doctor transplants them to the patient's depigmented skin patches. This procedure is currently experimental and is impractical for the routine care of people with vitiligo.

Additional Therapies

Sunscreens: People who have vitiligo, particularly those with fair skin, should use a sunscreen that provides protection from both the UVA and UVB forms of ultraviolet light. Sunscreen helps protect the skin from sunburn and long-term damage. Sunscreen also minimizes tanning, which makes the contrast between normal and depigmented skin less noticeable.

Cosmetics: Some patients with vitiligo cover depigmented patches with stains, makeup, or self-tanning lotions. These cosmetic products can be particularly effective for people whose vitiligo is limited to exposed areas of the body. Dermablend, Lydia O'Leary, Clinique, Fashion Flair, Vitadye, and Chromelin offer makeup or dyes that patients may find helpful for covering up depigmented patches.

Counseling and Support Groups

Many people with vitiligo find it helpful to get counseling from a mental health professional. People often find they can talk to their counselor about issues that are difficult to discuss with anyone else. A mental health counselor can also offer patients support and help in coping with vitiligo. In addition, it may be helpful to attend a vitiligo support group.

What research is being done on vitiligo?

For more than a decade, research on how melanocytes play a role in vitiligo has greatly increased. This includes research on autologous melanocyte transplants. At the University of Colorado, NIAMS supports a large collaborative project involving families with vitiligo in the United States and the United Kingdom. To date, over 2,400 patients are involved. It is hoped that genetic analysis of these families will uncover the location—and possibly the specific gene or genes—conferring susceptibility to the disease. Doctors and researchers continue to look for the causes of and new treatments for vitiligo.

Chapter 27

Pigmented Birthmarks and Vascular Skin Changes

Birthmarks are areas of flat or raised discolored skin that are often seen on the body at birth or may develop shortly after birth. While folk tales claim various reasons for these blemishes, the exact causes of birthmarks are unknown. However, most birthmarks are not inherited and are not caused by anything that happens to the mother during pregnancy.

They vary in color and may be brown, tan, or black to blue, pink or red. Some birthmarks are only stains on the surface of the skin, while others extend into the tissues under the skin or grow above the surface.

"Some birthmarks grow with the child and change little in color throughout a lifetime, while others fade or darken in time," said Sarah Chamlin, M.D., assistant professor of pediatrics and dermatology at Children's Memorial Hospital in Chicago.

Birthmarks are most often harmless; however. Dr. Chamlin said some troublesome birthmarks may require treatment.

Most birthmarks can be identified as either pigmented/brown lesions or vascular lesions.

Pigmented Birthmarks

Birthmarks that are flat but colorful include congenital nevi (commonly known as a mole), café-au-lait spots, and Mongolian spots.

"What Parents Should Know About Birthmarks," by Amy Gall, *Dermatology Insights*, Volume 4, Number 1. Reprinted with permission from the American Academy of Dermatology.

Congenital nevi are typically present at birth, brown or black in color, vary in size and location and can be either raised or flat. These common birthmarks most often require no treatment.

"Nevi with irregular color or borders, a nodular surface or bleeding should be evaluated by a dermatologist," said Dr. Chamlin. "Large nevi, particularly on the midline of the back or scalp, should also be evaluated."

Dr. Chamlin adds that surgical removal may be necessary for atypical appearing nevi due to a potential risk of skin cancer.

Café-au-lait spots are tan or light brown patches that are the result of too much pigment in the skin. These discolorations can sometimes appear in multiples, and about 10 to 20 percent of children and adults have one.

Café-au-lait spots may fade over a lifetime, but do not usually go away. A single spot is not typically serious, but numerous spots may suggest other health problems and a dermatologist should be consulted.

Mongolian spots are flat, gray-blue discolorations found on the back or buttocks of babies, and are commonly found in newborns with dark skin. Although they may never go away altogether, Mongolian spots usually disappear by school age without treatment.

Vascular Birthmarks

Vascular lesions are the result of an increase in the number of blood vessels in the skin. The most common types of vascular birthmarks are salmon patches, hemangiomas, and port-wine stains.

Salmon patches (nevus simplex) are the most frequently diagnosed vascular birthmark. They are flat, mild red, or pink and are sometimes called "angel's kisses" when they appear on the forehead, eyelids, nose or upper lip and "stork bites" when they are found on the back of the neck. Angel's kisses most often go away by age 1 to 2, but stork bites may last into adulthood. They are typically harmless and require no treatment.

Hemangiomas are a benign growth of blood vessels, and occur in as many as one out of 10 infants. They can be divided into two types: superficial (formerly referred to as strawberry hemangiomas) and deep (formerly referred to as cavernous hemangiomas).

Superficial hemangiomas are raised and bright red because the abnormal blood vessels are very close to the skin's surface.

Deep hemangiomas have a bluish-purple color because the abnormal vessels are deeper under the skin.

"[Deep hemangiomas] are most often not present at birth but slowly enlarge during the first six to nine months of life," said Dr. Chamlin. "They subsequently slowly resolve (improve in appearance) over several years."

After the first year, most hemangiomas stop growing. According to Dr. Chamlin, approximately 50 percent of hemangiomas resolve by age five, and 90 percent are flat by age nine. Texture change or superficial blood vessels may remain on the skin even after complete resolution.

The most commonly utilized treatments for hemangiomas include close observation, corticosteroids, and wound care when a lesion is ulcerated.

"When hemangiomas grow in locations that can threaten vision, damage cartilage around the nose or ear, or cause significant facial deformity, it is often necessary to treat the patient with oral steroids," said Dr. Chamlin.

Pulse-dye laser treatment may also be used to treat hemangiomas after or during involution (shrinking stage), but are only helpful for superficial hemangiomas. Hemangiomas with sores that will not heal may also benefit from the treatment of lasers.

"Surgery is sometimes performed during or after involution if a hemangioma leaves excess skin or tissue behind," said Dr. Chamlin. "Surgical removal is rarely performed on hemangiomas when they are actively growing."

Port-wine stains (capillary malformations) appear at birth in approximately three out of every 1,000 infants. They are flat, pink, red or purplish discolorations often found on the face, but can be present anywhere on the body. Unlike other birthmarks, port-wine stains grown proportionally as the child grows. While their texture and shade may change, they are permanent without treatment.

Specially designed cover-up makeup can be used to reduce the appearance of port-wine stains.

"The stain may also be lightened with pulsed-dye laser treatment," said Dr. Chamlin. "Treatments can start in infancy and need to be performed several times to achieve maximum lightening."

Combating Social Stigmas

Birthmarks, particularly facial hemangiomas, can cause significant psychological and social distress for both parents and children.

According to Ilona Frieden, M.D., clinical professor of dermatology and pediatrics at the University of California, it is normal for parents to feel a variety of emotions, including panic, sadness, guilt, and disbelief.

"Even when you tell parents their child's hemangioma will eventually disappear, it is not necessarily good news to them, especially when their infant's appearance was unflawed at birth but is now growing a bright red lesion," said Dr. Frieden.

Dealing with the reactions of strangers can also be stressful. When faced with stares or questions about their child's birthmark, Dr. Frieden recommends parents and children do what feels comfortable to them. For some, answering questions about the birthmark is fine, while others may choose to hand out a preprinted card with details on the condition. And some people simply choose to ignore insensitive comments altogether.

Parents and older children with birthmarks who are particularly distressed may benefit from talking to other children who have birthmarks and their parents. Ask your dermatologist if there is a birthmark support group near you.

Dermatologic Surgery for Kids: What Parents Should Consider

According to Children's Memorial Hospital dermatologist Annette Wagner, M.D., when faced with surgery for their child's birthmark removal, parents should ask themselves the following questions:

Question: Does the lesion need to come off?

Answer: Some lesions do not require excision, so it's important to first make sure you have the correct diagnosis and prognosis. Cosmetic removal of facial lesions can result in scars that are often more noticeable than the birthmark itself. If nature takes them away, don't trade lesions for lifelong scars, Dr. Wagner recommends.

Question: What is the appropriate age for a child to have surgery?

Answer: Many benign skin lesions can be removed safely with a local anesthetic at ages seven to 10. If there is no urgency to remove a birthmark, Dr. Wagner recommends postponing surgery until the child is a little older as pediatric patients are more active than other patients, increasing the risk of scar formation.

Question: Who should remove the birthmark?

Answer: Parents should select a surgeon with experience working with both birthmark removal and children.

Question: Will there be a scar?

Answer: All excisional surgery leaves a scar, even in the hands of the world's most talented plastic or reconstructive surgeons. The severity of scarring depends on the location and size of the birthmark, the activity of the patient post-operation and the skill of the surgeon.

Chapter 28

Skin Tags, Skin Discoloration, and Hyperpigmentation

Chapter Contents

Section 28.1

What Are Skin Tags?

Definition

Cutaneous skin tags are a skin condition involving small, generally benign skin growths.

Causes, Incidence, and Risk Factors

Cutaneous tags are very common, generally benign skin growths that occur most often after midlife. They are tiny skin protrusions and may have a small narrow stalk connecting the skin bump to the surface of the skin. They are usually painless and do not grow or change, except for occasional irritation from rubbing by clothing or other friction. Their origin is unknown.

Symptoms

- Skin growth
- Usually very small, but sometimes half an inch long
- Located on the neck, armpits, trunk, body folds, or other areas
- May have a narrow stalk
- Usually skin-colored, occasionally darker

Signs and Tests

Diagnosis is based primarily on the appearance of the skin growth.

Treatment

Treatment is usually not necessary unless the cutaneous tags are irritating or are cosmetically displeasing. The growths may be surgically removed, removed by freezing (cryotherapy), or electrically burning off (cautery).

Expectations (Prognosis)

Cutaneous tags are generally benign and usually not bothersome. They may become irritated or be cosmetically displeasing. There is usually no regrowth or scar formation when cutaneous tags are removed, although new growths may appear elsewhere on the body.

Complications

There are usually no complications. Occasionally, irritation and discomfort may occur. The skin tags may be cosmetically unsightly.

Calling Your Health Care Provider

Call your health care provider if cutaneous tags are present and you want them removed or if the appearance of a cutaneous tag changes.

Section 28.2

Acanthosis Nigricans

Definition

Acanthosis nigricans is a skin disorder characterized by dark, thick, velvety skin in body folds and creases.

Causes, Incidence, and Risk Factors

Acanthosis nigricans can affect otherwise healthy people, or it can be associated with medical problems. Some cases are genetically inherited. It is most common among people of African descent.

Obesity can lead to acanthosis nigricans, as can many endocrine disorders. It is frequently found in people with diabetes.

Some drugs, particularly hormones such as human growth hormone or oral contraceptives (the Pill), can also cause acanthosis nigricans.

People with cancers of the gastrointestinal or genitourinary tracts or with lymphoma can also develop severe cases of acanthosis nigricans.

Symptoms

Acanthosis nigricans usually appears slowly and doesn't cause any symptoms other than skin changes.

Eventually, dark, velvety skin with very visible markings and creases appears in the armpits, groin, and neck. Sometimes, the lips, palms, soles of feet, or other areas may be affected.

Signs and Tests

Your physician can usually diagnosis acanthosis nigricans by simply looking at your skin. A skin biopsy may be needed in unusual cases.

If no clear cause of acanthosis nigricans is obvious, it may be necessary to search for one. Your physician may order blood tests, endoscopy, or x-ray studies to eliminate the possibility of underlying diabetes or cancer.

Treatment

Because acanthosis nigricans itself usually only causes changes to the appearance of the skin, no particular treatment is needed.

It is important, however, to attempt to treat any underlying medical problem that may be causing these skin changes.

Expectations (Prognosis)

Acanthosis nigricans often fades if the cause can be found and treated.

Calling Your Health Care Provider

Call your physician if you develop areas of thick, dark, velvety skin.

Section 28.3

Hyperpigmentation

Reprinted with permission from the American Osteopathic College of Dermatology (AOCD), For additional information, visit the AOCD website at www.aocd.org.

Hyperpigmentation is a common, usually harmless condition in which patches of skin become darker in color than the normal surrounding skin. This darkening occurs when an excess of melanin, the brown pigment that produces normal skin color, forms deposits in the skin. Hyperpigmentation can affect the skin color of people of any race.

Age or "liver" spots are a common form of hyperpigmentation. They occur due to sun damage, and are referred to by doctors as solar lentigines. These small, darkened patches are usually found on the hands and face or other areas frequently exposed to the sun.

Melasma or chloasma spots are similar in appearance to age spots but are larger areas of darkened skin that appear most often as a result of hormonal changes. Pregnancy, for example, can trigger overproduction of melanin that causes the "mask of pregnancy" on the face and darkened skin on the abdomen and other areas. Women who take birth control pills may also develop hyperpigmentation because their bodies undergo similar kind of hormonal changes that occur during pregnancy. If one is really bothered by the pigment, the birth control pills should be stopped.

Changes in skin color can result from outside causes. For example, skin diseases such as acne may leave dark spots after the condition clears. Other causes of dark spots are injuries to the skin, including some surgeries. Freckles are small brown spots that can appear anywhere on the body, but are most common on the face and arms. Freckles are an inherited characteristic.

Freckles, age spots, and other darkened skin patches can become darker or more pronounced when skin is exposed to the sun. This happens because melanin absorbs the energy of the sun's harmful ultraviolet rays in order to protect the skin from overexposure.

The usual result of this process is skin tanning, which tends to darken areas that are already hyperpigmented. Wearing a sunscreen is a must. The sunscreen must be "broad spectrum" (i.e., it blocks both ultraviolet A and B rays). A single day of excess sun can undo months of treatment.

Most prescription creams used to lighten the skin contain hydroquinone. Bleaches lighten and fade darkened skin patches by slowing the production of melanin so those dark spots gradually fade to match normal skin coloration. Prescription bleaches contain twice the amount of hydroquinone, the active ingredient, as over-the-counter skin bleaches. In more severe cases prescription creams with tretinoin and a cortisone cream may be used. These may be somewhat irritating to sensitive skin and will take 3 to 6 months to produce improvement.

There are now several highly effective laser treatments. The q-switched ruby and other pigmented lesion lasers often remove pigment without scarring. A test spot in an inconspicuous place will need to be done as they sometimes make things worse instead of better.

Section 28.4

Progressive Pigmentary Purpura

Progressive pigmentary purpura (PPP) is a group of similar conditions (including Schamberg's disease, Lichenoid dermatitis of Gougerot-Blum, and purpura annularis telangiectodes of Majocchi and Lichen aureus). Schamberg's type is the most common, but many experts believe that dividing them into subgroups is artificial.

PPP results in a rusty brown skin discoloration. The brownish patches are unevenly scattered on both sides and may be few or many. Within the patches are tiny red dots that look as if someone lightly sprinkled cayenne pepper on the area. The area is flat, smooth, and not scaly. There are no internal symptoms or effects.

PPP usually starts in adult life, is more common in men, and may occur in children rarely. In it's most common form it first appears on the lower legs, then will often spread slowly up the legs eventually often going a little on the body and even the palms (hence the name progressive).

PPP really is a group of conditions, and the actual experience of any one patient is unique. PPP usually is only a cosmetic problem, but some people have severe itching. PPP can go away on its own within a few weeks, persist for years, or disappear only to recur again from time to time.

No one knows what causes it, but if a biopsy is done, inflammation is seen around the tiny capillaries in the skin. The blood leaking through the damaged walls forms the little red dots. The iron from the blood "rusts" (turns into hemosiderin), giving the distinct color. A biopsy may be done to confirm the diagnosis.

Occasionally PPP is caused by a reaction to a prescription drug, allergy to clothing dye and rubber, food preservatives and artificial coloring agents, or another skin disease. When it is limited to a few small patches, it may be due to abnormal veins or arteries underneath. Support stockings or surgery can clear it up.

Treatment is not always needed. Itching can usually be controlled with prescription steroid creams. In some cases, especially if fairly potent steroids are used, they may actually clear the PPP completely. More extensive cases can be treated with oral Trental (pentoxifylline). This takes several months and does not always work. Trental improves circulation, and aside from rare stomach upset, it is a very safe medication. Vitamins have been said to help also (vitamin C 500 milligrams twice daily and bioflavonoid complex with rutin).

Chapter 29

What You Need to Know about Moles and Dysplastic Nevi

Introduction

This information was written to help you learn more about common moles and unusual ones called dysplastic nevi or atypical moles. This chapter shows what moles look like and explains how they may be related to melanoma, a type of skin cancer. It describes the signs of melanoma and explains how you can check your skin for moles that might be cancerous. It also explains why and how you can protect your skin.

Cancer research has led to real progress against cancer—better survival and an improved quality of life. Through research, our knowledge about moles and cancers of the skin keeps increasing. We are finding new ways to prevent, detect, and treat cancer.

Moles

Moles are growths on the skin. Doctors call moles nevi (one mole is a nevus). These growths occur when cells in the skin, called melanocytes, grow in a cluster with tissue surrounding them. Moles are usually pink, tan, brown, or flesh-colored. Melanocytes are also spread evenly throughout the skin and produce the pigment that gives skin its natural color. When skin is exposed to the sun, melanocytes produce more pigment, causing the skin to tan, or darken.

Excerpted from the article by the National Cancer Institute, September 16, 2002. Available online at http://www.cancer.gov; accessed June 3, 2005.

Moles are very common. Most people have between 10 and 40 moles. A person may develop new moles from time to time, usually until about age 40. Moles can be flat or raised. They are usually round or oval and no larger than a pencil eraser. Many moles begin as a small, flat spot and slowly become larger in diameter and raised. Over many years, they may flatten again, become flesh-colored, and go away.

Dysplastic Nevi

About one out of every ten people has at least one unusual (or atypical) mole that looks different from an ordinary mole. The medical term for these unusual moles is dysplastic nevi.

Doctors believe that dysplastic nevi are more likely than ordinary moles to develop into a type of skin cancer called melanoma. Because of this, moles should be checked regularly by a doctor or nurse specialist, especially if they look unusual; grow larger; or change in color, outline, or in any other way.

Melanoma

Melanoma is a type of skin cancer—one of the most serious types because advanced melanomas have the ability to spread to other parts of the body. (Melanoma can also develop in the eye, called intraocular melanoma, or rarely in other parts of the body where pigment cells are found.) Melanoma begins when melanocytes (pigment cells) gradually become more abnormal and divide without control or order. These cells can invade and destroy the normal cells around them. The abnormal cells form a growth of malignant tissue (a cancerous tumor) on the surface of the skin. Melanoma can begin either in an existing mole or as a new growth on the skin. A doctor or nurse specialist can tell whether an abnormal-looking mole should be closely watched or should be removed and checked for melanoma cells. The purpose of routine skin exams is to identify and follow abnormal moles.

The removal of the entire mole or a sample of tissue for examination under a microscope is called a biopsy. If possible, it is best to remove moles by an excisional biopsy, rather than a shave biopsy.

If the biopsy results in a diagnosis of melanoma, the patient and the doctor should work together to make treatment decisions. In many cases, melanoma can be cured by minimal surgery if the tumor is discovered when it is thin (before it has grown downward from the skin surface) and before the cancer cells have begun to spread to other places in the body. However, if melanoma is not found early, the cancer cells can spread through the bloodstream and lymphatic system to form tumors in other parts of the body. Melanoma is much harder to control when it has spread. The spread of cancer is called metastasis.

Doctors and scientists believe that it is possible to prevent many melanomas and to detect most others early, when the disease is more likely to be cured with minimal surgery. In the past several decades, an increasing percentage of melanomas have been diagnosed at very early stages, when they are quite thin and unlikely to have spread. Learning about prevention and early detection, while important for everyone, is especially important for people who have an increased risk for melanoma. People who are at an increased risk include those who have dysplastic nevi or a very large number of ordinary moles.

It is important to remember that not everyone who has dysplastic nevi or other risk factors for melanoma gets the disease. In fact, most do not. Also, about half the people who develop melanoma do not have dysplastic nevi, and they may not have any other known risk factor for the disease. At this time, no one can explain why one person gets melanoma while another does not. Research has shown that sun exposure, especially excessive exposure that leads to bad, blistering sunburns, is an important and avoidable risk factor. Scientists are continuing their studies of risk factors for melanoma.

Prevention of Melanoma

The number of people in the world who develop melanoma is increasing each year. In the United States, the number has more than doubled in the past 20 years. Experts believe that much of the worldwide increase in melanoma is related to an increase in the amount of time people spend in the sun.

Ultraviolet (UV) radiation from the sun and from sunlamps and tanning booths damages the skin and can lead to melanoma and other types of skin cancer. Everyone, especially those who have dysplastic nevi or other risk factors, should try to reduce the risk of developing melanoma by protecting the skin from UV radiation. The intensity of UV radiation from the sun is greatest in the summer, particularly during midday hours. A simple rule is to avoid the sun or protect your skin whenever your shadow is shorter than you are.

People who work or play in the sun should wear protective clothing, such as a hat and long sleeves. Also, lotion, cream, or gel that contains sunscreen can help protect the skin. Many doctors believe sunscreens may help prevent melanoma, especially those that reflect, absorb, and/or scatter both types of ultraviolet radiation. Sunscreens are rated in strength according to a sun protection factor (SPF). The higher the SPF, the more sunburn protection is provided. Sunscreens with an SPF value of 2 to 11 provide minimal protection against sunburns. Sunscreens with an SPF of 12 to 29 provide moderate protection. Those with an SPF of 30 or higher provide high protection against sunburn. Sunglasses that have UV-absorbing lenses should also be worn. The label should specify that the lenses block at least 99 percent of UVA and UVB radiation.

Early Detection of Melanoma

Because melanoma usually begins on the surface of the skin, it often can be detected at an early stage with a total skin examination by a trained health care worker. Checking the skin regularly for any signs of the disease increases the chance of finding melanoma early. A monthly skin self-exam is very important for people who have any of the known risk factors, but doing skin self-exams routinely is a good idea for everyone.

Here is how to do a skin self-exam:

- After a bath or shower, stand in front of a full-length mirror in a well-lighted room. Use a hand-held mirror to look at hard-to-see areas.
- Begin with the face and scalp and work downward, checking the head, neck, shoulders, back, chest, and so on. Be sure to check the front, back, and sides of the arms and legs. Also, check the groin, the palms, the fingernails, the soles of the feet, the toenails, and the area between the toes.
- Be sure to check the hard-to-see areas of the body, such as the scalp and neck. A friend or relative may be able to help inspect these areas. Use a comb or a blow dryer to help move hair so you can see the scalp and neck better.
- Be aware of where your moles are and how they look. By checking your skin regularly, you will become familiar with what your moles look like. Look for any signs of change, particularly a new black mole or a change in outline, shape, size, color (especially a new black area), or feel of an existing mole. Also, note any new, unusual, or “ugly-looking” moles. If your doctor has taken photos of your skin, compare these pictures with the way your skin looks on self-examination.

- Check moles carefully during times of hormone changes, such as adolescence, pregnancy, and menopause. As hormone levels change, moles may change.
- It may be helpful to record the dates of your skin exams and to write notes about the way your skin looks. If you find anything unusual, see your doctor right away. Remember, the earlier a melanoma is found, the better the chance for a cure.

In addition to doing routine skin self-exams, people should have their skin checked regularly by a doctor or nurse specialist. A doctor can do a skin exam during visits for regular checkups. People who think they have dysplastic nevi should point them out to the doctor. It is also important to tell the doctor about any new, changing, or "ugly-looking" moles.

Sometimes it is necessary to see a specialist. A dermatologist (skin doctor) is likely to have the most training in diseases of the skin. Some plastic surgeons, general surgeons, oncologists, internists, and family doctors also have a special interest and training in moles and melanoma.

Melanoma may run in families, and members of these families are at high risk for the disease. In some of these families, certain members also have a large number (usually over 100) of dysplastic nevi. These people have an especially high risk of developing melanoma. When two or more family members develop melanoma, it is important for all of the patients' close relatives (parents, brothers, sisters, and children above the age of 10) to see a doctor and be examined carefully for dysplastic nevi or any signs of melanoma. The doctor can then decide how often each person needs to be seen. (Doctors may recommend that these family members have checkups every 6 months.) Anyone who has a large number of dysplastic nevi also should be examined regularly.

A doctor may want to watch a slightly abnormal mole closely to see whether it changes over time. Pictures taken at one visit may be compared with the appearance of the mole at the next visit. Sometimes a doctor decides that a mole should be removed so that the tissue can be examined under a microscope. The removal of a mole, called a biopsy, is usually done in the doctor's office using a local anesthetic. It generally takes only a few minutes. The patient may require stitches, and a small scar will remain after healing. A pathologist examines the tissue under a microscope to see whether the melanocytes are normal, dysplastic, or cancerous.

Because most moles, including most dysplastic nevi, do not develop into melanoma, removing all of them is not necessary. A doctor can recommend when and when not to remove moles. Usually, only moles that look like melanoma, those that change, or those that are both new and look abnormal need to be removed.

Ordinary Moles and Dysplastic Nevi

Ordinary Moles

- **Color:** Evenly tan or brown; all typical moles on one person tend to look similar.
- **Shape:** Round or oval, with a distinct edge that separates the mole from the rest of the skin.
- **Surface:** Begin as flat, smooth spots on skin; may become raised and form a smooth bump.
- **Size:** Usually less than 5 millimeters (about 1/4 inch) across (size of a pencil eraser).
- **Number:** Between 10 and 40 typical moles may be present on an adult's body.
- **Location:** Usually found above the waist on sun-exposed surfaces of the body. Scalp, breasts, and buttocks rarely have normal moles.

Dysplastic Nevi

- **Color:** Mixture of tan, brown, and red/pink. A person's moles often look quite different from one another.
- **Shape:** Have irregular, sometimes notched edges. May fade into the skin around it. The flat portion of the mole may be level with the skin.
- **Surface:** May have a smooth, slightly scaly, or rough, irregular, "pebbly" appearance.
- **Size:** Often larger than 5 millimeters (about 1/4 inch) across and sometimes larger than 10 millimeters (about 1/2 inch).
- **Number:** May be present in large numbers (more than 100 on the same person). However, some people have only a few dysplastic nevi.
- **Location:** May occur anywhere on the body but most frequently on the back and areas exposed to the sun. May also appear below the waist and on the scalp, breasts, and buttocks.

Chapter 30

Neurocutaneous Syndromes

Chapter Contents

Section 30.1

Overview of Neurocutaneous Syndromes

"Neurocutaneous Syndromes" was provided by KidsHealth, one of the largest resources online for medically reviewed health information written for parents, kids, and teens. For more articles like this one, visit www.KidsHealth.org, or www.TeensHealth.org. Reviewed by Marcy Yonker, M.D., October 2001.

Neurocutaneous syndromes is a term that refers to a group of genetic neurological (affecting the brain, spine, and peripheral nerves) disorders. The various kinds of neurocutaneous syndromes can cause tumors to grow inside the brain, spinal cord, organs, skin, and skeletal bones. The first symptoms most commonly noted in children are skin lesions, including birthmarks, tumors, and other growths.

The diseases are believed to arise from abnormal development of embryonic cells (primitive cells that are present in the earliest stages of an embryo's development) and can involve multiple organs in the body. Although there is no cure for these conditions, treatments are available that help to manage symptoms and complications.

What Are the Neurocutaneous Syndromes?

There are several neurocutaneous syndromes, but the most common ones that involve children include:

- neurofibromatosis, type 1 and 2 (NF1 and NF2)
- Sturge-Weber syndrome
- tuberous sclerosis (TS)
- ataxia-telangiectasia (A-T)
- von Hippel-Lindau disease (VHL)

Not only do symptoms vary widely from condition to condition, but they also vary widely from child to child. Because neurocutaneous syndromes affect children in different ways, the full extent of these diseases—even if detected at birth—may only be revealed as the child grows up. The conditions are always lifelong, which means that educational, social, and physical problems must be managed throughout a child's life.

Neurofibromatosis

Neurofibromatosis is one of the most common neurocutaneous syndromes. It primarily affects the growth and development of nerve cells. The disease can cause tumors to grow on nerves, producing skin changes, bone deformities, eye problems, and other complications, particularly in the brain.

Neurofibromatosis is usually inherited, but between 30% to 50% of new cases occur from changes (mutations) within a person's genes. Once this gene alteration has taken place, the changed (mutant) gene can then be passed on to succeeding generations. A parent with neurofibromatosis has a 50% chance of having a child with the disease.

Many years ago, medical experts classified the disorder into two different types, neurofibromatosis type 1 and type 2 (NF1 and NF2). We now know they are two totally separate disorders caused by two different genes. NF1 occurs far more frequently, accounting for approximately 90% of all cases.

Neurofibromatosis Type 1

NF1 is one of the most common genetic disorders, occurring in about one in 4,000 babies born in the United States. When diagnosing NF1 (also called von Recklinghausen disease), doctors will take a thorough medical history because children with NF1 often have a parent with the disease.

The classic sign of NF1 is a skin pigment problem known as "café-au-lait" spots. These light brown, coffee-colored patches may be present at birth, and may look like freckles at first but often increase in size and number during the first few years of life. A child diagnosed with NF1 will usually have at least six café-au-lait spots that are larger than freckles.

Another common sign of NF1 is Lisch nodules, tiny, benign (noncancerous) tumors found on the iris of the eye, and of no clinical significance except to help confirm the diagnosis. Tumors along the optic nerves can occur, rarely, and affect vision. Benign tumors called neurofibromas are found on or under the skin or along the nerves of the body. Often these do not start to appear until puberty. Bone deformities may also occur.

Treatment of a child with NF1 focuses on managing symptoms of the affected body system. Children who have complications involving the eye, nervous system, spine, or bones will be referred to an appropriate specialist for treatment. Surgical removal of neurofibromas is required if they are causing chronic pain, become infected, are pressing or growing into vital body organs, or for cosmetic reasons.

Children with NF1 also have a high incidence of seizures (30% to 40%), learning disabilities, attention deficit disorder, and speech problems and may require supportive therapies in those areas as well.

Neurofibromatosis Type 2

Neurofibromatosis type 2 is less common, occurring in about one in 40,000 births. People with this disease develop tumors on the auditory nerves (the nerves leading to the ear).

Hearing loss, ringing of the ears, and problems with balance generally become apparent in the teen years or early twenties. Several different treatment options are available for these tumors.

Tuberous Sclerosis

Tuberous sclerosis is a disorder that causes benign growths, called "tubers," to form on several different organs within the body, including the brain, eyes, kidneys, heart, skin, and lungs. It occurs in approximately one in 6,000 births. There is a 50% chance that a parent with TS will have a child with the disease.

The condition is often first recognized in children who experience epileptic seizures or who exhibit developmental delays. The severity of TS varies from mild skin abnormalities to very severe cases that cause mental retardation or kidney failure.

Treatment usually includes medication to prevent seizures, treatments to address skin problems, surgery to remove tumors (to reduce the risk of cancer as well as for cosmetic reasons), and the management of high blood pressure caused by kidney disease. As with all of the neurocutaneous syndromes, a child's prognosis depends on the severity of the case.

Sturge-Weber Syndrome

Sturge-Weber syndrome is a rare condition that affects the skin and the brain. It is caused by a spontaneous genetic mutation and is not passed down by parents who carry the disease. How often it occurs in babies is not known, and because it is not frequently diagnosed, it is difficult to estimate how many people currently have the disease.

According to the Sturge-Weber Foundation, the most apparent indication of the disease is a facial birthmark or "port-wine stain" present at birth, typically involving at least one upper eyelid and the forehead area. Every case of Sturge-Weber is unique and symptoms and skin abnormalities vary.

Neurological problems include unusual blood vessel growths on the brain called angiomas. Angiomas usually cause seizures, which begin before 1 year of age and may worsen with age. Convulsions usually appear on the side of the body opposite the port-wine stain and vary in severity.

About 30% of patients with Sturge-Weber also develop glaucoma (increased pressure inside the eye that impairs vision). Glaucoma is usually restricted to the eye that is affected by the port-wine stain. Enlarging of the eye (buphthalmos) can also occur in the eye that is involved with the stain. In some cases, strokes can occur.

Children as young as 1 month old who have Sturge-Weber may undergo laser treatment to reduce or remove port-wine stains. Anticonvulsant medication may be used to control seizures associated with the disorder, and surgery is available to control glaucoma and vision problems.

Ataxia-Telangiectasia

Ataxia-telangiectasia is a progressive degenerative disease that involves a large number of major body systems. According to the Ataxia-Telangiectasia Children's Project, A-T is a recessive genetic disease, meaning that both parents carry the gene that could combine to cause A-T in their children but do not have the disease themselves. Two parents with the mutated gene have a 25% chance of having a child affected by A-T.

A-T is usually noticed in the second year of life as a child develops problems with balance and slurred speech caused by ataxia (lack of muscle control). The onset of ataxia signifies that the cerebellum, the part of the brain that controls muscle movement, is degenerating. Eventually, the lack of muscle control becomes severe enough for the child to require a wheelchair.

Another symptom of A-T is the appearance of tiny, red, spiderlike veins in the corners of the eyes or on the ears and cheeks when exposed to sunlight. The veins are known as "telangiectases," and they are harmless.

About 70% of children with A-T also have immune system problems that make them more susceptible to chronic upper respiratory infections, lung infections, and pneumonia. In many children, these infections, when combined with a weakened immune system, can be fatal. Children with A-T are also very susceptible to developing certain cancers, such as leukemia and lymphoma.

There is currently no treatment available for A-T, and no way to stop the progression of the condition. At this time, the goals of treatment are to manage the child's symptoms and provide supportive care. Physical and occupational therapy may help maintain flexibility, and speech therapy can help address slurring and other speech problems. Special medications may be given to help enhance weakened immune systems.

Von Hippel-Lindau Disease

Von Hippel-Lindau disease is a genetic disorder involving the abnormal growth of blood vessels. It usually occurs in certain areas of the body, such as the brain and other parts of the central nervous system, the retina of the eye, the adrenal glands, the kidneys, or the pancreas. The prevalence of the disease is unknown, but a parent who carries the gene that causes VHL has a 50% chance of having a child with the disorder.

Blood vessels usually grow like branches on a tree, but in people with VHL, they form small tumors called angiomas. Doctors carefully monitor angiomas because depending on where they are located, they can cause other medical problems. For example, angiomas on the retina of the eye may lead to permanent vision loss.

VHL is diagnosed using a special imaging technique called magnetic resonance imaging (MRI) or a computerized tomography (CT) scan. A thorough physical examination and blood tests are also performed.

There are many symptoms of VHL, and they depend on the size and location of the angiomas. Symptoms include headaches, balance problems, dizziness, weakness, vision problems, and high blood pressure. Fluid-filled cysts or tumors (benign or cancerous) may develop around the angiomas, worsening these symptoms. People with this disorder have a higher risk of developing cancer, especially kidney cancer.

VHL is treated depending on the size and location of the angiomas. The goal of treatment is to treat the tumors while they are small in size and before they put pressure on any of the major organs, such as the brain and the spine. Surgery may be required to remove the tumors before they create severe problems.

The prognosis for VHL patients depends on the location and complications caused by the tumors. If untreated, VHL may result in blindness or permanent brain damage. Fortunately, early detection and treatment can improve a child's treatment outcome.

Caring for Your Child

It's normal to sometimes feel overwhelmed when caring for a child with a neurocutaneous syndrome. The illnesses associated with these syndromes can place enormous stress and emotional burdens on you and your child. Early intervention is important in helping your child achieve the best quality of life possible.

The focus of treatment is to prevent or minimize complications and maximize the child's strengths. Keep in mind the following tips:

- Positive reinforcement can strengthen your child's self-esteem and foster a sense of independence. Let your child find out what he is capable of, especially when performing daily living skills.
- Support groups for you and your child can be extremely beneficial, so seek out local chapters that address your child's particular illness (for a partial listing, click on the Additional Resources tab). Not only do these groups provide a supportive social environment, they also are a great way to share knowledge and resources.
- Psychotherapy or other supportive treatments can boost your child's self-esteem and coping skills, so ask your child's treatment team for appropriate referrals. Therapy can also help you and other family members to deal with the stress involved in caring for a child with a chronic illness or disability.
- Physical, occupational, or speech therapy can help your child improve some of the developmental delays caused by his specific illness.
- Check with your local hospital or university for seminars or informational classes about neurocutaneous syndromes. By educating yourself and your family members, you can become a valuable resource in your child's long-term treatment.

A number of medical professionals may care for your child throughout his diagnosis and treatment. These professionals include a family practitioner, pediatrician, neurologist, neurosurgeon, orthopedic surgeon, oncologist, and ophthalmologist. A genetic counselor may also be helpful in providing parents with information about genetic testing and the risk of passing the disease on to another child.

Remember that although each of these conditions is challenging, supportive therapies and treatments are available to help both you and your child.

Section 30.2

Incontinentia Pigmenti

"Incontinentia Pigmenti Information Page," National Institute of Neurological Disorders and Stroke (NINDS), December 3, 2004. Available online at http://www.ninds.nih.gov; accessed May 24, 2005.

Incontinentia pigmenti (IP) is one of a group of gene-linked diseases known as neurocutaneous disorders. These disorders cause characteristic patterns of discolored skin and also involve the brain, eyes, nails, and hair. In most cases, IP is caused by mutations in a gene called *NEMO* (NF-kappa B essential modulator).

Males are more severely affected than females. Discolored skin is caused by excessive deposits of melanin (normal skin pigment). Most newborns with IP will develop discolored skin within the first two weeks. The pigmentation involves the trunk and extremities, is slate-grey, blue or brown, and is distributed in irregular marbled or wavy lines. The discoloration fades with age. Neurological problems include cerebral atrophy, the formation of small cavities in the central white matter of the brain, and the loss of neurons in the cerebellar cortex. About 20% of children with IP will have slow motor development, muscle weakness in one or both sides of the body, mental retardation, and seizures. They are also likely to have visual problems, including crossed eyes, cataracts, and severe visual loss. Dental problems are also common, including missing or peg-shaped teeth. A related disorder, incontinentia pigmenti achromians, features skin patterns of light, unpigmented swirls and streaks that are the reverse of IP. Associated neurological problems are similar.

Is there any treatment?

The skin abnormalities of IP usually disappear by adolescence or adulthood without treatment. Diminished vision may be treated with corrective lenses, medication, or, in severe cases, surgery. A specialist may treat dental problems. Neurological symptoms such as seizures, muscle spasms, or mild paralysis may be controlled with medication and/or medical devices and with the advice of a neurologist.

What is the prognosis?

Although the skin abnormalities usually regress, and sometimes disappear completely, there may be residual neurological difficulties.

What research is being done?

Researchers have begun to use genetic linkage studies to map the location of genes associated with the neurocutaneous disorders. Research supported by the National Institute of Neurological Disorders and Stroke includes studies to understand how the brain and nervous system normally develop and function and how they are affected by genetic mutations. These studies contribute to a greater understanding of gene-linked disorders such as IP, and have the potential to open promising new avenues of treatment.

Part Five

Malignant Skin Growths and Dermatological Side Effects of Cancer Treatment

Chapter 31

Actinic Keratoses: Precursors to Skin Cancer

You have surely seen an actinic keratosis. The name may be unfamiliar, but the appearance is commonplace. Anyone who spends time in the sun runs a high risk of developing one or more.

What is it?

An actinic keratosis (AK), also known as a solar keratosis, is a scaly or crusty bump that arises on the skin surface. The base may be light or dark, tan, pink, red, or a combination of these or the same color as your skin. The scale or crust is horny, dry, and rough, and is often recognized by touch rather than sight. Occasionally it itches or produces a pricking or tender sensation. It can also become inflamed and surrounded by redness. In rare instances, actinic keratoses can even bleed.

The skin abnormality or lesion develops slowly and generally reaches a size from an eighth to a quarter of an inch. Early on, it may disappear only to reappear later. You will often see several AKs at a time.

An AK is most likely to appear on the face, ears, scalp, neck, backs of the hands and forearms, shoulders, and lips—the parts of the body most often exposed to sunshine. The growths may be flat and pink or raised and rough.

"Actinic Keratosis: What You Should Know About This Common Precancer," reprinted with permission from The Skin Cancer Foundation, NY, NY, www.skin cancer.org.

Why is it dangerous?

AK can be the first step in the development of skin cancer. It is thus a precursor of cancer or a precancer.

If treated early, almost all AKs can be eliminated without becoming skin cancers. But untreated, about two to five percent of these lesions may progress to squamous cell carcinomas. In fact, some scientists now believe that AK is the earliest form of SCC [squamous cell carcinoma]. These cancers are usually not life threatening, provided they are detected and treated in the early stages. However, if this is not done, they can grow large and invade the surrounding tissues and, on rare occasions, metastasize or spread to the internal organs.

Another form of AK, actinic cheilitis, develops on the lips and may evolve into a type of SCC that can spread rapidly to other parts of the body.

If you have AKs, it indicates that you have sustained sun damage and could develop any kind of skin cancer—not just squamous cell carcinoma. The more keratoses that you have, the greater the chance that one or more may turn into skin cancer. People may also have up to 10 times as many subclinical (invisible) lesions as visible, surface lesions.

What does it look like?

Common forms of actinic keratoses are listed here in the locations where they most often develop. Examine your skin to find any lesions that look like these. If you spot them, consult your doctor promptly.

- Back of hand with scattered, thickened red, scaly patches
- Cheek and ear with multiple crusted lesions, ranging in color from red to brown
- Sun-damaged forehead and bald scalp with multiple keratoses seen as small red bumps and small tan crusts
- Lower lip filled with fissures filled with dried blood and large keratosis covered with horny scale

What is the cause?

Chronic sun exposure is the cause of almost all AKs. Sun damage to the skin accumulates over time, so that even a brief exposure adds to the lifetime total.

The likelihood of developing AK is highest in regions near the equator. However, regardless of climate, everyone is exposed to the sun. About 80 percent of solar UV [ultraviolet] rays can pass through clouds. These rays can also bounce off sand, snow, and other reflective surfaces, giving you extra exposure.

AKs can also appear on skin that has been frequently exposed to artificial sources of UV light (such as tanning devices). More rarely, they may be caused by extensive exposure to x-rays or specific industrial chemicals.

Who is at greatest risk?

People who have fair skin, blonde or red hair, and/or blue, green, or gray eyes are at greatest risk. Because their skin has little protective pigment, they are most susceptible to sunburn. But even darker-skinned people can develop AKs if exposed to the sun without protection.

Individuals whose immune systems are weakened as a result of cancer, chemotherapy, AIDS, or organ transplantation are also at higher risk.

How common is it?

AK is the most common type of precancerous skin lesion. Older people are more likely than younger ones to develop these lesions, because cumulative sun exposure increases with the years. Some experts believe that the majority of people who live to the age of 80 will have AK.

On average, however, more than half of our lifetime sun exposure occurs before age 20. Thus, AKs also appear in people in their early twenties who have spent too much time in the sun with little or no protection.

How is it treated?

There are many effective methods for eliminating AKs. All cause a certain amount of reddening, and some may cause scarring, while other approaches are less likely to do so. You and your doctor should decide together the best course of treatment, based on the nature of the lesion and your age and health.

Cryosurgery: The most common treatment for AK, it is especially effective when a limited number of lesions exist. No cutting or anesthesia is required. Liquid nitrogen is applied to the growths with a spray device or cotton-tipped applicator to freeze them. They subsequently shrink or become crusted and fall off. Some temporary swelling may occur after treatment, and in dark-skinned patients, some pigment may be lost.

Curettage and Desiccation: This is a valuable procedure for lesions suspected to be early cancers. To test for malignancy, the physician takes a biopsy specimen, either by shaving off the top of the lesion with a scalpel or scraping it off with a curette. Then the curette is used to remove the base of the lesion. Bleeding is stopped with an electrocautery needle, and local anesthesia is required.

Topical Medications: Medicated creams and solutions are especially useful in removing both visible and invisible AKs when the lesions are numerous. The patient applies the medication according to a schedule worked out by the physician. The doctor will also regularly check progress. After treatment, some discomfort may result from skin breakdown.

5-fluorouracil (5-FU) cream or solution, in concentrations from 0.5 to 5 percent, is the most widely used topical treatment for AK. It works especially well on the face, ears, and neck. Some swelling and crusting may occur.

For those who are oversensitive to 5-FU or other topical treatments, a gel combining hyaluronic acid and the anti-inflammatory drug diclofenac also may prove effective.

Another preparation, imiquimod cream, is also being used by physicians for multiple keratoses. FDA-approved as a genital wart treatment, it causes cells to produce interferon, a chemical that destroys cancerous and precancerous cells.

Chemical Peeling: This method makes use of trichloroacetic acid (TCA) or a similar agent applied directly to the skin. The top skin layers slough off, usually replaced within seven days by new epidermis (the skin's outermost layer). This technique requires local anesthesia and can cause temporary discoloration and irritation.

Laser Surgery: A carbon dioxide or erbium YAG [Yttrium Aluminum Garnet] laser is focused onto the lesion, removing epidermis and different amounts of deeper skin. This finely controlled treatment is a good option for lesions in small or narrow areas; it can be particularly effective for keratoses on the face and scalp, as well as actinic cheilitis on the lips. However, local anesthesia may be necessary, and some pigment loss can occur.

Photodynamic Therapy (PDT): PDT may be used to treat lesions on the face and scalp. Topical 5-aminolevulinic acid (5-ALA) is applied to the lesions by the physician. The next day, the medicated areas are exposed to strong light, which activates the 5-ALA. The treatment selectively destroys actinic keratoses, causing little damage to surrounding normal skin, although some swelling often occurs.

How can it be prevented?

The best way to prevent actinic keratosis is to protect yourself from the sun. The Skin Cancer Foundation recommends that these sun safety habits be part of everyone's daily health care:

- Avoid unnecessary sun exposure, especially during the sun's peak hours (10 A.M. to 4 P.M.).
- Seek the shade.
- Cover up with clothing, including a broad-brimmed hat, long pants, a long-sleeved shirt, and UV-blocking sunglasses.
- Wear a broad-spectrum sunscreen with a sun protection factor (SPF) of 15 or higher.
- Avoid tanning parlors and artificial tanning devices.
- Keep newborns out of the sun. Sunscreens can be used on babies over the age of six months.
- Teach children good sun-protective practices.
- Examine your skin from head to toe once every month.
- Have a professional skin examination annually.

Chapter 32

What You Need to Know about Skin Cancer

The Skin

The skin is the body's outer covering. It protects us against heat, light, injury, and infection. It regulates body temperature and stores water, fat, and vitamin D. Weighing about 6 pounds, the skin is the body's largest organ. It is made up of two main layers: the outer epidermis and the inner dermis.

The epidermis (outer layer of the skin) is mostly made up of flat, scale-like cells called squamous cells. Under the squamous cells are round cells called basal cells. The deepest part of the epidermis also contains melanocytes. These cells produce melanin, which gives the skin its color.

The dermis (inner layer of skin) contains blood and lymph vessels, hair follicles, and glands. These glands produce sweat, which helps regulate body temperature, and sebum, an oily substance that helps keep the skin from drying out. Sweat and sebum reach the skin's surface through tiny openings called pores.

What Is Cancer?

Cancer is a group of more than 100 diseases. Although each type of cancer differs from the others in many ways, every cancer is a disease of some of the body's cells.

From the National Cancer Institute, September 16, 2002. Available online at http://www.cancer.gov; accessed June 1, 2005.

Healthy cells that make up the body's tissues grow, divide, and replace themselves in an orderly way. This process keeps the body in good repair. Sometimes, however, normal cells lose their ability to limit and direct their growth. They divide too rapidly and grow without any order. Too much tissue is produced, and tumors begin to form. Tumors can be benign or malignant.

- Benign tumors are not cancer. They do not spread to other parts of the body and are seldom a threat to life. Often, benign tumors can be removed by surgery, and they are not likely to return.
- Malignant tumors are cancer. They can invade and destroy nearby healthy tissues and organs. Cancer cells also can spread, or metastasize, to other parts of the body and form new tumors.

Types of Skin Cancer

The two most common kinds of skin cancer are basal cell carcinoma and squamous cell carcinoma. (Carcinoma is cancer that begins in the

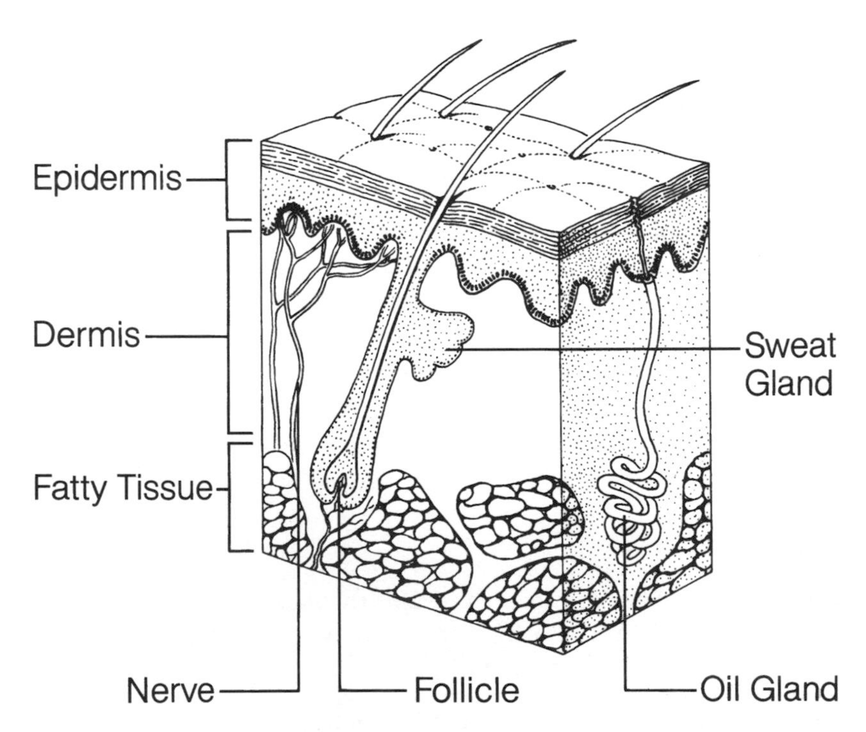

Figure 32.1. *Epidermis and Dermis*

cells that cover or line an organ.) Basal cell carcinoma accounts for more than 90 percent of all skin cancers in the United States. It is a slow-growing cancer that seldom spreads to other parts of the body. Squamous cell carcinoma also rarely spreads, but it does so more often than basal cell carcinoma. However, it is important that skin cancers be found and treated early because they can invade and destroy nearby tissue.

Basal cell carcinoma and squamous cell carcinoma are sometimes called nonmelanoma skin cancer. Another type of cancer that occurs in the skin is melanoma, which begins in the melanocytes.

Cause and Prevention

Skin cancer is the most common type of cancer in the United States. According to current estimates, 40 to 50 percent of Americans who live to age 65 will have skin cancer at least once. Although anyone can get skin cancer, the risk is greatest for people who have fair skin that freckles easily—often those with red or blond hair and blue or light-colored eyes.

Ultraviolet (UV) radiation from the sun is the main cause of skin cancer. Artificial sources of UV radiation, such as sunlamps and tanning booths, can also cause skin cancer.

The risk of developing skin cancer is affected by where a person lives. People who live in areas that get high levels of UV radiation from the sun are more likely to get skin cancer. In the United States, for example, skin cancer is more common in Texas than it is in Minnesota, where the sun is not as strong. Worldwide, the highest rates of skin cancer are found in South Africa and Australia, areas that receive high amounts of UV radiation.

In addition, skin cancer is related to lifetime exposure to UV radiation. Most skin cancers appear after age 50, but the sun's damaging effects begin at an early age. Therefore, protection should start in childhood to prevent skin cancer later in life.

Whenever possible, people should avoid exposure to the midday sun (from 10 a.m. to 2 p.m. standard time, or from 11 a.m. to 3 p.m. daylight saving time). Keep in mind that protective clothing, such as sun hats and long sleeves, can block out the sun's harmful rays. Also, lotions that contain sunscreens can protect the skin. Sunscreens are rated in strength according to a sun protection factor (SPF), which ranges from 2 to 30 or higher. Those rated 15 to 30 block most of the sun's harmful rays.

The National Cancer Institute is supporting research to try to find new ways to prevent skin cancer. This research involves people who have a high risk of developing skin cancer—those who have already had the disease and those who have certain other rare skin diseases that increase their risk of skin cancer.

Symptoms

The most common warning sign of skin cancer is a change on the skin, especially a new growth or a sore that doesn't heal. Skin cancers don't all look the same. For example, the cancer may start as a small, smooth, shiny, pale, or waxy lump. Or it can appear as a firm red lump. Sometimes, the lump bleeds or develops a crust. Skin cancer can also start as a flat, red spot that is rough, dry, or scaly.

Both basal and squamous cell cancers are found mainly on areas of the skin that are exposed to the sun—the head, face, neck, hands, and arms. However, skin cancer can occur anywhere.

Actinic keratosis, which appears as rough, red or brown scaly patches on the skin, is known as a precancerous condition because it sometimes develops into squamous cell cancer. Like skin cancer, it usually appears on sun-exposed areas but can be found elsewhere.

Changes in the skin are not sure signs of cancer; however, it is important to see a doctor if any symptom lasts longer than 2 weeks. Don't wait for the area to hurt—skin cancers seldom cause pain.

Detection

The cure rate for skin cancer could be 100 percent if all skin cancers were brought to a doctor's attention before they had a chance to spread. Therefore, people should check themselves regularly for new growths or other changes in the skin. Any new, colored growths or any changes in growths that are already present should be reported to the doctor without delay.

Doctors should also look at the skin during routine physical exams. People who have already had skin cancer should be sure to have regular exams so that the doctor can check the skin—both the treated areas and other places where cancer may develop.

Diagnosis

Basal cell carcinoma and squamous cell carcinoma are generally diagnosed and treated in the same way. When an area of skin does not look normal, the doctor may remove all or part of the growth. This is called a biopsy. To check for cancer cells, the tissue is examined

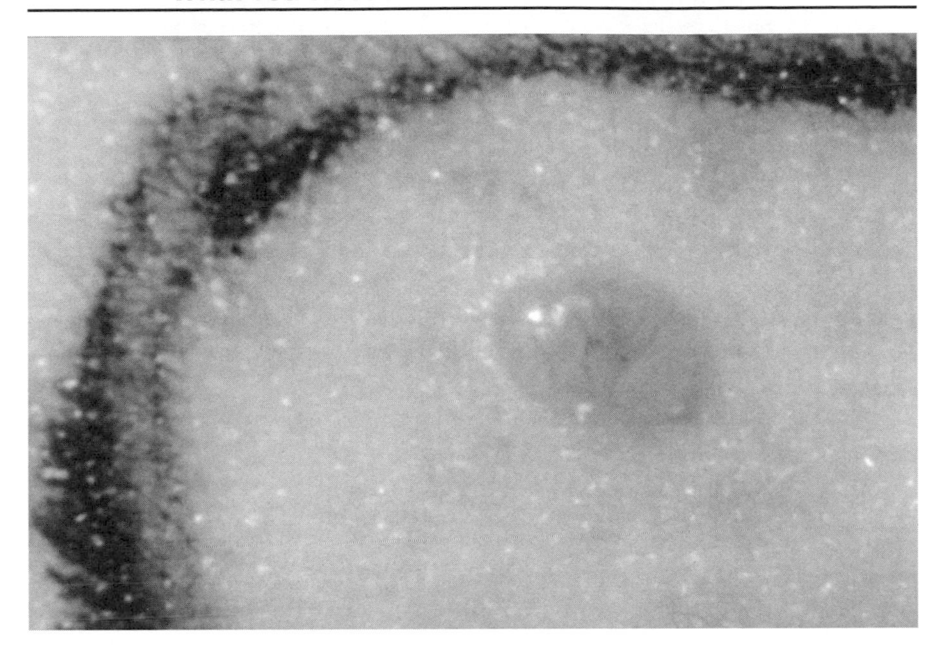

Figure 32.2. *Skin cancer can appear as a small, smooth, shiny, pale, or waxy lump.*

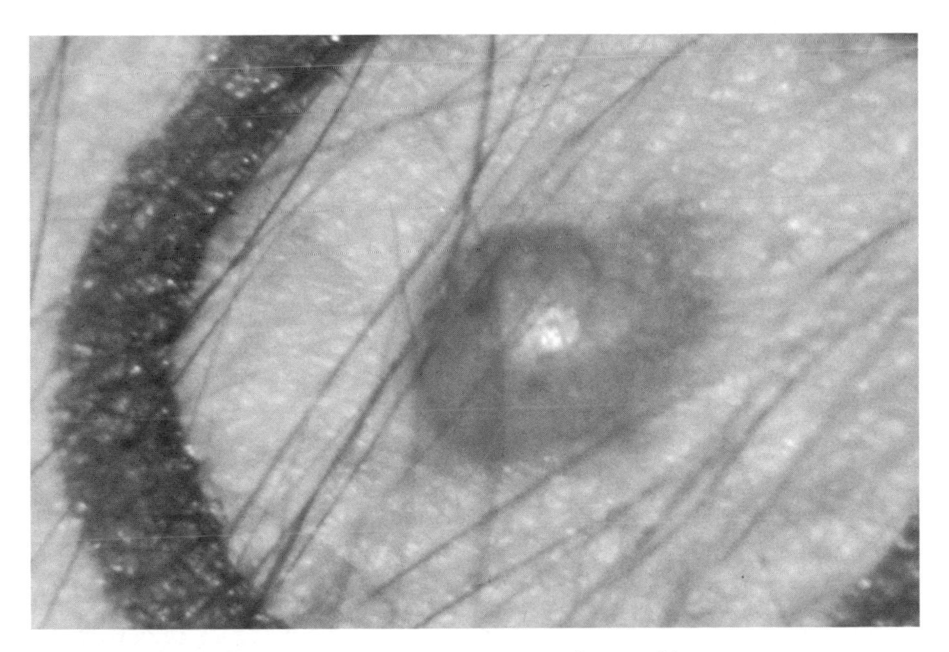

Figure 32.3. *Skin cancer can appear as a firm red lump*

under a microscope by a pathologist or a dermatologist. A biopsy is the only sure way to tell if the problem is cancer.

Doctors generally divide skin cancer into two stages: local (affecting only the skin) or metastatic (spreading beyond the skin). Because skin cancer rarely spreads, a biopsy often is the only test needed to determine the stage. In cases where the growth is very large or has been present for a long time, the doctor will carefully check the lymph nodes in the area. In addition, the patient may need to have additional tests, such as special x-rays, to find out whether the cancer has spread to other parts of the body. Knowing the stage of a skin cancer helps the doctor plan the best treatment

Treatment Planning

In treating skin cancer, the doctor's main goal is to remove or destroy the cancer completely with as small a scar as possible. To plan the best treatment for each patient, the doctor considers the location and size of the cancer, the risk of scarring, and the person's age, general health, and medical history.

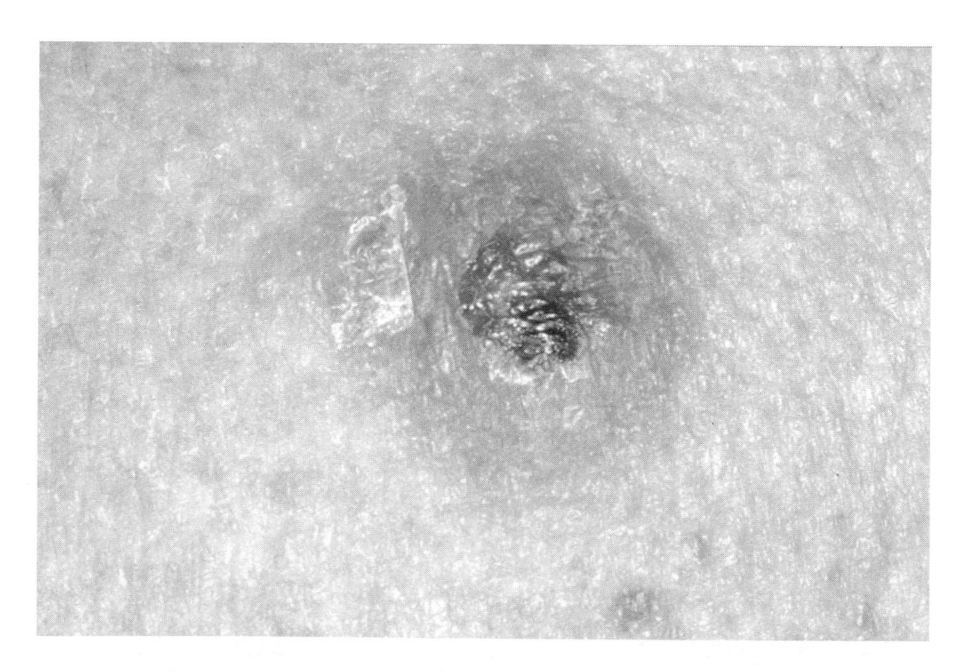

Figure 32.4. *Skin cancer can appear as a lump that bleeds or develops a crust.*

It is sometimes helpful to have the advice of more than one doctor before starting treatment. It may take a week or two to arrange for a second opinion, but this short delay will not reduce the chance that treatment will be successful. There are a number of ways to find a doctor for a second opinion:

- The patient's doctor may be able to suggest a doctor, such as a dermatologist or a plastic surgeon, who has a special interest in skin cancer.
- The Cancer Information Service, at (800) 4-CANCER, can tell callers about treatment facilities, including cancer centers and other programs that are supported by the National Cancer Institute. Patients can get the names of doctors from local and national medical societies, a nearby hospital, or a medical school.
- The American Board of Medical Specialties (ABMS) has a list of doctors who have met certain education and training requirements and have passed specialty examinations. *The Official ABMS Directory of Board Certified Medical Specialists* lists doctors'

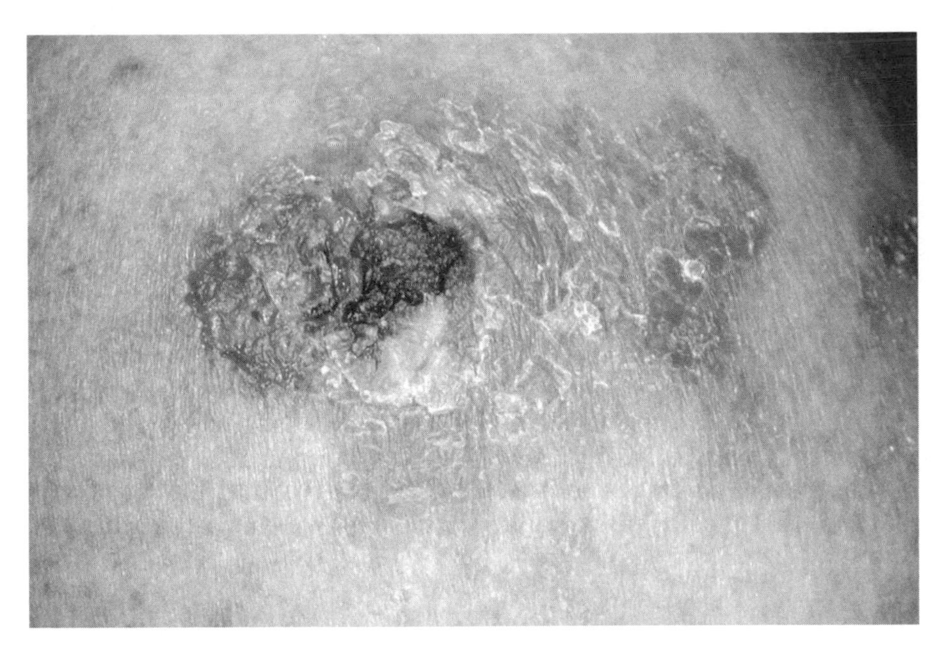

Figure 32.5. *Skin cancer can appear as a flat, red spot that is rough, dry, or scaly.*

names along with their specialty and their educational background. The directory is available in most public libraries. Also, ABMS offers this information on the Internet at http://www.abms.org.

Treating Skin Cancer

Treatment for skin cancer usually involves some type of surgery. In some cases, doctors suggest radiation therapy or chemotherapy. Sometimes a combination of these methods is used.

Surgery

Many skin cancers can be cut from the skin quickly and easily. In fact, the cancer is sometimes completely removed at the time of the biopsy, and no further treatment is needed.

Curettage and Electrodesiccation

Doctors commonly use a type of surgery called curettage. After a local anesthetic numbs the area, the cancer is scooped out with a curette, an instrument with a sharp, spoon-shaped end. The area is also treated by electrodesiccation. An electric current from a special machine is used to control bleeding and kill any cancer cells remaining around the edge of the wound. Most patients develop a flat, white scar.

Mohs' Surgery

Mohs' technique is a special type of surgery used for skin cancer. Its purpose is to remove all of the cancerous tissue and as little of the healthy tissue as possible. It is especially helpful when the doctor is not sure of the shape and depth of the tumor. In addition, this method is used to remove large tumors, those in hard-to-treat places, and cancers that have recurred. The patient is given a local anesthetic, and the cancer is shaved off one thin layer at a time. Each layer is checked under a microscope until the entire tumor is removed. The degree of scarring depends on the location and size of the treated area. This method should be used only by doctors who are specially trained in this type of surgery.

Cryosurgery

Extreme cold may be used to treat precancerous skin conditions, such as actinic keratosis, as well as certain small skin cancers. In cryosurgery, liquid nitrogen is applied to the growth to freeze and kill the abnormal cells. After the area thaws, the dead tissue falls off. More than one freezing may be needed to remove the growth completely. Cryosurgery usually does not hurt, but patients may have pain and swelling after the area thaws. A white scar may form in the treated area.

Laser Therapy

Laser therapy uses a narrow beam of light to remove or destroy cancer cells. This approach is sometimes used for cancers that involve only the outer layer of skin.

Grafting

Sometimes, especially when a large cancer is removed, a skin graft is needed to close the wound and reduce the amount of scarring. For this procedure, the doctor takes a piece of healthy skin from another part of the body to replace the skin that was removed.

Radiation

Skin cancer responds well to radiation therapy (also called radiotherapy), which uses high-energy rays to damage cancer cells and stop them from growing. Doctors often use this treatment for cancers that occur in areas that are hard to treat with surgery. For example, radiation therapy might be used for cancers of the eyelid, the tip of the nose, or the ear. Several treatments may be needed to destroy all of the cancer cells. Radiation therapy may cause a rash or make the skin in the area dry or red. Changes in skin color and/or texture may develop after the treatment is over and may become more noticeable many years later.

Topical Chemotherapy

Topical chemotherapy is the use of anticancer drugs in a cream or lotion applied to the skin. Actinic keratosis can be treated effectively with the anticancer drug fluorouracil (also called 5-FU). This treatment is also useful for cancers limited to the top layer of skin. The 5-FU is applied daily for several weeks. Intense inflammation is common during treatment, but scars usually do not occur.

Clinical Trials

In clinical trials (research studies with cancer patients), doctors are studying new treatments for skin cancer. For example, they are exploring photodynamic therapy, a treatment that destroys cancer cells with a combination of laser light and drugs that make the cells sensitive to light. Biological therapy (also called immunotherapy) is a form of treatment to improve the body's natural ability to fight cancer. Interferon and tumor necrosis factor are types of biological therapy under study for skin cancer.

Follow-Up Care

Even though most skin cancers are cured, the disease can recur in the same place. Also, people who have been treated for skin cancer have a higher-than-average risk of developing a new cancer elsewhere on the skin. That's why it is so important for them to continue to examine themselves regularly, to visit their doctor for regular checkups, and to follow the doctor's instructions on how to reduce the risk of developing skin cancer again.

Questions to Ask the Doctor

Skin cancer has a better prognosis, or outcome, than most other types of cancer. Although skin cancer is the most common type of cancer in this country, it accounts for much less than 1 percent of all cancer deaths. It is cured in 85 to 95 percent of all cases. Still, any diagnosis of cancer can be frightening, and it's natural to have concerns about medical tests, treatments, and doctors' bills.

Patients have many important questions to ask about cancer, and their doctor is the best person to provide answers. Most people want to know exactly what kind of cancer they have, how it can be treated, and how successful the treatment is likely to be. The following are some other questions that patients might want to ask their doctor:

- What types of treatment are available?
- Are there any risks or side effects of treatment?
- Will there be a scar?
- Will I have to change my normal activities?
- How can I protect myself from getting skin cancer again?
- How often will I need a checkup?

Some patients become concerned that treatment may change their appearance, especially if the skin cancer is on their face. Patients should discuss this important concern with their doctor. And they may want to have a second opinion before treatment.

Skin Cancer Research

Scientists at hospitals and research centers are studying the causes of skin cancer and looking for new ways to prevent the disease. They are also exploring ways to improve treatment.

When laboratory research shows that a new prevention or treatment method has promise, doctors use it with people in clinical trials. These trials are designed to answer scientific questions and to find out whether the new approach is both safe and effective. People who take part in clinical trials make an important contribution to medical science and may have the first chance to benefit from improved methods.

People interested in taking part in a trial should discuss this option with their doctor.

How to Do a Skin Self-Exam

You can improve your chances of finding skin cancer promptly by performing a simple skin self-exam regularly.

The best time to do this self-exam is after a shower or bath. You should check your skin in a well-lighted room using a full-length mirror and a handheld mirror. It's best to begin by learning where your birthmarks, moles, and blemishes are and what they usually look like. Check for anything new—a change in the size, texture, or color of a mole, or a sore that does not heal.

Check **all** areas, including the back, the scalp, between the buttocks, and the genital area.

1. Look at the front and back of your body in the mirror, then raise your arms and look at the left and right sides.

2. Bend your elbows and look carefully at your palms; forearms, including the undersides; and the upper arms.

3. Examine the back and front of your legs. Also look between your buttocks and around your genital area.

4. Sit and closely examine your feet, including the soles and the spaces between the toes.

5. Look at your face, neck, and scalp. You may want to use a comb or a blow dryer to move hair so that you can see better.

By checking your skin regularly, you will become familiar with what is normal. If you find anything unusual, see your doctor right away. Remember, the earlier skin cancer is found, the better the chance for cure.

Chapter 33

Nonmelanoma Skin Cancer

Chapter Contents

Section 33.1

Basal Cell Carcinoma

"Basal Cell Carcinoma: The Most Common Skin Cancer" is reprinted with permission from The Skin Cancer Foundation, NY, NY, www.skincancer.org.

Basal cell carcinoma (BCC) is the most common form of skin cancer, affecting more than 800,000 Americans each year. In fact, it is the most common of all cancers. More than one out of every three new cancers are skin cancers, and the vast majority are BCCs. These cancers arise in the basal cells, which are at the bottom of the epidermis (outer skin layer).

The Major Cause

Chronic exposure to sunlight is the cause of almost all BCCs, which occur most frequently on exposed parts of the body—the face, ears, neck, scalp, shoulders, and back. On rare occasions, however, tumors develop on unexposed areas. In a few cases, contact with arsenic, exposure to radiation, open sores that resist healing, chronic inflammatory skin conditions, and complications of burns, scars, infections, vaccinations, or even tattoos are contributing factors.

Who Gets It?

Anyone with a history of sun exposure can develop BCC. However, people who are at highest risk have fair skin, blond or red hair, and blue, green, or grey eyes. Those most often affected are older people, but as the number of new cases has increased sharply each year in the last few decades, the average age of onset of the disease has steadily decreased. The disease is rarely seen in children, but occasionally a teenager is affected. Dermatologists report that more and more people in their twenties and thirties are being treated for this skin cancer.

Men with BCC have outnumbered women with the disease, but more women are getting BCCs than in the past. Workers in occupations that require long hours outdoors and people who spend their leisure time in the sun are particularly susceptible. Geographic location is also a factor: The closer to the equator, the higher the number of cases, particularly among fair-skinned individuals.

What to Look For

The five most typical characteristics of BCC include:

- An open sore that bleeds, oozes, or crusts and remains open for three or more weeks. A persistent non-healing sore is a very common sign of an early BCC.
- A reddish patch or irritated area, frequently occurring on the chest, shoulders, arms, or legs. Sometimes the patch crusts. It may also itch or hurt. At other times, it persists with no noticeable discomfort.
- A pink growth with a slightly elevated rolled border and a crusted indentation in the center. As the growth slowly enlarges, tiny blood vessels may develop on the surface.
- A shiny bump, or nodule, that is pearly or translucent and is often pink, red, or white. The bump can also be tan, black, or brown, especially in dark-haired people, and can be confused with a mole.
- A scar-like area that is white, yellow or waxy, and often has poorly defined borders; the skin itself appears shiny and taut. This warning sign can indicate the presence of an aggressive tumor.

Frequently, two or more features are present in one tumor. In addition, BCC sometimes resembles non-cancerous skin conditions such as psoriasis or eczema. Only a trained physician, usually a specialist in diseases of the skin, can decide for sure.

Learn the signs of BCC, and examine your skin regularly—once a month, or even more often if you are at high risk. Be sure to include the scalp, backs of ears, neck, and other hard-to-see areas. If you observe any of the warning signs or some other worrisome change in your skin, consult your physician immediately.

The Skin Cancer Foundation advises people to have a total-body skin exam by a dermatologist at regular intervals. The physician will suggest the correct time frame for follow-up visits, depending on your specific risk factors, such as skin type and history of sun exposure.

Types of Treatment

After the physician's examination, the diagnosis of BCC is confirmed with a biopsy. In this procedure, a small piece of tissue is removed and examined in the laboratory under a microscope. If tumor cells are present, treatment—usually surgery—is required. Fortunately, there are several effective methods for eradicating BCC. Choice of treatment is based on the type, size, location, and depth of penetration of the tumor, as well as the patient's age and general health. Treatment can almost always be performed on an outpatient basis in the physician's office or at a clinic. With the various surgical techniques, a local anesthetic is commonly used. Pain or discomfort during the procedure is minimal, and pain afterward is rare.

Excisional Surgery

Using a scalpel, the physician removes the entire growth along with a surrounding border of normal skin as a safety margin. The surgical site is then closed with stitches, and the excised tissue is sent to the laboratory for microscopic examination to verify that all the malignant cells have been removed.

Curettage and Electrodesiccation

The cancerous growth is scraped off with a curette (a sharp, ring-shaped instrument). The heat produced by an electrocautery needle destroys residual tumor and controls bleeding. This technique may be repeated twice or more to ensure that all cancer cells are eliminated.

Cryosurgery

Tumor tissue is destroyed by freezing with liquid nitrogen, without the need for cutting or anesthesia. The growth becomes crusted and scabbed, and usually falls off within days. The procedure may be repeated to ensure total destruction of the malignant cells. Cryosurgery is effective for the most common tumors and is the treatment of choice for patients with bleeding disorders or an intolerance to anesthesia.

Radiation

X-ray beams are directed at the tumor. Total destruction generally requires several treatments a week for a few weeks. Radiation may be used for tumors that are hard to manage surgically and for elderly patients or others who are in poor health.

Mohs Micrographic Surgery

The physician removes the tumor with a curette or scalpel, and then removes very thin layers of the surrounding skin one layer at a time. Each layer is checked thoroughly under a microscope, and the procedure is repeated until the last layer viewed is cancer-free. This technique saves the greatest amount of healthy tissue and has the highest cure rate. It is frequently used for tumors that have recurred or are in hard-to-treat places such as the head, neck, hands, and feet.

Laser Surgery

The skin's outer layer and variable amounts of deeper skin are removed using a carbon dioxide or erbium YAG laser. Lasers give the doctor good control over the depth of tissue removed, and are sometimes used as a secondary therapy when other techniques are unsuccessful.

Photodynamic Therapy (PDT)

PDT can be especially useful when patients have multiple BCCs. Topical 5-aminolevulinic acid (5-ALA) is applied to the growths at the physician's office. The next day, the patient returns, and those medicated areas are activated by a strong light. This treatment selectively destroys BCCs while causing minimal damage to surrounding normal tissue.

Imiquimod

FDA-approved for the treatment of genital warts, this topical cream is used by some physicians to treat precancerous skin growths called actinic keratoses. In clinical trials, it has shown promise in treating superficial and thin BCCs, and it may soon become more widely available for this purpose. Imiquimod may be especially useful for BCCs in skin areas where other treatments might leave an unacceptable scar.

5-Fluorouracil (5-FU)

The most commonly used topical medication for actinic keratoses, it is also sometimes used for the treatment of superficial BCCs. Side effects may include redness, swelling, and crusting.

Not a Trivial Cancer

When removed promptly, BCCs are easily treated in their early stages. The larger the tumor has grown, however, the more extensive the treatment needed. Although this skin cancer seldom spreads, or metastasizes, to vital organs, it can damage surrounding tissues, sometimes causing considerable destruction and even the loss of an eye, ear, or nose. When small skin cancers are removed, the scars are usually cosmetically acceptable. If the tumors are very large, a skin graft or flap may be used to cover the defect.

Risk of Recurrence

People who have had one BCC are at risk of developing others over the years, either in the same area or elsewhere on the body. Therefore, regular visits to a dermatologist should become a routine part of health maintenance; and it is important at these visits to examine not only the site(s) previously treated, but the entire skin surface.

BCCs on the scalp and nose are especially troublesome, with recurrences typically taking place within the first two years following surgery.

Should a cancer recur, the physician may recommend a different type of treatment. Some methods, such as Mohs micrographic surgery, may be highly effective for recurrences.

Preventing Skin Cancer

While BCCs and other skin cancers are almost always curable when detected and treated early, the surest line of defense is to prevent them in the first place. Here are some sun safety habits that should be part of everyone's daily health care:

- Avoid unnecessary sun exposure, especially during the sun's peak hours (10 A.M. to 4 P.M.).
- Seek the shade.
- Cover up with clothing, including a broad-brimmed hat, long pants, a long-sleeved shirt, and UV-blocking sunglasses.
- Wear a broad-spectrum sunscreen with a sun protection factor (SPF) of 15 or higher.
- Avoid tanning parlors and artificial tanning devices.

- Examine your skin head to toe every month.
- Have a professional skin examination annually.

Section 33.2

Squamous Cell Carcinoma

Squamous cell carcinoma (SCC), the second most common skin cancer after basal cell carcinoma, afflicts more than 200,000 Americans each year. It arises from the epidermis and resembles the squamous cells that comprise most of the upper layers of skin. SCCs may occur on all areas of the body including the mucous membranes, but are most common in areas exposed to the sun.

Although SCCs usually remain confined to the epidermis for some time, they eventually penetrate the underlying tissues if not treated. When this happens, they can be disfiguring. In a small percentage of cases, they spread (metastasize) to distant tissues and organs and can become fatal. SCCs that metastasize most often arise on sites of chronic inflammatory skin conditions or on the mucous membranes or lips.

What Causes It?

Chronic exposure to sunlight causes most cases of SCC. That is why tumors appear most frequently on sun-exposed parts of the body: the face, neck, bald scalp, hands, shoulders, arms, and back. The rim of the ear and the lower lip are especially vulnerable to the development of these cancers.

SCCs may also occur where skin has suffered certain kinds of injury: burns, scars, infections, long-standing sores, and sites previously exposed to X-rays or certain chemicals (such as arsenic and petroleum by-products). In addition, chronic skin inflammation or medical conditions that suppress the immune system over an extended period of time may encourage development of SCC.

In some cases, SCC arises spontaneously on what appears to be normal, healthy, undamaged skin. Some researchers believe that a tendency to develop this cancer may sometimes be inherited.

Who Gets It?

Anyone with a substantial history of sun exposure can develop SCC. But people who have fair skin, light hair, and blue, green, or grey eyes are at highest risk. Those whose occupations require long hours outdoors or who spend extensive leisure time in the sun are in particular jeopardy.

More than two thirds of the skin cancers that individuals of African descent develop are SCCs, usually arising on the sites of preexisting inflammatory skin conditions or burn injuries. Although dark-skinned individuals of any background are less likely than fair-skinned individuals to develop skin cancer, it is still essential for them to practice sun protection.

Precancerous Conditions

Certain precursor conditions, some of which result from extensive sun damage, are worth noting. They are sometimes associated with the later development of SCC. They include the following:

Actinic, or Solar, Keratosis

Actinic keratoses are rough, scaly, slightly raised growths that range in color from brown to red and may be up to one inch in diameter. They appear most often in older people. Some experts believe that actinic keratosis is the earliest form of SCC.

Actinic cheilitis is a type of actinic keratosis occurring on the lips. It causes them to become dry, cracked, scaly, and pale or white. It mainly affects the lower lip, which typically receives more sun exposure than the upper lip.

Leukoplakia

These white patches or plaques on the tongue or inside of the mouth, arising in the mucous membranes, have the potential to develop into SCC. They are caused by sources of chronic irritation, including smoking or other tobacco use, and rough teeth or rough edges on dentures and fillings. Leukoplakia on the lips is mainly caused by sun damage.

Bowen Disease

This is generally considered to be a superficial SCC that has not yet spread. It appears as a persistent red-brown, scaly patch, which may resemble psoriasis or eczema. It untreated, it may invade deeper structures.

Regardless of appearance, any change in a preexisting skin growth, or the development of a new growth or open sore that fails to heal, should prompt an immediate visit to a physician. If it is a precursor condition, early treatment will prevent it from developing into SCC. Often, all that is needed is a simple surgical procedure or application of a topical chemotherapeutic agent.

What to Look For

SCCs occur most frequently on areas of the body that have been exposed to the sun for prolonged periods. Usually, the skin in these areas reveals telltale signs of sun damage, such as wrinkling, changes in pigmentation, and loss of elasticity.

- A persistent, scaly red patch with irregular borders that sometimes crusts or bleeds.
- An elevated growth with a central depression that occasionally bleeds. A growth of this type may rapidly increase in size.
- A wart-like growth that crusts and occasionally bleeds.
- An open sore that bleeds and crusts and persists for weeks.

These growths usually appear as thickened, rough scaly patches that can bleed if bumped. They often look like warts and sometimes appear as open sores with a raised border and a crusted surface over an elevated pebbly base.

Types of Treatment

After a physician's examination, a biopsy will be performed to confirm the diagnosis of SCC. This involves removing a piece of the affected tissue and examining it under a microscope. If tumor cells are present, treatment (usually surgery) is required.

Fortunately, there are several effective ways to eradicate SCC. The choice of treatment is based on the type, size, location, and depth of penetration of the tumor, as well as the patient's age and general state of health.

Treatment can almost always be performed on an outpatient basis in a physician's office or at a clinic. A local anesthetic is used during most procedures. Pain or discomfort is usually minimal with most techniques, and there is rarely much pain afterward.

Excisional Surgery

The physician uses a scalpel to remove the entire growth along with a surrounding border of apparently normal skin as a safety margin. The incision is then closed with sutures and the growth is sent to the laboratory, where it is examined microscopically to verify that all the malignant cells have been removed.

Curettage and Electrodesiccation

The physician scrapes off the growth with a sharp, ring-shaped instrument called a curette, then uses an electrocautery needle to burn the scraped area and a margin of normal skin around it to control bleeding. This two-step procedure may be repeated several times, a deeper layer of tissue being scraped and burned each time, until the physician determines that no tumor cells remain.

Cryosurgery

The physician applies liquid nitrogen to the growths with a cotton-tipped applicator or spray device. This freezes them without requiring any cutting or anesthesia. They subsequently shrink or become crusted or fall off. The procedure may be repeated several times at the same visit to ensure total destruction of malignant cells. Easy to administer, cryosurgery is favored for patients with bleeding disorders or intolerance to anesthesia. Redness, swelling, blistering, and crusting can occur following this treatment. In dark-skinned patients, some pigment may be lost.

Mohs Micrographic Surgery

The physician removes the tumor with a curette or scalpel and then removes very thin layers of the remaining surrounding skin one layer at a time. Each layer is checked under a microscope, and the procedure is repeated until the last layer viewed is cancer-free. This technique saves the greatest amount of healthy tissue and may reduce the rate of local recurrence. It is often used for tumors that have recurred or are in hard-to-treat places such as the head, neck, hands, and feet.

Radiation

A radiation therapist directs x-ray beams at the tumor. Total destruction generally requires several treatments a week for one to four weeks. Radiation therapy is ideal for tumors that are hard to manage surgically and for elderly patients or other individuals who are in poor overall health.

Laser Surgery

The skin's outer layer and variable amounts of deeper skin are removed using a carbon dioxide or erbium YAG laser. Lasers give the doctor good control over the depth of tissue removed, much like chemical peels. Lasers are also used as a secondary therapy when other techniques are unsuccessful. But the risks of scarring and pigment loss are slightly greater than with other techniques, and local anesthesia may be required. One advantage of this technique is that it seals blood vessels as it cuts, making it useful for patients with bleeding disorders.

Preventing Skin Cancer

While SCCs and other skin cancers are almost always curable when detected and treated early, the surest line of defense is to prevent them in the first place. Here are some sun safety habits that should be part of everyone's daily health care:

- Avoid unnecessary sun exposure, especially during the sun's peak hours (10 A.M. to 4 P.M.).
- Seek the shade.
- Cover up with clothing, including a broad-brimmed hat, long pants, a long-sleeved shirt, and UV-blocking sunglasses.
- Wear a broad-spectrum sunscreen with a sun protection factor (SPF) of 15 or higher.
- Avoid tanning parlors and artificial tanning devices.
- Examine your skin head to toe every month.
- Have a professional skin examination annually.

Chapter 34

Melanoma

Introduction

Melanoma is the most serious type of cancer of the skin. Each year in the United States, more than 53,600 people learn they have melanoma.

In some parts of the world, especially among Western countries, melanoma is becoming more common every year. In the United States, for example, the percentage of people who develop melanoma has more than doubled in the past 30 years.

Research continues to teach us more about melanoma. Scientists are learning more about its causes. They are exploring new ways to prevent, find, and treat this disease. Because of research, people with melanoma can look forward to a better quality of life and less chance of dying from this disease.

What Is Melanoma?

Melanoma is a type of skin cancer. It begins in cells in the skin called melanocytes. To understand melanoma, it is helpful to know about the skin and about melanocytes—what they do, how they grow, and what happens when they become cancerous.

Excerpted from "What You Need To Know About Melanoma," National Cancer Institute (NCI), March 31, 2003. Available online at http://www.cancer.gov; accessed May 4, 2005.

The Skin

The skin is the body's largest organ. It protects against heat, sunlight, injury, and infection. It helps regulate body temperature, stores water and fat, and produces vitamin D.

The skin has two main layers: the outer epidermis and the inner dermis.

- The epidermis is mostly made up of flat, scalelike cells called squamous cells. Round cells called basal cells lie under the squamous cells in the epidermis. The lower part of the epidermis also contains melanocytes.
- The dermis contains blood vessels, lymph vessels, hair follicles, and glands. Some of these glands produce sweat, which helps regulate body temperature. Other glands produce sebum, an oily substance that helps keep the skin from drying out. Sweat and sebum reach the skin's surface through tiny openings called pores.

Melanocytes and Moles

Melanocytes produce melanin, the pigment that gives skin its natural color. When skin is exposed to the sun, melanocytes produce more pigment, causing the skin to tan, or darken.

Sometimes, clusters of melanocytes and surrounding tissue form noncancerous growths called moles. (Doctors also call a mole a nevus; the plural is nevi.) Moles are very common. Most people have between 10 and 40 moles. Moles may be pink, tan, brown, or a color that is very close to the person's normal skin tone. People who have dark skin tend to have dark moles. Moles can be flat or raised. They are usually round or oval and smaller than a pencil eraser. They may be present at birth or may appear later on—usually before age 40. They tend to fade away in older people. When moles are surgically removed, they normally do not return.

Understanding Cancer

Cancer begins in cells, the building blocks that make up tissues. Tissues make up the organs of the body. Normally, cells grow and divide to form new cells as the body needs them. When cells grow old, they die, and new cells take their place.

Sometimes this orderly process goes wrong. New cells form when the body does not need them, and old cells do not die when they should.

These extra cells can form a mass of tissue called a growth or tumor. Not all tumors are cancer.

Tumors can be benign or malignant:

- Benign tumors are not cancer:
    - They are rarely life threatening.
    - Usually, benign tumors can be removed, and they seldom grow back.
    - Cells from benign tumors do not spread to tissues around them or to other parts of the body.
- Malignant tumors are cancer:
    - They are generally more serious and may be life threatening.
    - Malignant tumors usually can be removed, but they can grow back.
    - Cells from malignant tumors can invade and damage nearby tissues and organs. Also, cancer cells can break away from a malignant tumor and enter the bloodstream or lymphatic system. That is how cancer cells spread from the original cancer (the primary tumor) to form new tumors in other organs. The spread of cancer is called metastasis. Different types of cancer tend to spread to different parts of the body.

Melanoma

Melanoma occurs when melanocytes (pigment cells) become malignant. Most pigment cells are in the skin; when melanoma starts in the skin, the disease is called cutaneous melanoma. Melanoma may also occur in the eye (ocular melanoma or intraocular melanoma). Rarely, melanoma may arise in the meninges, the digestive tract, lymph nodes, or other areas where melanocytes are found.

Melanoma is one of the most common cancers. The chance of developing it increases with age, but this disease affects people of all ages. It can occur on any skin surface. In men, melanoma is often found on the trunk (the area between the shoulders and the hips) or the head and neck. In women, it often develops on the lower legs. Melanoma is rare in black people and others with dark skin. When it does develop in dark-skinned people, it tends to occur under the fingernails or toenails, or on the palms or soles.

When melanoma spreads, cancer cells may show up in nearby lymph nodes. Groups of lymph nodes are found throughout the body. Lymph nodes trap bacteria, cancer cells, or other harmful substances that may be in the lymphatic system. If the cancer has reached the lymph nodes, it may mean that cancer cells have spread to other parts of the body such as the liver, lungs, or brain. In such cases, the cancer cells in the new tumor are still melanoma cells, and the disease is called metastatic melanoma, not liver, lung, or brain cancer.

Melanoma: Who's at Risk?

No one knows the exact causes of melanoma. Doctors can seldom explain why one person gets melanoma and another does not.

However, research has shown that people with certain risk factors are more likely than others to develop melanoma. A risk factor is anything that increases a person's chance of developing a disease. Still, many who do get this disease have no known risk factors.

Studies have found the following risk factors for melanoma:

- **Dysplastic nevi:** Dysplastic nevi are more likely than ordinary moles to become cancerous. Dysplastic nevi are common, and many people have a few of these abnormal moles. The risk of melanoma is greatest for people who have a large number of dysplastic nevi. The risk is especially high for people with a family history of both dysplastic nevi and melanoma.
- **Many (more than 50) ordinary moles:** Having many moles increases the risk of developing melanoma.
- **Fair skin:** Melanoma occurs more frequently in people who have fair skin that burns or freckles easily (these people also usually have red or blond hair and blue eyes) than in people with dark skin. White people get melanoma far more often than do black people, probably because light skin is more easily damaged by the sun.
- **Personal history of melanoma or skin cancer:** People who have been treated for melanoma have a high risk of a second melanoma. Some people develop more than two melanomas. People who had one or more of the common skin cancers (basal cell carcinoma or squamous cell carcinoma) are at increased risk of melanoma.
- **Family history of melanoma:** Melanoma sometimes runs in families. Having two or more close relatives who have had this

disease is a risk factor. About 10 percent of all patients with melanoma have a family member with this disease. When melanoma runs in a family, all family members should be checked regularly by a doctor.

- **Weakened immune system:** People whose immune system is weakened by certain cancers, by drugs given following organ transplantation, or by HIV are at increased risk of developing melanoma.
- **Severe, blistering sunburns:** People who have had at least one severe, blistering sunburn as a child or teenager are at increased risk of melanoma. Because of this, doctors advise that parents protect children's skin from the sun. Such protection may reduce the risk of melanoma later in life. Sunburns in adulthood are also a risk factor for melanoma.
- **Ultraviolet (UV) radiation:** Experts believe that much of the worldwide increase in melanoma is related to an increase in the amount of time people spend in the sun. This disease is also more common in people who live in areas that get large amounts of UV radiation from the sun. In the United States, for example, melanoma is more common in Texas than in Minnesota, where the sun is not as strong. UV radiation from the sun causes premature aging of the skin and skin damage that can lead to melanoma. Artificial sources of UV radiation, such as sunlamps and tanning booths, also can cause skin damage and increase the risk of melanoma. Doctors encourage people to limit their exposure to natural UV radiation and to avoid artificial sources.

Doctors recommend that people take steps to help prevent and reduce the risk of melanoma caused by UV radiation:

- Avoid exposure to the midday sun (from 10 a.m. to 4 p.m.) whenever possible. When your shadow is shorter than you are, remember to protect yourself from the sun.
- If you must be outside, wear long sleeves, long pants, and a hat with a wide brim.
- Protect yourself from UV radiation that can penetrate light clothing, windshields, and windows.
- Protect yourself from UV radiation reflected by sand, water, snow, and ice.

- Help protect your skin by using a lotion, cream, or gel that contains sunscreen. Many doctors believe sunscreens may help prevent melanoma, especially sunscreens that reflect, absorb, and/or scatter both types of ultraviolet radiation. These sunscreen products will be labeled with "broad-spectrum coverage." Sunscreens are rated in strength according to a sun protection factor (SPF). The higher the SPF, the more sunburn protection is provided. Sunscreens with an SPF value of 2 to 11 provide minimal protection against sunburns. Sunscreens with an SPF of 12 to 29 provide moderate protection. Those with an SPF of 30 or higher provide the most protection against sunburn.
- Wear sunglasses that have UV-absorbing lenses. The label should specify that the lenses block at least 99 percent of UVA and UVB radiation. Sunglasses can protect both the eyes and the skin around the eyes.

People who are concerned about developing melanoma should talk with their doctor about the disease, the symptoms to watch for, and an appropriate schedule for checkups. The doctor's advice will be based on the person's personal and family history, medical history, and other risk factors.

Signs and Symptoms

Often, the first sign of melanoma is a change in the size, shape, color, or feel of an existing mole. Most melanomas have a black or blue-black area. Melanoma also may appear as a new mole. It may be black, abnormal, or "ugly looking."

If you have a question or concern about something on your skin, see your doctor. Do not use the following pictures to try to diagnose it yourself. Pictures are useful examples, but they cannot take the place of a doctor's examination.

Thinking of ABCD can help you remember what to watch for:

- **Asymmetry**—The shape of one half does not match the other.
- **Border**—The edges are often ragged, notched, blurred, or irregular in outline; the pigment may spread into the surrounding skin.
- **Color**—The color is uneven. Shades of black, brown, and tan may be present. Areas of white, grey, red, pink, or blue also may be seen.

- **Diameter**—There is a change in size, usually an increase. Melanomas are usually larger than the eraser of a pencil (1/4 inch or 5 millimeters).

Melanomas can vary greatly in how they look. Many show all of the ABCD features. However, some may show changes or abnormalities in only one or two of the ABCD features.

Melanomas in an early stage may be found when an existing mole changes slightly, for example, when a new black area forms. Newly formed fine scales and itching in a mole also are common symptoms of early melanoma. In more advanced melanoma, the texture of the mole may change. For example, it may become hard or lumpy. Melanomas may feel different from regular moles. More advanced tumors may itch, ooze, or bleed. But melanomas usually do not cause pain.

A skin examination is often part of a routine checkup by a health care provider. People also can check their own skin for new growths or other changes. Changes in the skin, such as a change in a mole, should be reported to the health care provider right away. The person may be referred to a dermatologist, a doctor who specializes in diseases of the skin.

Melanoma can be cured if it is diagnosed and treated when the tumor is thin and has not deeply invaded the skin. However, if a melanoma is not removed at its early stages, cancer cells may grow downward from the skin surface and invade healthy tissue. When a melanoma becomes thick and deep, the disease often spreads to other parts of the body and is difficult to control.

People who have had melanoma have a high risk of developing a new melanoma. People at risk for any reason should check their skin regularly and have regular skin exams by a health care provider.

Dysplastic Nevi

Some people have certain abnormal-looking moles (called dysplastic nevi or atypical moles) that are more likely than normal moles to develop into melanoma. Most people with dysplastic nevi have just a few of these abnormal moles; some people have many. People with dysplastic nevi and their health care provider should examine these moles regularly to watch for changes. Dysplastic nevi often look very much like melanoma. Doctors with special training in skin diseases are in the best position to decide whether an abnormal-looking mole should be closely watched or removed and checked for cancer.

In some families, many members have a large number of dysplastic nevi, and some have had melanoma. Members of these families have a very high risk of melanoma. Doctors often recommend that they have frequent checkups (every 3 to 6 months) so that any problems can be detected early. The doctor may take pictures of a person's skin to help show when changes occur.

Diagnosis

If the doctor suspects that a spot on the skin is melanoma, the patient will need to have a biopsy. A biopsy is the only way to make a definite diagnosis. In this procedure, the doctor tries to remove all of the suspicious-looking growth. This is an excisional biopsy. If the growth is too large to be removed entirely, the doctor removes a sample of the tissue. The doctor will never "shave off" or cauterize a growth that might be melanoma.

A biopsy can usually be done in the doctor's office using local anesthesia. A pathologist then examines the tissue under a microscope to check for cancer cells. Sometimes it is helpful for more than one pathologist to check the tissue for cancer cells.

Staging

If the diagnosis is melanoma, the doctor needs to learn the extent, or stage, of the disease before planning treatment. Staging is a careful attempt to learn how thick the tumor is, how deeply the melanoma has invaded the skin, and whether melanoma cells have spread to nearby lymph nodes or other parts of the body. The doctor may remove nearby lymph nodes to check for cancer cells. (Such surgery may be considered part of the treatment because removing cancerous lymph nodes may help control the disease.) The doctor also does a careful physical exam and, if the tumor is thick, may order chest x-rays, blood tests, and scans of the liver, bones, and brain.

Stages of Melanoma

The following stages are used for melanoma:

- Stage 0: In stage 0, the melanoma cells are found only in the outer layer of skin cells and have not invaded deeper tissues.
- Stage I: Melanoma in stage I is thin:
    - The tumor is no more than 1 millimeter (1/25 inch) thick. The outer layer (epidermis) of skin may appear scraped. (This is called an ulceration).

- Or, the tumor is between 1 and 2 millimeters (1/12 inch) thick. There is no ulceration.
- The melanoma cells have not spread to nearby lymph nodes.

- Stage II: The tumor is at least 1 millimeter thick:
  - The tumor is between 1 and 2 millimeters thick. There is ulceration.
  - Or, the thickness of the tumor is more than 2 millimeters. There may be ulceration.
  - The melanoma cells have not spread to nearby lymph nodes.
- Stage III: The melanoma cells have spread to nearby tissues:
  - The melanoma cells have spread to one or more nearby lymph nodes.
  - Or, the melanoma cells have spread to tissues just outside the original tumor but not to any lymph nodes.
- Stage IV: The melanoma cells have spread to other organs, to lymph nodes, or to skin areas far away from the original tumor.
- Recurrent: Recurrent disease means that the cancer has come back (recurred) after it has been treated. It may have come back in the original site or in another part of the body.

Treatment

The doctor can describe treatment choices and discuss the results expected with each treatment option. The doctor and patient can work together to develop a treatment plan that fits the patient's needs. Treatment for melanoma depends on the extent of the disease, the patient's age and general health, and other factors.

People with melanoma are often treated by a team of specialists. The team may include a dermatologist, surgeon, medical oncologist, radiation oncologist, and plastic surgeon.

Methods of Treatment

People with melanoma may have surgery, chemotherapy, biological therapy, or radiation therapy. Patients may have a combination of treatments.

At any stage of disease, people with melanoma may have treatment to control pain and other symptoms of the cancer, to relieve the side effects of therapy, and to ease emotional and practical problems. This kind of treatment is called symptom management, supportive care, or palliative care.

The doctor is the best person to describe the treatment choices and discuss the expected results.

A patient may want to talk to the doctor about taking part in a clinical trial, a research study of new treatment methods.

Surgery

Surgery is the usual treatment for melanoma. The surgeon removes the tumor and some normal tissue around it. This procedure reduces the chance that cancer cells will be left in the area. The width and depth of surrounding skin that needs to be removed depends on the thickness of the melanoma and how deeply it has invaded the skin:

- The doctor may be able to completely remove a very thin melanoma during the biopsy. Further surgery may not be necessary.
- If the melanoma was not completely removed during the biopsy, the doctor takes out the remaining tumor. In most cases, additional surgery is performed to remove normal-looking tissue around the tumor (called the margin) to make sure all melanoma cells are removed. This is often necessary, even for thin melanomas. If the melanoma is thick, the doctor may need to remove a larger margin of tissue.

If a large area of tissue is removed, the surgeon may do a skin graft. For this procedure, the doctor uses skin from another part of the body to replace the skin that was removed.

Lymph nodes near the tumor may be removed because cancer can spread through the lymphatic system. If the pathologist finds cancer cells in the lymph nodes, it may mean that the disease has also spread to other parts of the body. Two procedures are used to remove the lymph nodes:

- Sentinel lymph node biopsy—The sentinel lymph node biopsy is done after the biopsy of the melanoma but before the wider excision of the tumor. A radioactive substance is injected near the melanoma. The surgeon follows the movement of the substance on a computer screen. The first lymph node(s) to take up the substance is called the sentinel lymph node(s). (The imaging study is called lymphoscintigraphy. The procedure to identify the sentinel node(s) is called sentinel lymph node mapping.) The surgeon removes the sentinel node(s) to check for cancer cells. If a sentinel node contains cancer cells, the surgeon removes the rest of the lymph nodes in the area. However, if a sentinel node does not contain cancer cells, no additional lymph nodes are removed.

- Lymph node dissection—The surgeon removes all the lymph nodes in the area of the melanoma.

Therapy may be given after surgery to kill cancer cells that remain in the body. This treatment is called adjuvant therapy. The patient may receive biological therapy.

Surgery is generally not effective in controlling melanoma that has spread to other parts of the body. In such cases, doctors may use other methods of treatment, such as chemotherapy, biological therapy, radiation therapy, or a combination of these methods.

Chemotherapy

Chemotherapy, the use of drugs to kill cancer cells, is sometimes used to treat melanoma. The drugs are usually given in cycles: a treatment period followed by a recovery period, then another treatment period, and so on. Usually a patient has chemotherapy as an outpatient (at the hospital, at the doctor's office, or at home). However, depending on which drugs are given and the patient's general health, a short hospital stay may be needed.

People with melanoma may receive chemotherapy in one of the following ways:

- By mouth or injection—Either way, the drugs enter the bloodstream and travel throughout the body.
- Isolated limb perfusion (also called isolated arterial perfusion)—For melanoma on an arm or leg, chemotherapy drugs are put directly into the bloodstream of that limb. The flow of blood to and from the limb is stopped for a while. This allows most of the drug to reach the tumor directly. Most of the chemotherapy remains in that limb.

The drugs may be heated before injection. This type of chemotherapy is called hyperthermic perfusion.

Biological Therapy

Biological therapy (also called immunotherapy) is a form of treatment that uses the body's immune system, either directly or indirectly, to fight cancer or to reduce side effects caused by some cancer treatments. Biological therapy for melanoma uses substances called cytokines. The body normally produces cytokines in small amounts in response to infections and other diseases. Using modern laboratory techniques, scientists can produce cytokines in large amounts. In some cases, biological therapy given after surgery can help prevent melanoma from recurring. For patients with metastatic melanoma or a high risk of recurrence, interferon alpha and interleukin-2 (also called IL-2 or aldesleukin) may be recommended after surgery.

Radiation Therapy

Radiation therapy (also called radiotherapy) uses high-energy rays to kill cancer cells. A large machine directs radiation at the body. The patient usually has treatment at a hospital or clinic, five days a week for several weeks. Radiation therapy may be used to help control melanoma that has spread to the brain, bones, and other parts of the body. It may shrink the tumor and relieve symptoms.

Treatment Choices by Stage

The following are brief descriptions of the treatments most often used for each stage. (Other treatments may sometimes be appropriate.)

- Stage 0: People with Stage 0 melanoma may have minor surgery to remove the tumor and some of the surrounding tissue.
- Stage I: People with Stage I melanoma may have surgery to remove the tumor. The surgeon may also remove as much as 2 centimeters (3/4 inch) of tissue around the tumor. To cover the wound, the patient may have skin grafting.
- Stage II or Stage III: People with Stage II or Stage III melanoma may have surgery to remove the tumor. The surgeon may also remove as much as 3 centimeters (1 1/4 inches) of nearby tissue. Skin grafting may be done to cover the wound. Sometimes the surgeon removes nearby lymph nodes.
- Stage IV: People with Stage IV melanoma often receive palliative care. The goal of palliative care is to help the patient feel

better—physically and emotionally. This type of treatment is intended to control pain and other symptoms and to relieve the side effects of therapy (such as nausea), rather than to extend life. The patient may have one of the following: surgery to remove lymph nodes that contain cancer cells or to remove tumors that have spread to other areas of the body and radiation therapy, biological therapy, or chemotherapy to relieve symptoms.

- Recurrent Melanoma: Treatment for recurrent melanoma depends on where the cancer came back, which treatments the patient has already received, and other factors. As with Stage IV melanoma, treatment usually cannot cure melanoma that recurs. Palliative care is often an important part of the treatment plan. Many patients have palliative care to ease their symptoms while they are getting anticancer treatments to slow the progress of the disease. Some receive only palliative care to improve their quality of life by easing pain, nausea, and other symptoms. The patient may have one of the following:
  - Surgery to remove the tumor
  - Radiation therapy, biological therapy, or chemotherapy to relieve symptoms
  - Heated chemotherapy drugs injected directly into the tumor

Followup Care

Melanoma patients have a high risk of developing new melanomas. Some also are at risk of a recurrence of the original melanoma in nearby skin or in other parts of the body.

To increase the chance of detecting a new or recurrent melanoma as early as possible, patients should follow their doctor's schedule for regular checkups. It is especially important for patients who have dysplastic nevi and a family history of melanoma to have frequent checkups. Patients also should examine their skin monthly. They should follow their doctor's advice about how to reduce their chance of developing another melanoma.

The chance of recurrence is greater for patients whose melanoma was thick or had spread to nearby tissue than for patients with very thin melanomas. Followup care for those who have a high risk of recurrence may include x-rays, blood tests, and scans of the chest, liver, bones, and brain.

The Promise of Cancer Research

Doctors all over the country are conducting many types of clinical trials. These are research studies in which people take part voluntarily. Studies include new ways to treat melanomas. Research already has led to advances, and researchers continue to search for more effective approaches.

Patients who join these studies have the first chance to benefit from treatments that have shown promise in earlier research. They also make an important contribution to medical science by helping doctors learn more about the disease. Although clinical trials may pose some risks, researchers take very careful steps to protect their patients.

Researchers are testing new anticancer drugs. They are looking at combining chemotherapy with radiation therapy. Other studies are combining chemotherapy with biological therapy. Scientists also are studying several cancer vaccines and a type of gene therapy designed to help the immune system kill cancer cells.

Patients who are interested in being part of a clinical trial should talk with their doctor. The National Cancer Institute's (NCI) website includes a section on clinical trials at http://cancer.gov/clinical_trials. This section of the website provides general information about clinical trials.

It also offers detailed information about ongoing studies of melanoma treatment by linking to PDQ®, a cancer information database developed by the NCI. The Cancer Information Service at (800) 4-CANCER can answer questions and provide information from the database.

How to Do a Skin Self-Exam

Your doctor or nurse may recommend that you do a regular skin self-exam. If your doctor has taken photos of your skin, comparing your skin to the photos can help you check for changes.

The best time to do a skin self-exam is after a shower or bath. You should check your skin in a well-lighted room using a full-length mirror and a hand-held mirror. It's best to begin by learning where your birthmarks, moles, and blemishes are and what they usually look and feel like.

Check for anything new:

- A new mole (that looks abnormal)

- A change in the size, shape, color, or texture of a mole
- A sore that does not heal

Check yourself from head to toe. Don't forget to check all areas of the skin, including the back, the scalp, between the buttocks, and the genital area.

1. Look at your face, neck, ears, and scalp. You may want to use a comb or a blow dryer to move your hair so that you can see better. You also may want to have a relative or friend check through your hair because this is difficult to do yourself.
2. Look at the front and back of your body in the mirror, then raise your arms and look at your left and right sides.
3. Bend your elbows and look carefully at your fingernails, palms, forearms (including the undersides), and upper arms.
4. Examine the back, front, and sides of your legs. Also look between your buttocks and around your genital area.
5. Sit and closely examine your feet, including the toenails, the soles, and the spaces between the toes.

By checking your skin regularly, you will become familiar with what is normal for you. It may be helpful to record the dates of your skin exams and to write notes about the way your skin looks. If you find anything unusual, see your doctor right away.

Chapter 35

Mycosis Fungoides and the Sézary Syndrome

Introduction

Mycosis fungoides and the Sézary syndrome are diseases in which lymphocytes (a type of white blood cell) become malignant (cancerous) and affect the skin.

Lymphocytes are made in the bone marrow and fight infection and disease. There are three types of lymphocytes:

- **B-cell lymphocytes** that make antibodies to help fight infection.
- **T-cell lymphocytes** that help B-lymphocytes make the antibodies that help fight infection.
- **Natural killer cells** that attack cancer cells and viruses.

In mycosis fungoides, T-cell lymphocytes become cancerous and affect the skin. In the Sézary syndrome, cancerous T-cell lymphocytes affect the skin and the peripheral blood.

Excerpted from the PDQ® Cancer Information Summary. National Cancer Institute; Bethesda, MD. Mycosis Fungoides and the Sézary Syndrome (PDQ®): Treatment—Patient. Updated 04/2005. Available at: http://cancer.gov. Accessed June 9, 2005.

Mycosis fungoides and the Sézary syndrome are types of cutaneous T-cell lymphoma.

This chapter describes the two most common types of cutaneous T-cell lymphomas: mycosis fungoides and the Sézary syndrome.

A possible sign of mycosis fungoides and the Sézary syndrome is a red rash on the skin.

Mycosis fungoides and the Sézary syndrome may move through the following phases:

- **Premycotic phase:** A scaly, red rash in areas of the body that usually are not exposed to the sun. This rash does not cause symptoms and may last for months or years. It is hard to diagnose the rash as mycosis fungoides during this phase.
- **Patch phase:** Thin, reddened, eczema-like rash.
- **Plaque phase:** Thickened, red patches or reddened skin.
- **Tumor phase:** Tumors form on the skin. These tumors may develop ulcers and the skin may get infected.

Sézary syndrome is an advanced form of mycosis fungoides.

In the Sézary syndrome, skin all over the body is reddened, itchy, peeling, and painful. There may also be patches, plaques, or tumors on the skin. Cancerous T-cells are found in the blood. Mycosis fungoides does not always progress to the Sézary syndrome.

Certain factors affect prognosis (chance of recovery) and treatment options.

The prognosis (chance of recovery) and treatment options depend on the following:

- The stage of the cancer (the amount of skin affected and whether cancer has spread to the lymph nodes, the blood, or other places in the body).
- The type of lesion (patches, plaques, or tumors).
- The number of cutaneous T-cell lymphocytes in the blood.

Mycosis fungoides and the Sézary syndrome are difficult to cure. Treatment is usually palliative, to relieve symptoms and improve the quality of life. Patients can live many years with this disease.

Stages of Mycosis Fungoides and the Sézary Syndrome

After mycosis fungoides and the Sézary syndrome have been diagnosed, tests are done to find out if cancer cells have spread from the skin to other parts of the body.

The process used to find out if cancer has spread from the skin to other parts of the body is called staging. The information gathered from the staging process determines the stage of the disease. It is important to know the stage in order to plan treatment. The following procedures may be used in the staging process:

- **Chest x-ray:** An x-ray of the organs and bones inside the chest. An x-ray is a type of energy beam that can go through the body and onto film, making a picture of areas inside the body.
- **CT scan (CAT scan):** A procedure that makes a series of detailed pictures of areas inside the body, such as the lymph nodes, chest, abdomen, and pelvis, taken from different angles. The pictures are made by a computer linked to an x-ray machine. A dye may be injected into a vein or swallowed to help the organs or tissues show up more clearly. This procedure is also called computed tomography, computerized tomography, or computerized axial tomography.
- **MRI (magnetic resonance imaging):** A procedure that uses a magnet, radio waves, and a computer to make a series of detailed pictures of areas inside the body, such as the lymph nodes, chest, abdomen, and pelvis. This procedure is also called nuclear magnetic resonance imaging (NMRI).
- **Lymph node biopsy:** The removal of all or part of a lymph node. A pathologist views the tissue under a microscope to look for cancer cells.

Recurrent Mycosis Fungoides and the Sézary Syndrome

Recurrent mycosis fungoides and the Sézary syndrome are cancers that have recurred (come back) after they have been treated. The cancer may come back in the skin or in other parts of the body.

Treatment Option Overview

There are different types of treatment for patients with mycosis fungoides and the Sézary syndrome cancer.

Different types of treatment are available for patients with mycosis fungoides and the Sézary syndrome. Some treatments are standard (the currently used treatment), and some are being tested in clinical trials. Before starting treatment, patients may want to think about taking part in a clinical trial. A treatment clinical trial is a research study meant to help improve current treatments or obtain information on new treatments for patients with cancer. When clinical trials show that a new treatment is better than the standard treatment, the new treatment may become the standard treatment.

Clinical trials are taking place in many parts of the country. Information about ongoing clinical trials is available from the National Cancer Institute website. Choosing the most appropriate cancer treatment is a decision that ideally involves the patient, family, and health care team.

Five types of standard treatment are used:

Photodynamic therapy: Photodynamic therapy is a cancer treatment that uses a drug and a certain type of laser light to kill cancer cells. A drug that is not active until it is exposed to light is injected into a vein. The drug collects more in cancer cells than in normal cells. Fiberoptic tubes are then used to deliver the laser light to the cancer cells, where the drug becomes active and kills the cells. Photodynamic therapy causes little damage to healthy tissue. It is used mainly to treat tumors on or just under the skin or in the lining of internal organs, such as the lungs and the esophagus. Patients undergoing photodynamic therapy will need to limit the amount of time spent in sunlight.

In one type of photodynamic therapy, called psoralen and ultraviolet A (PUVA) therapy, the patient receives a drug called psoralen and then ultraviolet radiation is directed to the skin. In another type of photodynamic therapy, called extracorporeal photochemotherapy, the patient is given drugs and then some blood cells are taken from the body, put under a special ultraviolet A light, and put back into the body.

Radiation therapy: Radiation therapy is a cancer treatment that uses high-energy x-rays or other types of radiation to kill cancer cells.

There are two types of radiation therapy. External radiation therapy uses a machine outside the body to send radiation toward the cancer. Internal radiation therapy uses a radioactive substance sealed in needles, seeds, wires, or catheters that are placed directly into or near the cancer.

Sometimes, total skin electron beam (TSEB) radiation therapy is used to treat mycosis fungoides and the Sézary syndrome. In this type of radiation treatment, the skin over the whole body is treated with special rays of tiny particles called electrons.

The way the radiation therapy is given depends on the type and stage of the cancer being treated.

Chemotherapy: Chemotherapy is a cancer treatment that uses drugs to stop the growth of cancer cells, either by killing the cells or by stopping the cells from dividing. When chemotherapy is taken by mouth or injected into a vein or muscle, the drugs enter the bloodstream and can reach cancer cells throughout the body (systemic chemotherapy).

When chemotherapy is placed directly into the spinal column, an organ, or a body cavity such as the abdomen, the drugs mainly affect cancer cells in those areas (regional chemotherapy). Sometimes the chemotherapy is topical (applied to the skin in a cream or lotion.)

The way the chemotherapy is given depends on the type and stage of the cancer being treated.

Other drug therapy: Retinoids are drugs related to vitamin A that can slow the growth of certain types of cancer cells. The retinoids may be taken by mouth or applied to the skin.

Biologic therapy: Biologic therapy is a treatment that uses the patient's immune system to fight cancer. Substances made by the body or made in a laboratory are used to boost, direct, or restore the body's natural defenses against cancer. This type of cancer treatment is also called biotherapy or immunotherapy.

Specific types of biologic therapy used in treating mycosis fungoides and the Sézary syndrome include the following:

- *Monoclonal antibody therapy:* A cancer treatment that uses antibodies made in the laboratory, from a single type of immune system cell. These antibodies can identify substances on cancer cells or normal substances that may help cancer cells grow. The antibodies attach to the substances and kill the cancer cells, block their growth, or keep them from spreading. Monoclonal antibodies are given by infusion. They may be used alone or to carry drugs, toxins, or radioactive material directly to cancer cells.

- *Interferon alfa:* A substance that interferes with the division of cancer cells and can slow tumor growth.
- *Interleukin-2:* A substance that can improve the body's natural response to infection and disease.

Other types of treatment are being tested in clinical trials. These include the following:

High-dose chemotherapy and radiation therapy with stem cell transplant: This treatment is a method of giving high doses of chemotherapy and radiation therapy and replacing blood-forming cells destroyed by the cancer treatment. Stem cells (immature blood cells) are removed from the bone marrow or blood of the patient or a donor and are frozen and stored. After therapy is completed, the stored stem cells are thawed and given back to the patient through an infusion. These reinfused stem cells grow into (and restore) the body's blood cells.

This chapter refers to specific treatments under study in clinical trials, but it may not mention every new treatment being studied. Information about ongoing clinical trials is available from the National Cancer Institute website (http://www.cancer.gov).

Chapter 36

Kaposi Sarcoma

What Is Kaposi Sarcoma?

Kaposi sarcoma (KS) is a disease in which cancer (malignant) cells are found in the tissues under the skin or mucous membranes that line the mouth, nose, and anus. KS causes red or purple patches (lesions) on the skin and/or mucous membranes and spreads to other organs in the body, such as the lungs, liver, or intestinal tract.

Until the early 1980s, Kaposi sarcoma was a very rare disease that was found mainly in older men, patients who had organ transplants, or African men. With the acquired immunodeficiency syndrome (AIDS) epidemic in the early 1980s, doctors began to notice more cases of Kaposi sarcoma in Africa and in gay men with AIDS. Kaposi sarcoma usually spreads more quickly in these patients.

If there are signs of KS, a doctor will examine the skin and lymph nodes carefully (lymph nodes are small bean-shaped structures that are found throughout the body; they produce and store infection-fighting cells). The doctor also may order other tests to see if the patient has other diseases.

The chance of recovery (prognosis) depends on what type of Kaposi sarcoma the patient has, the patient's age and general health, and whether the patient has AIDS.

Excerpted from the PDQ® Cancer Information Summary. National Cancer Institute; Bethesda, MD. Kaposi's Sarcoma (PDQ®): Treatment—Patient. Updated 06/2003. Available at: http://cancer.gov. Accessed June 1, 2005.

There is no accepted staging system for Kaposi sarcoma. Patients are grouped depending on which type of Kaposi sarcoma they have.

There are three types of Kaposi sarcoma:

Classic

Classic Kaposi sarcoma usually occurs in older men of Jewish, Italian, or Mediterranean heritage. This type of Kaposi sarcoma progresses slowly, sometimes over 10 to 15 years. As the disease gets worse, the lower legs may swell and the blood may not be able to flow properly. After some time, the disease may spread to other organs. Many patients with classic Kaposi sarcoma may develop another type of cancer later on in their lives.

Immunosuppressive Treatment Related

Kaposi sarcoma may occur in people who are taking drugs to make their immune systems weaker (immunosuppressants). The immune system helps the body fight off infection. People who have had an organ transplant (such as a liver or kidney transplant) have to take drugs to prevent their immune system from attacking the new organ.

Epidemic

Kaposi sarcoma in patients who have acquired immunodeficiency syndrome (AIDS) is called epidemic Kaposi sarcoma. AIDS is caused by a virus called the human immunodeficiency virus (HIV), which attacks and weakens the immune system. Infections and other diseases can then invade the body, and the immune system cannot fight against them. Kaposi sarcoma in people with AIDS usually spreads more quickly than other kinds of Kaposi sarcoma and often is found in many parts of the body.

Recurrent

Recurrent disease means that the KS has come back (recurred) after it has been treated. It may come back in the area where it first started or in another part of the body.

How Kaposi Sarcoma Is Treated

There are treatments for all patients with Kaposi sarcoma. Four kinds of treatment are used:

- Radiation therapy (using high-dose x-rays to kill cancer cells).
- Surgery (taking out the cancer).
- Chemotherapy (using drugs to kill cancer cells).
- Biological therapy (using the body's immune system to fight cancer).

Radiation therapy is a common treatment of Kaposi sarcoma. Radiation therapy uses high-dose x-rays or other high-energy rays to kill cancer cells and shrink tumors. Radiation for Kaposi sarcoma comes from a machine outside the body (external beam radiation therapy).

Surgery means taking out the cancer. A doctor may remove the cancer using one of the following:

- Local excision cuts out the lesion and some of the tissue around it.
- Electrodesiccation and curettage burns the lesion and removes it with a sharp instrument.
- Cryotherapy freezes the tumor and kills it.

Chemotherapy uses drugs to kill cancer cells. Chemotherapy may be taken by pill, or it may be put into the body by a needle in a vein or muscle. Chemotherapy is called a systemic treatment because the drug enters the bloodstream, travels through the body, and can kill cancer cells outside the original site. Chemotherapy for Kaposi sarcoma also may be injected into the lesion (intralesional chemotherapy).

Biological therapy tries to get the body to fight the cancer. It uses materials made by the body or made in a laboratory to boost, direct, or restore the body's natural defenses against disease. Biological therapy is sometimes called biological response modifier (BRM) therapy or immunotherapy.

Treatment by Stage

Treatment of Kaposi sarcoma depends on the type of Kaposi sarcoma the patient has, and the patient's age and general health. Standard treatment may be considered because of its effectiveness in patients in past studies, or participation in a clinical trial may be considered. Not all patients are cured with standard therapy and some standard treatments may have more side effects than are desired. For these reasons, clinical trials are designed to find better ways to treat cancer patients and are based on the most up-to-date information. Clinical trials are ongoing in most parts of the country for most stages of Kaposi sarcoma. To learn more about clinical trials, call the Cancer Information Service at (800) 4-CANCER (800-422-6237) or visit the National Cancer Institute website at http://cancer.gov.

Chapter 37

Merkel Cell Carcinoma

What Is Merkel Cell Carcinoma?

Merkel cell carcinoma, also called neuroendocrine cancer of the skin, is a rare type of disease in which malignant (cancer) cells are found on or just beneath the skin and in hair follicles. Merkel cell carcinoma usually appears as firm, painless, shiny lumps of skin. These lumps or tumors can be red, pink, or blue in color and vary in size from less than a quarter of an inch to more than two inches. Merkel cell carcinoma is usually found on the sun-exposed areas of the head, neck, arms, and legs. This type of cancer occurs mostly in whites between 60 and 80 years of age, but it can occur in people of other races and ages as well.

Merkel cell carcinoma grows rapidly and often metastasizes (spreads) to other parts of the body. Even relatively small tumors are capable of metastasizing. When the disease spreads, it tends to spread to the regional (nearby) lymph nodes and may also spread to the liver, bone, lungs, and brain. Lymph nodes are small, bean-shaped structures that are found throughout the body. They produce and store infection-fighting cells.

Treatment of Merkel cell carcinoma depends on the stage of the disease and the patient's age and overall condition.

Excerpted from the PDQ® Cancer Information Summary. National Cancer Institute; Bethesda, MD. Merkel Cell Carcinoma (PDQ®): Treatment—Patient. Updated 06/2003. Available at: http://cancer.gov. Accessed June 3, 2005.

Stages of Merkel Cell Carcinoma

After Merkel cell carcinoma has been diagnosed (found), more tests will be done to find out if cancer cells have spread from the place the cancer started to other parts of the body. The process used to find out whether the cancer has spread to other parts of the body is called staging. It is important to know the stage of the disease to plan the best treatment. The following stages are used for Merkel cell carcinoma:

Stage I

The primary tumor has not spread to lymph nodes or other parts of the body. Lymph nodes are small, bean-shaped structures that are found throughout the body. They produce and store infection-fighting cells.

Stage II

The cancer has spread to nearby lymph nodes, but has not spread to other parts of the body.

Stage III

The cancer has spread beyond nearby lymph nodes and to other parts of the body.

Recurrent

Recurrent disease means that the cancer has recurred (come back) after it has been treated. It may come back in the same part of the body or in another part of the body.

How Merkel Cell Carcinoma Is Treated

There are treatments for all patients with Merkel cell carcinoma. Three kinds of treatment are used:

- Surgery (taking out the cancer).
- Radiation therapy (using high-dose x-rays or other high-energy rays to kill cancer cells).
- Chemotherapy (using drugs to kill cancer cells).

There are several different types of surgery that may be used to remove the tumor. These include:

- Wide surgical excision takes out the cancer and some of the skin around the tumor.
- Cryosurgery freezes the tumor and then removes it.
- Micrographic surgery is a tissue-sparing technique that removes only the tumor.

Radiation therapy uses high-energy x-rays to kill cancer cells and shrink tumors. Radiation may come from a machine outside the body (external radiation therapy) or from putting materials that produce radiation (radioisotopes) through thin plastic tubes in the area where the cancer cells are found (internal radiation therapy).

Chemotherapy uses drugs to kill cancer cells. Chemotherapy may be taken by pill, or it may be put into the body by a needle in a vein or muscle. Chemotherapy is called a systemic treatment because the drugs enter the bloodstream, travel through the body, and can kill cancer cells throughout the body.

If a doctor removes all the cancer that can be seen at the time of the operation, a patient may be given chemotherapy after surgery to kill any cancer cells that are left. Chemotherapy given after an operation to a person who has no cancer cells that can be found is called adjuvant chemotherapy.

Chapter 38

The Effect of Cancer Treatment on the Skin, Hair, and Nails

Because cancer cells may grow and divide more rapidly than normal cells, many anticancer drugs are made to kill growing cells. But certain normal, healthy cells also multiply quickly, and chemotherapy can affect these cells, too. This damage to normal cells causes side effects. The fast-growing, normal cells most likely to be affected are blood cells forming in the bone marrow and cells in the digestive tract (mouth, stomach, intestines, esophagus), reproductive system (sexual organs), and hair follicles. Some anticancer drugs may affect cells of vital organs, such as the heart, kidney, bladder, lungs, and nervous system.

You may have none of these side effects or just a few. The kinds of side effects you have and how severe they are, depend on the type and dose of chemotherapy you get and how your body reacts. Before starting chemotherapy, your doctor will discuss the side effects that you are most likely to get with the drugs you will be receiving. Before starting the treatment, you will be asked to sign a consent form. You should be given all the facts about treatment including the drugs you will be given and their side effects before you sign the consent form.

How Long Do Side Effects Last?

Normal cells usually recover when chemotherapy is over, so most side effects gradually go away after treatment ends, and the healthy

---

Excerpted from "Chemotherapy and You: A Guide to Self-Help During Cancer Treatment," National Cancer Institute, updated: June 1999; reprinted: September 2003. Reviewed by David A. Cooke, M.D., on April 27, 2005.

cells have a chance to grow normally. The time it takes to get over side effects depends on many things, including your overall health and the kind of chemotherapy you have been taking.

Most people have no serious long-term problems from chemotherapy. However, on some occasions, chemotherapy can cause permanent changes or damage to the heart, lungs, nerves, kidneys, reproductive, or other organs. And certain types of chemotherapy may have delayed effects, such as a second cancer, that show up many years later. Ask your doctor about the chances of any serious, long-term effects that can result from the treatment you are receiving (but remember to balance your concerns with the immediate threat of your cancer).

Great progress has been made in preventing and treating some of chemotherapy's common as well as rare serious side effects. Many new drugs and treatment methods destroy cancer more effectively while doing less harm to the body's healthy cells.

The side effects of chemotherapy can be unpleasant, but they must be measured against the treatment's ability to destroy cancer. Medicines can help prevent some side effects such as nausea. Sometimes people receiving chemotherapy become discouraged about the length of time their treatment is taking or the side effects they are having. If that happens to you, talk to your doctor or nurse. They may be able to suggest ways to make side effects easier to deal with or reduce them.

Below you will find suggestions for dealing with some of the more common dermatological side effects of chemotherapy.

Hair Loss

Hair loss (alopecia) is a common side effect of chemotherapy, but not all drugs cause hair loss. Your doctor can tell you if hair loss might occur with the drug or drugs you are taking. When hair loss does occur, the hair may become thinner or fall out entirely. Hair loss can occur on all parts of the body, including the head, face, arms and legs, underarms, and pubic area. The hair usually grows back after the treatments are over. Some people even start to get their hair back while they are still having treatments. Sometimes, hair may grow back a different color or texture.

Hair loss does not always happen right away. It may begin several weeks after the first treatment or after a few treatments. Many people say their head becomes sensitive before losing hair. Hair may fall out gradually or in clumps. Any hair that is still growing may become dull and dry.

How Can I Care for My Scalp and Hair during Chemotherapy?

- Use a mild shampoo.
- Use a soft hairbrush.
- Use low heat when drying your hair.
- Have your hair cut short. A shorter style will make your hair look thicker and fuller. It also will make hair loss easier to manage if it occurs.
- Use a sunscreen, sun block, hat, or scarf to protect your scalp from the sun if you lose hair on your head.
- Avoid brush rollers to set your hair.
- Avoid dyeing, perming, or relaxing your hair.

Some people who lose all or most of their hair choose to wear turbans, scarves, caps, wigs, or hairpieces. Others leave their head uncovered. Still others switch back and forth, depending on whether they are in public or at home with friends and family members. There are no right or wrong choices; do whatever feels comfortable for you.

If you choose to cover your head:

- Get your wig or hairpiece before you lose a lot of hair. That way, you can match your current hairstyle and color. You may be able to buy a wig or hairpiece at a specialty shop just for cancer patients. Someone may even come to your home to help you. You also can buy a wig or hairpiece through a catalog or by phone.
- You may also consider borrowing a wig or hairpiece, rather than buying one. Check with the nurse or social work department at your hospital about resources for free wigs in your community.
- Take your wig to your hairdresser or the shop where it was purchased for styling and cutting to frame your face.
- Some health insurance policies cover the cost of a hairpiece needed because of cancer treatment. It is also a tax-deductible expense. Be sure to check your policy and ask your doctor for a "prescription."

Losing hair from your head, face, or body can be hard to accept. Feeling angry or depressed is common and perfectly all right. At the same time, keep in mind that it is a temporary side effect. Talking about your feelings can help. If possible, share your thoughts with someone who has had a similar experience.

Effects on Skin and Nails

You may have minor skin problems while you are having chemotherapy, such as redness, rashes, itching, peeling, dryness, acne, and increased sensitivity to the sun. Certain anticancer drugs, when given intravenously, may cause the skin all along the vein to darken, especially in people who have very dark skin. Some people use makeup to cover the area, but this can take a lot of time if several veins are affected. The darkened areas will fade a few months after treatment ends.

Your nails may also become darkened, yellow, brittle, or cracked. They also may develop vertical lines or bands.

While most of these problems are not serious and you can take care of them yourself, a few need immediate attention. Certain drugs given intravenously (IV) can cause serious and permanent tissue damage if they leak out of the vein. Tell your doctor or nurse right away if you feel any burning or pain when you are getting IV drugs. These symptoms do not always mean there is a problem, but they must always be checked at once. Don't hesitate to call your doctor about even the less serious symptoms.

Some symptoms may mean you are having an allergic reaction that may need to be treated at once. Call your doctor or nurse right away if:

- you develop sudden or severe itching.
- your skin breaks out in a rash or hives.
- you have wheezing or any other trouble breathing.

How Can I Cope with Skin and Nail Problems?

Acne

- Try to keep your face clean and dry.
- Ask your doctor or nurse if you can use over-the-counter medicated creams or soaps.

Itching and Dryness

- Apply cornstarch as you would a dusting powder.

- To help avoid dryness, take quick showers or sponge baths. Do not take long, hot baths. Use a moisturizing soap.
- Apply cream and lotion while your skin is still moist.
- Avoid perfume, cologne, or after-shave lotion that contains alcohol.
- Use a colloidal oatmeal bath or diphenhydramine for generalized pruritus.

Nail Problems

- You can buy nail-strengthening products in a drugstore. Be aware that these products may bother your skin and nails.
- Protect your nails by wearing gloves when washing dishes, gardening, or doing other work around the house.
- Be sure to let your doctor know if you have redness, pain, or changes around the cuticles.

Sunlight Sensitivity

- Avoid direct sunlight as much as possible, especially between 10 a.m. and 4 p.m. when the sun's rays are the strongest.
- Use a sunscreen lotion with a skin protection factor (SPF) of 15 or higher to protect against sun damage. A product such as zinc oxide, sold over the counter, can block the sun's rays completely.
- Use a lip balm with a sun protection factor.
- Wear long-sleeve cotton shirts, pants, and hats with a wide brim (particularly if you are having hair loss), to block the sun.
- Even people with dark skin need to protect themselves from the sun during chemotherapy.

Radiation Recall

Some people who have had radiation therapy develop "radiation recall" during their chemotherapy. During or shortly after certain anticancer drugs are given, the skin over an area that had received radiation turns red—a shade anywhere from light to very bright. The skin may blister and peel. This reaction may last hours or even days. Report radiation recall reactions to your doctor or nurse. You can soothe the itching and burning by:

- Placing a cool, wet compress over the affected area.
- Wearing soft, non-irritating fabrics. Women who have radiation for breast cancer following lumpectomy often find cotton bras the most comfortable.

Part Six

Skin Trauma, Ulcering, and Blistering Disorders

Chapter 39

Bites and Stings

Chapter Contents

Section 39.1

Human Bites

Definition

Human bites are usually caused by one person biting another, although they may result from a situation in which one person comes into contact with another person's teeth. In a fight, for example, one person's knuckles may come into contact with another person's teeth, and if the impact breaks the skin, the injury would be considered a bite.

Considerations

Human bites that break the skin, like all puncture wounds, have a high risk of infection. They also pose a risk of injury to tendons and joints.

Bites are very common among young children. Children often bite to express anger or other negative feelings.

Symptoms

Bites may produce symptoms ranging from mild to severe:

- Skin breaks with or without bleeding
- Puncture wounds
- Major cuts
- Crushing injuries

First Aid

1. Calm and reassure the person. Wash your hands thoroughly with soap.
2. If the bite is **not** bleeding severely, wash the wound with mild soap and running water for 3 to 5 minutes and then cover the bite with a clean dressing.

3. If the bite is actively bleeding, apply direct pressure with a clean, dry cloth until the bleeding subsides. Elevate the area.
4. Get medical attention.

Do Not

- **Do not** ignore any human bite, especially if it is bleeding.
- **Do not** put the wound into your mouth.

Call Immediately for Emergency Medical Assistance If

All human bites that break the skin should be promptly evaluated by a doctor. Bites may be especially serious when:

- There is swelling, redness, pus draining from the wound, or pain.
- The bite occurred near the eyes or involved the face, hands, wrists, or feet.
- The person who was bitten has a weakened immune system (for example, from HIV or receiving chemotherapy for cancer). The person is at a higher risk for the wound to become infected.

Prevention

- Teach young children not to bite others.
- NEVER put your hand near or in the mouth of someone who is having a seizure.

Section 39.2

Animal Bites

Each year millions of people in the United States—most of them children—are bitten by animals. Most animal bites are from dogs; cat bites are second most common. However, the risk of infection from a cat bite is much higher than that from a dog bite. Most bites occur on the fingers of the dominant hand, but children may also be bitten about the head and neck area.

A major concern about an animal bite is the possibility of rabies. Because most pets in the United States are vaccinated, most cases of rabies result from the bite of a wild animal such as a skunk, bat or raccoon. However, in other countries, dog bites are the most common source of rabies. If you are bitten by a dog outside the United States, consult a doctor immediately.

Signs and Symptoms

In some cases, the bite will not break the skin but may cause damage to underlying tendons and joints. If the skin is broken, there is the additional possibility of infection as well as injury to tendons and nerves. Dogs have powerful jaws and can cause crushing injuries to bone, muscles, tendons, ligaments and nerves.

Signs of an infection include:

- Warmth around the wound;
- Swelling;
- Pain;
- A pus discharge;
- Redness around the puncture wound.

Signs of damage to tendons or nerves include:

- An inability to bend or straighten the finger;
- A loss of sensation over the tip of the finger.

First Aid

1. Don't put the bitten area in your mouth! You will just be adding the bacteria in your mouth to that already in the wound.
2. If the wound is superficial, wash the area thoroughly. Use soap and water or an antiseptic such as hydrogen peroxide or alcohol. Apply an antibiotic ointment and cover with a non-stick bandage. Watch the area carefully to see if there are signs of damaged nerves or tendons. Some bruising may develop, but the wound should heal within a week to 10 days. If it does not, or if you see signs of infection or damage to nerves and tendons, seek medical help.
3. If there is bleeding, apply direct pressure with a clean dry cloth. Elevate the area. Do not clean a wound that is actively bleeding. Cover the wound with a clean sterile dressing and always seek medical help.
4. If the wound is to the face and/or head and neck area, seek medical help immediately.
5. Contact your physician to see whether additional treatment is needed.
6. Report the incident to your public health department. They may ask your assistance in locating the animal so that it can be confined and observed for symptoms of rabies.

Medical Assistance

Tell your doctor how you got the bite. Your physician will wash the wound area thoroughly and check for signs of nerve or tendon damage. The doctor may examine your arm to see if there are signs of a spreading infection. Your physician will probably leave the wound open (without stitches), unless you have a facial wound. You may need to get x-rays and a blood test. You may also need to get a tetanus shot and a prescription for antibiotics. If the tendons or nerves have been injured, you may need to see a specialist for additional treatment.

More about Rabies

Rabies is a disease that affects only mammals (such as raccoons, bats, dogs, horses, and humans). It is caused by a virus that attacks the nervous system. Without treatment, it is 100 percent fatal. Rabies develops in two stages. During the first stage, which can last up to 10 days, the individual may have a headache, fever, decreased appetite, vomiting and general malaise, along with pain, itching, and tingling at the wound site. Symptoms of stage two include difficulty in swallowing, agitation, disorientation, paralysis, and coma. At this point, there is no known effective treatment.

If rabies is identified early, a series of highly effective vaccinations can be administered. That's why it's important to capture and observe the animal that bit you. If the animal cannot be captured, but must be killed, the head should be kept intact so the brain can be examined for signs of rabies.

Preventing Animal Bites

Follow these recommendations to prevent animal bites and rabies.

1. Do not try to separate fighting animals.
2. Avoid animals that appear sick or act strangely. Call animal control.
3. Leave animals, even pets or other animals you know, alone when they are eating or sleeping.
4. Keep pets on a leash when out in public.
5. Never leave a young child alone with a pet. Don't allow children to tease an animal by waving sticks, throwing stones, or pulling a tail.
6. Be sure your pet is vaccinated.
7. Do not approach or play with any kind of wild animal. Teach children not to pet strange animals, even pets on a leash, without asking permission of the owner first.

Section 39.3

Insect Stings

Most people are not allergic to insect stings and should recognize the difference between an allergic reaction and a normal reaction. This will reduce anxiety and prevent unnecessary medical expense.

More than 500,000 people enter hospital emergency rooms every year suffering from insect stings. A severe allergic reaction known as anaphylaxis occurs in 0.5 percent to 5 percent of the U.S. population as a result of insect stings. At least 40 deaths per year result from insect sting anaphylaxis.

The majority of insect stings in the United States come from wasps, yellow jackets, hornets, and bees. The red or black imported fire ant now infests more than 260 million acres in the southern United States, where it has become a significant health hazard and may be the number one agent of insect stings.

What is a normal reaction to an insect sting and how is it treated?

The severity of an insect sting reaction varies from person to person. A normal reaction will result in pain, swelling, and redness confined to the sting site. Simply disinfect the area (washing with soap and water will do) and apply ice to reduce the swelling.

A large local reaction will result in swelling that extends beyond the sting site. For example, a sting on the forearm could result in the entire arm swelling to twice its normal size. Although alarming in appearance, this condition is often treated the same as a normal reaction. An unusually painful or very large local reaction may need medical attention. Because this condition may persist for two to three days, antihistamines and corticosteroids are sometimes prescribed to lessen the discomfort.

Fire ants, yellow jackets, hornets, and wasps can sting repeatedly. Honeybees have barbed stingers that are left behind in their victim's skin. These stingers are best removed by a scraping action, rather than a pulling motion, which may actually squeeze more venom into the skin.

Almost all people stung by fire ants develop an itchy, localized hive or lump at the sting site, which usually subsides within 30 to 60 minutes. This is followed by a small blister within four hours. This usually appears to become filled with pus by 8 to 24 hours. However, the material seen is really dead tissue and the blister has little chance of being infected unless it is opened. When healed, these lesions may leave scars.

Treatment for fire ant stings is aimed at preventing secondary bacterial infection, which may occur if the pustule is scratched or broken. Clean the blisters with soap and water to prevent secondary infection. Do not break the blister. Topical corticosteroid ointments and oral antihistamines may relieve the itching associated with these reactions.

What are symptoms of insect sting allergy?

The most serious reaction to an insect sting is an allergic one. This condition requires immediate medical attention. Symptoms of an allergic reaction may include one or more of the following:

- Hives, itching, and swelling in areas other than the sting site.
- Tightness in the chest and difficulty in breathing.
- Hoarse voice or swelling of the tongue.

An even more severe allergic reaction, or anaphylaxis, can occur within minutes after the sting and may be life threatening. Symptoms may include:

- Dizziness or a sharp drop in blood pressure.
- Unconsciousness or cardiac arrest.

People who have experienced an allergic reaction to an insect sting have a 60 percent chance of a similar or worse reaction if stung again.

How are allergic reactions to insect stings treated?

Insect sting allergy is treated in a two-step approach. The first step is the emergency treatment of the symptoms of a serious reaction; the second step is preventive treatment of the underlying allergy with venom immunotherapy.

Life-threatening allergic reactions can progress very rapidly and require immediate medical attention. Emergency treatment usually includes administration of certain drugs, such as epinephrine, antihistamines, and in some cases, corticosteroids, intravenous fluids, oxygen, and other treatments. Once stabilized, these patients are sometimes required to stay overnight at the hospital under close observation.

Injectable epinephrine for self-administration is often prescribed as emergency rescue medication for treating an allergic reaction. People who have had previous allergic reactions and rely on epinephrine must remember to carry it with them at all times. Also, because one dose may not be enough to reverse the reaction, immediate medical attention following an insect sting is recommended.

What is venom immunotherapy?

The long-term treatment of insect sting allergy is called venom immunotherapy, a highly effective program administered by an allergist-immunologist, which can prevent future allergic reactions to insect stings.

Venom immunotherapy involves administering gradually increasing doses of venom, which stimulate the patient's own immune system to reduce the risk of a future allergic reaction to the same as the general population. In a matter of weeks to months, people who previously lived under the constant threat of severe reactions to insect stings can return to leading normal lives.

Ask your doctor to send a consult to an allergist-immunologist, a physician who is a specialist in the diagnosis and treatment of allergic disease. Based on your past history and certain tests, the allergist will determine if you are a candidate for skin testing and immunotherapy.

How can I avoid insect stings?

Knowing how to avoid stings from fire ants, bees, wasps, hornets, and yellow jackets leads to a more enjoyable summer for everyone. Stinging insects are most active during the summer and early fall, when nest populations can exceed 60,000 insects. Insect repellents do not work against stinging insects.

Yellow jackets will nest in the ground and in walls. Hornets and wasps will nest in bushes, trees, and on buildings. Use extreme caution when working or playing in these areas. Avoid open garbage cans and exposed food at picnics. Also, try to reduce the amount of exposed skin when outdoors.

Effective methods for insecticide treatment of fire ant mounds use attractant baits consisting of soybean oil, corn grits, or chemical agents. The bait is picked up by the worker ants and taken deeper into the mound to the queen. It can take weeks for these insecticides to work.

Allergists-immunologists recommend the following additional precautions to avoid insect stings:

- Avoid wearing sandals or walking barefoot in the grass. Honeybees and bumblebees forage on white clover, a weed that grows in lawns throughout the country.
- Never swat at a flying insect. If need be, gently brush it aside or patiently wait for it to leave.
- Do not drink from open beverage cans. Stinging insects will crawl inside a can attracted by the sweet beverage.
- When eating outdoors, try to keep food covered at all times.
- Garbage cans stored outside should be covered with tight-fitting lids.
- Avoid sweet-smelling perfumes, hair sprays, colognes, and deodorants.
- Avoid wearing bright-colored clothing.
- Yard work and gardening should be done with caution.
- Keep window and door screens in good repair. Drive with car windows closed.
- Keep prescribed medications handy at all times and follow the attached instructions if you are stung. These medications are for immediate emergency use while en route to a hospital emergency room for observation and further treatment.
- If you have had an allergic reaction to an insect sting, it's important that you see an allergist-immunologist.

For more medical information, please contact an allergist in your area.

Section 39.4

Removing a Tick from the Skin

A tick's mouth parts have reverse harpoon-like barbs, designed to penetrate and attach to skin. Ticks secrete a cement-like substance that helps them adhere firmly to the host. If you find that you or your pet has been bitten by a tick, it is important to remove it properly.

Tick Removal Procedure

1. Use fine-point tweezers to grasp the tick at the place of attachment, as close to the skin as possible.
2. Gently pull the tick straight out.
3. Place the tick in a small vial labeled with the victim's name, address, and the date.
4. Wash your hands and disinfect the tweezers and bite site.
5. Mark your calendar with the victim's name, place of tick attachment on the body, and general health at the time.
6. Call your doctor to determine if treatment is warranted.
7. Watch the tick-bite site and your general health for signs or symptoms of a tick-borne illness. Make sure you mark any changes in your health status on your calendar.
8. If possible, have the tick identified/tested by a lab, your local health department, or veterinarian.

If the Mouth Parts Break off in the Skin, Should I Dig Them out?

We have heard two competing opinions about this. One viewpoint states that the mouth parts can cause a secondary infection, and should be removed as if it was a splinter. Another viewpoint was shared with us by a pediatrician in a hyperendemic area. He states that parents can do more harm by trying to hold down a child and dig out the mouth parts with a needle. He instructs his families to leave the mouth parts and that they will come out on their own as the skin sloughs off.

Cautions

- Children should be taught to seek adult help for tick removal.
- If you must remove the tick with your fingers, use a tissue or leaf to avoid contact with infected tick fluids.
- Do not prick, crush, or burn the tick as it may release infected fluids or tissue.
- Do not try to smother the tick (e.g., with petroleum jelly or nail polish) as the tick has enough oxygen to complete the feeding.

Chapter 40

Common Types of Skin Trauma

Chapter Contents

Section 40.1

Corns and Calluses

"Common Foot Ailments: What Is a Callus/Corn?" is reprinted with permission from the American Podiatric Medical Association, www.apma.org.

What Is a Callus/Corn?

A callus or corn is a buildup of skin that forms at points of pressure or over bony prominences. Calluses form on the bottom side of the foot. Corns form on the top of the foot and between the toes.

Statistics

- 65 out of 1,000 people are afflicted with calluses or corns.
- 37 out of 1,000 males are afflicted.
- 91 out of 1,000 females are afflicted.

Causes of Calluses/Corns

- Repeated friction and pressure from skin rubbing against bony areas or against an irregularity in a shoe
- Heredity disorders

What Can You Do?

- Wear supportive shoes with a wide toe box and a low heel.
- Use over-the-counter creams, avoiding any acid preparations.
- Use pumice stone or file to treat if you're not diabetic.

What Will a Podiatric Physician Do for You?

- Perform a physical examination.
- Perform x-ray evaluation if needed.

- Perform trimming or padding of the lesions.
- Perform surgery as indicated.

Section 40.2

Blisters

"Common Foot Ailments: What Is a Blister?" is reprinted with permission from the American Podiatric Medical Association, www.apma.org.

What Is a Blister?

Blisters are painful, fluid-filled lesions, often caused by friction and pressure.

Causes of Blisters

- Ill-fitting shoes
- Stiff shoes
- Wrinkled socks against the skin
- Excessive moisture
- Foot deformities

What Can You Do?

- Keep your feet dry.
- Always wear socks as a cushion between your feet and shoes.
- Wear properly fitting shoes.
- If a blister does occur, do not pop it.
- Cut a hole in a 1/4" piece of foam or felt, forming a "doughnut" over the blister; tape the foam or felt in place or cover with a soft gel-type dressing.

- Treat an open blister with mild soap and water; cover it with an antiseptic ointment and protective soft gel dressing to prevent infection and speed up the healing process.

What Will a Podiatric Physician Do?

- Remove the blister surface if needed.
- Prescribe appropriate medications, topical or oral.
- Recommend paddings, dressings, and friction-reducing measures.

Section 40.3

Burns

This information was provided by KidsHealth, one of the largest resources online for medically reviewed health information written for parents, kids, and teens. For more articles like this one, visit www.KidsHealth.org, or www.TeensHealth.org. Reviewed by Barbara P. Homeier, M.D., September 2004.

Whether your little one washes up under a too-hot faucet or tips over your favorite coffee cup, burns are a potential hazard in every home. In fact, burns, especially scalds from hot water and liquids, are some of the most common childhood accidents. Babies and young children may be more susceptible than adults are—they're curious, small, and have sensitive skin that needs extra protection.

Although some minor burns aren't cause for concern and can be safely treated at home, other more serious burns require medical care. But, many times, burns can be prevented by taking some simple precautions to make your home more safe.

Common Causes

The first step in helping to prevent your child from being burned is to understand the common causes of burns in kids:

- scalds, the number-one culprit (from steam, hot bath water, tipped-over coffee cups, cooking fluids, etc.)
- contact with flames or hot objects (from the stove, fireplace, curling iron, etc.)
- chemical burns (from swallowing things like drain cleaner or watch batteries or spilling chemicals, such as bleach, onto the skin)
- electrical burns (from biting on electrical cords or sticking fingers or objects in electrical outlets, etc.)
- overexposure to the sun

Types of Burns

Burns are often categorized as first-, second-, or third-degree burns, depending on how badly the skin is damaged. Any of the injuries above can cause any type of burn. But both the type of burn and its cause will determine how the burn is treated. All burns should be treated quickly to reduce the temperature of the burned area and reduce damage to the skin and underlying tissue (if the burn is severe).

First-degree burns, the mildest of the three, are limited to the top layer of skin.

- *Signs and symptoms:* These burns produce redness, pain, minor swelling, but no blistering. The skin often turns white when you press on the burned area.
- *Healing time:* Healing time is about 3 to 6 days; the superficial skin layer over the burn may peel off in 1 or 2 days.

Second-degree burns are more serious and involve the skin layers beneath the top layer.

- *Signs and symptoms:* These burns produce blisters, severe pain, and redness. The skin can appear blotchy white to cherry red.
- *Healing time:* Healing time varies depending on the severity of the burn.

Third-degree burns are the most serious type of burn and involve all the layers of the skin and underlying tissue.

- *Signs and symptoms:* The remaining surface can look waxy, leathery, or charred. There may be little or no pain at first because of nerve damage.
- *Healing time:* Healing time depends on the severity of the burn. Deep second- and third-degree burns (called full-thickness burns) will likely need to be treated with skin grafts, in which healthy skin is taken from another part of the body and surgically placed over the burn wound to help the area heal.

What to Do

Seek Medical Help Immediately If

- You think your child has a second- or third-degree burn.
- The burned area is large, even if it seems like a minor burn. For any burn that appears to cover more than 15% to 20% of the body, call for medical assistance. And don't use wet compresses because they can cause the child's body temperature to drop. Instead, cover the area with a clean, soft cloth or towel.
- The burn comes from a fire, an electrical wire or socket, or chemicals.
- The burn is on the face, scalp, hands, joint surfaces, or genitals.
- The burn looks infected (with swelling, pus, increasing redness, or red streaking of the skin near the wound).

For First-Degree Burns

- Remove clothing from the burned area immediately.
- Run cool (not cold) water over the burned area (if water isn't available, any cold, drinkable fluid can be used) or hold a clean, cold compress on the burn until pain subsides (do not use ice, as it may cause the burn to take longer to heal).
- Do not apply butter, grease, powder, or any other remedies to the burn, as these increase the risk of infection.
- If the burned area is small, loosely cover it with a sterile gauze pad or bandage.
- Give your child acetaminophen or ibuprofen for pain.
- If the area affected is small (the size of a quarter or smaller), keep the area clean and continue to use cool compresses and a

loose dressing over the next 24 hours. You can also apply antibiotic cream two to three times a day, although this isn't absolutely necessary.

For Second- and Third-Degree Burns

Seek emergency medical care, then follow these steps until medical personnel arrive:

- Keep your child lying down with the burned area elevated.
- Follow the instructions for first-degree burns.
- Remove all jewelry and clothing from around the burn (in case there's any swelling after the injury), except for clothing that's stuck to the skin. If you're having difficulty removing clothing, you may need to cut it off or wait until medical assistance arrives.
- Do not break any blisters.
- Put wet, sterile bandages on the burned area until help arrives.

For Flame Burns

- Extinguish the flames by having your child roll on the ground.
- Cover him or her with a blanket or jacket.
- Remove smoldering clothing and any jewelry around the burned area.
- Call for medical assistance, then follow instructions for second- and third-degree burns.

For Electrical and Chemical Burns

- Flush the burned area with lots of running water for 5 minutes or more.
- If the burned area is large, use a tub, shower, buckets of water, or a garden hose.
- Do not remove any of your child's clothing before you've begun flushing the burn with water. As you continue flushing the burn, you can then remove clothing from the burned area.
- If the burned area is small, flush for another 10 to 20 minutes, apply a sterile gauze pad or bandage, and call your child's doctor.

- Chemical burns to the mouth or eyes require immediate medical evaluation after thorough flushing with water.

Although both chemical and electrical burns might not always be visible, they can be serious because of potential damage to the child's internal organs. Symptoms may vary, depending on the type and severity of the burn and what caused it and may include abdominal pain.

If you think your child may have swallowed a chemical substance or an object that could be harmful (i.e., a watch battery) first call poison control and then the emergency department. It's a good idea to have the number for poison control, (800) 222-1222, in an easily accessible place, such as on the refrigerator.

Preventing Burns

Although you can't keep your child free from injuries all the time, taking some simple precautions can reduce the chances that your child will be burned unnecessarily in your own home.

In General

- Keep matches, lighters, chemicals, and lit candles out of your child's reach.
- Put child-safety covers on all electrical outlets.
- Get rid of equipment and appliances with old or frayed cords and extension cords that look damaged.
- If you need to use a humidifier or vaporizer, use a cool-mist model rather than a hot-steam one.
- Don't use fireworks or sparklers.
- Choose sleepwear that's labeled flame retardant (either polyester or treated cotton). Cotton sweatshirts or pants that aren't labeled as sleepwear generally aren't flame retardant.
- Make sure older children are especially careful when using irons or curling irons.
- Don't smoke inside, especially in bed.
- Prevent house fires by making sure that you have a smoke alarm on every level of your home and in each bedroom.

Bathroom

- Set the thermostat on your hot water heater to 120 degrees Fahrenheit (49 degrees Celsius) or lower, or use the "low-medium setting." A child can be scalded in 2 to 3 seconds if the temperature is only 5 degrees higher than 120 degrees Fahrenheit (49 degrees Celsius). If you're unable to control the water temperature (if you live in an apartment, for example), install an antiscald device, which is relatively inexpensive and can be installed yourself or by a plumber.
- Always test bath water with your elbow before putting your child in it.
- Always turn the cold water on first and turn it off last when running water in the bathtub or sink.

Kitchen/Dining Room

- Turn pot handles toward the back of the stove every time you cook.
- Avoid using tablecloths or large place mats. A small child can pull on them and overturn a hot drink or plate of food.
- Keep hot drinks and foods out of reach of children.
- Screen fireplaces and woodstoves. Radiators and electric baseboard heaters may need to be screened as well.
- Block access to the stove as much as possible.
- Never let a child use a walker in the kitchen (the American Academy of Pediatrics strongly discourages the use of walkers overall).
- Never drink hot beverages or soup with a child sitting on your lap or carry hot liquids or dishes around your child. If you have to walk with hot liquid in the kitchen (like a pot of soup or cup of coffee), make sure you know where your child is, so you don't trip over him or her.
- Never hold a baby or small child while cooking.
- Never warm baby bottles in the microwave oven. The liquid may heat unevenly, resulting in pockets of breast milk or formula that can scald your baby's mouth.

Outside/In the Car

- Use playground equipment with caution. If it's very hot outside, use the equipment only in the morning, when it's had a chance to cool down during the night.
- Remove your child's safety seat or stroller from the hot sun when not in use, because children can get burns from hot vinyl and metal. If you must leave your car seat or stroller in the sun, cover it with a blanket or towel.
- Before leaving your parked car on a hot day, hide the seatbelts' metal latch plates in the seats to prevent the sun from hitting them directly.

Section 40.4

Helping Burn Wounds Heal

"Helping Wounds Heal," by Linda Bren, U.S. Food and Drug Administration, *FDA Consumer* magazine, May 2002. Available online at http://www.fda.gov; accessed June 1, 2005.

When Darren Benton leaned over to light a homemade firecracker a few days before the Fourth of July in 2000, all he was expecting was a sizzle and a loud noise. But what he got was a flash fire that burned 90 percent of his face.

"I didn't feel anything at first," says Darren. But after looking at himself in the mirror, he got very scared. The 13-year-old's face was completely black, and his right hand and knee also were burned.

Darren's parents rushed him to the hospital. Two days later, after the swelling from his burns went down, surgeons at Children's Hospital in Washington, D.C., anesthetized Darren, scrubbed the dead skin off, and gently applied a wound dressing made of human cells and synthetic material.

For several days afterward, Darren stared out of two small eye slits cut in the bandages that swathed his face to hold the wound dressing in place. He sipped liquid food through a straw poked into another small slit in the bandages.

The surgeons couldn't predict whether his face would be scarred or discolored, says Darren's mother, Patricia Benton. "Children's Hospital hadn't been using [the wound dressing] very long, and they had never used it on a child's face, but they were very positive."

Darren left the hospital after a week, and six months later, he had "completely healed," says Bruce Benton, Darren's father. Except for the loss of a few freckles on the redheaded boy's face and a slightly paler color, "it was as if nothing had happened," he says. "It was a miracle," adds Darren's mother.

The skin covering used on Darren, called TransCyte, is one of several cellular wound dressings approved by the Food and Drug Administration. These products are helping to transform the treatment of burns and chronic wounds by decreasing the risk of infection, protecting against fluid loss, requiring fewer skin grafts, and promoting and speeding the healing process.

Each year, about 45,000 Americans are hospitalized for burn treatments and 4,500 deaths occur from fire and burns, according to the American Burn Association (ABA). Twenty years ago, burns covering half the body were routinely fatal, but today, even people with extensive and severe burns have a good chance of survival, says the ABA. Essential to survival is the process of quickly removing dead tissue and immediately covering the wound.

Surgeons discovered many years ago that dead tissue was a breeding ground for bacterial infections, says Charles Durfor, Ph.D., a chemist in the FDA's Plastic and Reconstructive Surgery Devices Branch. "So there was a tremendous advance in surgical care of burns when they started cutting off that dead tissue. All of a sudden the survivability rate went way up."

But once the dead skin has been removed, the blood and fluids that the skin holds within the body start evaporating and weeping, says Phillip Noguchi, M.D., director of the FDA's Division of Cellular and Gene Therapies. "People literally can dehydrate and die from exposure."

This is where the cellular wound dressings come in. "They provide a cover that keeps fluids from evaporating and prevents blood from oozing out," says Noguchi. "And some of these products grow in place and expand much like your own skin would do when you heal."

Is It Really Skin?

As the largest organ of the body, skin protects our internal organs and tissues from toxins, disease-carrying bacteria and viruses, bumps and bruises, and extreme heat and cold. Skin has a sensory function, too. Nerve endings near the surface give us a sense of touch and the ability to feel sensations such as hot and cold.

Two layers make up the skin: the epidermis, which is the thin top layer of tissue, and the dermis, which is the thicker bottom layer. The outermost surface of the epidermis is a tough, protective coating of dead cells called keratinocytes. Underneath these dead cells are live keratinocytes, which divide and replenish the outer layer as the dead cells fall off. Also found within the epidermis are cells that give skin its color (melanocytes) and cells that help protect the body against infection (Langerhans' cells).

The dermis, the lower layer of skin, consists of cells called fibroblasts. These fibroblasts produce collagen, the most common protein in the body, which gives structure and flexibility to the skin. The dermis also contains blood vessels, nerves, hair follicles, and oil and sweat glands.

Cellular wound dressings are sometimes called "artificial skin" or "skin substitutes," but FDA scientists prefer to avoid these labels. "Although they may look and feel like skin, these products do not function totally like skin," says Durfor. "Unlike real skin, they are missing hair follicles, sweat glands, melanocytes and Langerhans' cells."

In some respects, cellular wound dressings try to simulate the two layers of real skin. Some have a synthetic top layer structured like an epidermis. Over time, it peels away or is replaced with healthy skin through skin grafting. The bottom layer usually consists of a scaffold, or matrix, which supports cells that help promote the growth of new skin. Blood vessels, fibroblasts, and nerve fibers from healthy tissue surrounding a burn or wound cross into the matrix to mix with the wound dressing's cells. The matrix eventually disappears as a new dermis forms.

"No one has a full understanding of how these products work," says Durfor. "How they are involved in wound repair is a subject of great scientific interest."

"We do know that they promote a higher rate of healing," says Stephen Rhodes, head of the FDA's Plastic and Reconstructive Surgery Devices Branch. "More patients heal with these devices than with the standard of care, which includes compression bandages and gauze."

Skin Deep

How a burn is treated and the type of cellular wound dressing used depends on the depth and extent of the burn and the overall health of the person burned.

Traditionally classified as first-, second-, or third-degree, burns are frequently classified by health professionals as superficial, partial thickness, or full thickness, depending on their depth and the amount of tissue damage. Superficial burns, such as a sunburn, redden the skin and damage only the epidermis, making it possible for the body to repair itself. Healthy cells from the dermis reproduce and migrate to the epidermis to heal the damaged skin.

Partial thickness burns cause blisters and damage all of the epidermis and part of the underlying dermis. Although these burns usually heal on their own when treated with cleaning and bandaging, if they are extensive or in a sensitive area, such as the face, they may benefit from the use of cellular wound dressings.

Full-thickness burns completely damage both the epidermis and the dermis, and may even destroy the underlying flesh and bones. The body is unable to heal itself properly because there are no healthy cells to regenerate. These burns require surgery to replace damaged skin with healthy skin, a process known as grafting. If these wounds are not treated, the body attempts to close them by forming scar tissue that contracts over time, leading to disfigurement and loss of motion in nearby joints.

In grafting of burn wounds, surgeons use healthy skin from another part of the person's own body (autografting) as a permanent treatment. But when the skin damage is so extensive that there is not enough healthy skin available to graft initially, surgeons may use cellular wound dressings. These temporary coverings help prevent infection and fluid loss until autografting can be performed. "And these products may allow surgeons to take thinner grafts because not as much dermis in the autograft is required," says Durfor.

An alternative to autografting is to use skin from another person (allograft) or from another species (xenograft) as a temporary covering to protect the wound.

Allografting uses skin from cadaver donors, and xenografting uses skin from animals. "Allografts provide the natural protection of human skin and are used most commonly. Xenografts of pigskin are sometimes used if allografts are not available," says Steven Boyce, Ph.D., director of the department of tissue engineering at Shriners Burns Hospital in Cincinnati. "Xenografts of pigskin are in plentiful supply and it's the closest anatomically to human skin."

Allografts and xenografts are temporary measures because, within several weeks, both types will be rejected and must be replaced with an autograft. "The immune system recognizes that the foreign cells do not belong to the patient," says Boyce. "Immune cells, called T-cells, will attack and destroy foreign cells in the grafts."

Grafts may not be necessary for partial-thickness burns, such as those suffered by Darren Benton; cellular wound dressings are more commonly used. "Almost 80 percent of burns in children are partial thickness," says Martin Eichelberger, M.D., director of emergency trauma and burn services at Children's Hospital in Washington, D.C., where Darren was treated. "The largest volume is from scalding."

Since the introduction of the cellular wound dressing TransCyte, Children's Hospital has used it to treat several hundred children, says Eichelberger. "It's changed our entire paradigm of care for partial thickness burns in children. The mean length of stay used to be 14 days; it's now down to one to two days." Before cellular wound dressings, when gauze was the traditional wound treatment, the pain could be so intense that the patient had to be sedated with morphine or another painkiller just to change the dressing, says Eichelberger. The development of advanced wound dressings such as TransCyte and Integra have changed that. "We're doing fewer skin grafts and we've cut our utilization of morphine by almost 80 percent," he says.

Types of Cellular Wound Dressings

Biobrane and Integra were the first FDA-approved biologically based wound dressings. Biobrane is a temporary dressing for a variety of wounds including ulcers, lacerations, and full-thickness burns. It may also be used on wounds that develop on donor sites—the areas from which healthy skin is transplanted to cover damaged skin. Made by Bertek Pharmaceuticals, Research Triangle Park, N.C., Biobrane uses an ultrathin silicone film and nylon fabric, which is partially imbedded into the film. The nylon material contains a gelatin derived from pig tissue that interacts with clotting factors in the wound. Biobrane is trimmed away as the wound heals or until autografting becomes possible.

Integra Dermal Regeneration Template was approved in 1996 to treat full-thickness and some partial-thickness burns. Made by Integra LifeSciences Corp., Plainsboro, N.J., Integra is a two-layer membrane. The bottom layer, made of shark cartilage and collagen from cow tendons, acts as a matrix onto which a person's own cells migrate over two to three weeks. The cells gradually absorb the cartilage and collagen to create a new dermis, or "neo-dermis." This bottom layer is a permanent cover. The top layer is a protective silicone sheet that is peeled off after several weeks. A very thin layer of the person's own skin is then grafted onto the neo-dermis.

Both Biobrane and Integra use animal tissue; the more recently approved cellular wound dressings are made with human tissue. One of these products is OrCel®, made by Ortec International Inc. of New York. Approved by the FDA in 2001 to treat donor sites in burn patients, OrCel is made of living human skin cells grown on a cow collagen matrix. OrCel was also approved the same year to help treat epidermolysis bullosa, a rare skin condition in children.

TransCyte is made by Advanced Tissue Sciences Inc. of La Jolla, Calif., and was approved by the FDA in 1997. "TransCyte was the first product that FDA approved that delivered nonviable (dead) cellular material," says Rhodes. The product starts with living cells, but these cells die when frozen. TransCyte consists of human cells grown on nylon mesh, combined with a synthetic epidermal layer.

TransCyte is packaged and shipped in a frozen state to burn treatment facilities. The surgeon then thaws the product and stretches it over a burn site. In about one to two weeks, the TransCyte starts peeling off, not unlike a sunburn, and the surgeon trims it away as it peels.

TransCyte can be used as a temporary covering over full thickness and some partial-thickness burns until autografting is possible. It's also a temporary covering for some burn wounds that heal without autografting, as in Darren's case.

In addition to burn patients, people with chronic wounds can benefit from cellular wound dressings. Apligraf and Dermagraft are two products used for the treatment of diabetic foot ulcers. People with diabetes are particularly at risk for foot ulcers because of poor blood circulation in the legs and feet. If these ulcers do not heal, amputation of the foot may be required.

Apligraf, made by Organogenesis Inc., of Canton, Mass., was approved by the FDA in 1998 for leg ulcers caused by blood flow problems and in 2000 for treating the hard-to-heal diabetic foot ulcers. Apligraf is a two-layer wound dressing that contains live human skin cells combined with cow collagen.

"Apligraf is unique in that it's the first product approval that delivered live cells from a different donor," says Rhodes. As with OrCel and TransCyte, the donor cells come from circumcised infant foreskin. One small patch of cells, about the size of a postage stamp, from a single donor can be grown in the laboratory to produce tens of thousands of pieces of Apligraf.

Dermagraft, approved by the FDA in 2001, is a product of Advanced Tissue Sciences. Dermagraft is made from human cells placed on a dissolvable mesh material. Once placed on the wound or ulcer, the mesh material is gradually absorbed and the human cells grow and replace the damaged skin.

The Future of Wound Care

The technology of burn and wound care using cellular wound dressings and grafts continues to make tremendous strides forward. But most surgeons agree that nothing seems to work as well as a person's own skin.

Boyce of Shriners Burns Hospital and other researchers are experimenting with cultured skin grown from a burned person's own skin cells. With this method, cells are taken from a small patch of skin, grown in the laboratory, and combined with a collagen matrix. After this cultured skin is placed on the burned area, the matrix dissolves, and the transplanted cells reform skin tissue to heal the wound.

Boyce has found this method to be especially valuable for people who have burns over more than 50 percent of their bodies, which limits the amount of healthy skin available for grafting.

Boyce envisions other future efforts to be focused on improving cosmetic outcome after burn injury. "Smoothness and pliability may have been restored completely," says Boyce, "but better color matching to uninjured skin is needed." Also needed is new technology to make wound treatment faster, and to restore hair and glands of the skin that do not regenerate from grafts.

"Researchers continue to make advances, but the field is in its infancy," says Rhodes.

Becoming a Skin Donor

On April 17, 2001, Health and Human Services Secretary Tommy G. Thompson launched a national organ donor initiative to encourage Americans to "Donate the Gift of Life." "Fifteen Americans die each day while waiting for an organ to become available," says Thompson. "More than 75,000 men, women, and children now wait for a transplant . . . Every 16 minutes, another person joins the waiting list."

Many people don't realize that skin is an organ, but in fact it's the body's largest organ. And like other organ donations, skin donations are critically needed, says Phil Walters, director of the skin bank at Boston Shriners Hospital. Walters says the two most frequently asked questions he fields about skin donation are: is skin taken from a living donor, and can tissue surgically removed from a patient by procedures such as those performed to reduce obesity be donated? "The answer to both questions is no," says Walters. "Skin is procured from a deceased organ donor, just like any other donated organ."

No charge is made to the donor's family for donating organs. And it does not change the appearance of the donor's body or cause a delay in funeral arrangements.

For a downloadable donor card and brochure on organ and tissue donation, visit www.organdonor.gov, or call the Health Resources and Services Administration (HRSA) Information Center at 1-888-ASK-HRSA (1-888-275-4772).

Section 40.5

Cuts, Abrasions, and Lacerations

"Bleeding" was provided by KidsHealth, one of the largest resources online for medically reviewed health information written for parents, kids, and teens. For more articles like this one, visit www.KidsHealth.org, or www.TeensHealth.org. Reviewed by Steven Dowshen, M.D., September 2004.

Most small cuts don't present any danger to your child. But bleeding from large cuts may require immediate medical treatment. Depending on the type of wound and its location, there can be damage to tendons and nerves.

What to Do

For Minor Bleeding from a Small Cut or Abrasion (Scrape)

- Rinse the wound thoroughly with water to clean out dirt and debris.
- Then wash the wound with a mild soap and rinse thoroughly. (For minor wounds, it isn't necessary to use an antiseptic solution to prevent infection, and some can cause allergic skin reactions).

- Cover the wound with a sterile adhesive bandage or sterile gauze and adhesive tape.
- Examine the wound daily. If the bandage gets wet, remove it and apply a new one. After the wound forms a scab, a bandage is no longer necessary.
- Call your child's doctor if the wound is red, swollen, tender, warm, or draining pus.

For Bleeding from a Large Cut or Laceration

- Wash the wound thoroughly with water. This will allow you to see the wound clearly and assess its size.
- Place a piece of sterile gauze or a clean cloth over the entire wound. If available, use clean latex or rubber gloves to protect yourself from exposure to possible infection from the blood of a child who isn't your own. If you can, raise the bleeding body part above the level of your child's heart. Do not apply a tourniquet.
- Using the palm of your hand on the gauze or cloth, apply steady, direct pressure to the wound for 5 minutes. (During the 5 minutes, do not stop to check the wound or remove blood clots that may form on the gauze.)
- If blood soaks through the gauze, do not remove it. Apply another gauze pad on top and continue applying pressure.
- Call your child's doctor or seek immediate medical attention for all large cuts or lacerations, or if:
  - you're unable to stop the bleeding after 5 minutes of pressure, or if the wound begins bleeding again (Continue applying pressure until help arrives.)
  - you're unable to clean out dirt and debris thoroughly, or there's something else stuck in the wound
  - the wound is on your child's face or neck
  - the injury was caused by an animal or human bite, burn, electrical injury, or puncture wound (e.g., a nail)
  - the cut is more than half an inch long or appears to be deep. Large or deep wounds can result in nerve or tendon damage. (If you have any doubt about whether stitches are needed, phone your child's doctor.)

Chapter 41

Keloids, Hypertrophic Scars, and Pyogenic Granuloma

Chapter Contents

Section 41.1

Keloids and Hypertrophic Scars

Keloids are raised, reddish nodules that develop at the site of an injury. After a wound has occurred to the skin, both skin cells and connective tissue cells (fibroblasts) begin multiplying to repair the damage. A scar is made up of connective tissue, gristle-like fibers deposited in the skin by the fibroblasts to hold the wound closed. With keloids, the fibroblasts continue to multiply even after the wound is filled in. Thus keloids project above the surface of the skin and form large mounds of scar tissue.

Keloids may form on any part of the body, although the upper chest, shoulders, and upper back are especially prone to keloid formation. Symptoms include pigmentation of the skin, itchiness, redness, unusual sensations and pain.

It is estimated that keloids occur in about 10% of people. While most people never form keloids, others develop them after minor injuries, even insect bites or pimples. Darkly pigmented people seem to be more prone to forming keloids. Men and women are equally affected.

A hypertrophic scar looks similar to a keloid. Hypertrophic scars are more common. They don't get a big as keloids and may fade with time. They occur in all racial groups. Keloids are considered a benign tumor, but they are mainly a cosmetic nuisance and never become malignant. Operating on a keloid usually stimulates more scar tissue to form, so people with keloids may have been told that there is nothing that can be done to get rid of them.

Keloids may be often be prevented by using a pressure dressing, silicone gel pad or paper tape over the injury site. These are left on for 23 of 24 hours each day. This treatment is after healing of the wound or injury, usually within a month. Once they have formed, there is no completely satisfactory treatment for keloids. Treatments include cryosurgery (freezing), excision, laser, x-rays, and steroid injections.

The best initial treatment is to inject long-acting cortisone (steroid) into the keloid once a month. After several injections with cortisone, the keloid usually becomes less noticeable and flattens in three to six month's time. Hypertrophic scars often respond completely, but keloids and are notoriously difficult to treat, with recurrences commonly seen. People who have a family history of keloids have a higher rate of recurrence after treatment.

Cryosurgery is an excellent treatment for keloids that are small and occur on lightly pigmented skin. It is often combined with monthly cortisone injections. Earlobe keloids are often surgically excised and followed with several steroid injections. In addition, a drug called alpha-interferon has been injected into the scar immediately after keloid removal with very promising results. Laser treatment is very good at improving skin texture and color, but doesn't always flatten out the keloid.

For severe cases, the keloid can surgically excised and given x-ray treatments to the site immediately afterward, usually the on the same day. This works in about 85% of the most severe cases. Electron beam radiation can be used, which will not go deep enough to affect internal organs. Orthovoltage radiation is more penetrating and slightly more effective. There have not been any reports of this causing any form of cancer in many years of use, but it is very expensive. Silicone pads and creams are sold over the counter for use on keloids. These do benefit hypertrophic scars but will not cure a true keloid. However, they can reduce pain, swelling, and itching from a keloid. They usually take 3 months or more to work.

Section 41.2

Pyogenic Granuloma

Definition

Pyogenic granulomas are small, reddish bumps on the skin that bleed easily due to an abnormally high concentration of blood vessels. These lesions often appear at sites of previous trauma.

Causes, Incidence, and Risk Factors

The exact cause of pyogenic granulomas is unknown, but they frequently appear following injury. They often occur on the hands and arms or face.

Because these lesions bleed easily, they can be quite annoying. Pyogenic granulomas are common in children.

Symptoms

- Small red vascular lump that bleeds easily
- Often occurs at site of recent trauma
- Seen most frequently on hands, arms, and face

Signs and Tests

Physical examination is usually sufficient for your health care provider to diagnose pyogenic granuloma. A skin biopsy may be necessary to confirm the diagnosis.

Treatment

Small pyogenic granulomas may go away suddenly. Larger lesions are treated with surgery, electrocautery, freezing, or lasers. The recurrence rate is high if the entire lesion is not destroyed.

Expectations (Prognosis)

Most pyogenic granulomas can be removed, but scarring may appear after treatment. Recurrences at the same site are not infrequent.

Complications

- Bleeding from the lesion
- Reappearance of treated lesions

Calling Your Health Care Provider

Call for an appointment with your health care provider if you have a skin lesion that bleeds easily or that changes appearance.

Chapter 42

Bedsores (Pressure Sores)

Chapter Contents

Section 42.1

What Are Bedsores?

"Treating Pressure Sores: Consumer Guide" is from the Agency for Healthcare Research and Quality, Publication No. 95-0654, December 1994. Reviewed by David A. Cooke, M.D., on April 27, 2005.

What Is a Pressure Sore?

A pressure sore (or bed sore) is an injury to the skin and tissue under it. Pressure sores are usually caused by unrelieved pressure. If you sit or lie in the same position for a long time, the pressure on a small area of the body can squeeze shut tiny blood vessels that normally supply tissue with oxygen and nutrients. If tissue is starved of these "fuels" for too long, it begins to die, and a pressure sore starts to form.

Pressure sores are called pressure ulcers and decubitus ulcers as well as bed sores. How serious they are depends on the amount of damage to skin and tissue. Damage can range from a change in the color of unbroken skin (Stage I) to severe, deep wounds down to muscle or bone (Stage IV). In light-skinned people, a Stage I sore may change skin color to a dark purple or red area that does not become pale under fingertip pressure. In dark-skinned people, this area may become darker than normal. The affected area may feel warmer than surrounding tissue.

Treatment

Healing a pressure sore is a team effort. A team of health care professionals will work with you to prepare a treatment plan. Your team may include doctors, nurses, dietitians, social workers, pharmacists, and occupational and physical therapists. However, you and your caregiver are the most important team members. Feel free to ask questions or share concerns with other team members.

Your Role

You and your caregiver need to:

- Know your roles in the treatment program.
- Learn how to perform the care.
- Know what to report to the doctor or nurse.
- Know how to tell if the treatment works.
- Help change the treatment plan when needed.
- Know what questions you want to ask.
- Get answers you understand.

Treatment Plan

To develop a treatment plan that meets your needs, the doctor or nurse must know about:

- Your general health.
- Illnesses that might slow healing (such as diabetes or hardening of the arteries).
- Prescription or over-the-counter medicines you take.
- The emotional support and physical assistance available from family, friends, and others.

Your doctor or nurse will perform a physical exam and check the condition of your pressure sore to decide how to care for it. If you have had a pressure sore before, tell the doctor or nurse what helped it heal and what didn't help.

Your emotional health is also important. Be sure to share information about stresses in your life as well as health beliefs and practices. This will help your care team design a treatment plan that meets your personal needs.

The treatment plan will be based on the results of your physical exam, health history, personal circumstances, and the condition of the sore (how it looks). This plan will include specific instructions for:

- Taking pressure off the sore.
- Caring for the pressure sore by cleaning the wound, removing dead tissue and debris, and dressing or bandaging the area to protect it while it heals.
- Aiding healing by making sure you get enough calories, protein, vitamins, and minerals.

Note to Caregivers

Although patients should be as active in their care as possible, you may need to provide much or all of their care. As a result, you may find you have questions or problems. If so, ask for help. Call doctors, nurses, and other professionals for answers and other support.

Remember that patients who must be in a bed or chair for long periods don't have to get pressure sores. Pressure sores can be prevented. And sores that have formed can be healed.

Helping Pressure Sores Heal

Healing pressure sores depends on three principles: pressure relief, care of the sore, and good nutrition.

Pressure Relief

Pressure sores form when there is constant pressure on certain parts of the body. Long periods of unrelieved pressure cause or worsen pressure sores and slow healing once a sore has formed. Taking pressure off the sore is the first step toward healing.

Pressure sores usually form on parts of the body over bony prominences (such as hips and heels) that bear weight when you sit or lie down for a long time.

You can relieve or reduce pressure by:

- Using special surfaces to support your body.
- Putting your body in certain positions.
- Changing positions often.

Support surfaces: Support surfaces are special beds, mattresses, mattress overlays, or seat cushions that support your body in bed or in a chair. These surfaces reduce or relieve pressure. By relieving pressure, you can help pressure sores heal and prevent new ones from forming.

You can get different kinds of support surfaces. The best kind depends on your general health, if you are able to change positions, your body build, and the condition of your sore. You and your doctor or nurse can choose the surface best for you.

One way to see if a support surface reduces pressure enough is for the caregiver to do a "hand check" under the person. The caregiver places his or her hand under the support surface, beneath the pressure point, with the palm up and fingers flat. If there is less than 1 inch of support surface between the pressure point of the body and the caregiver's hand, the surface does not give enough support. If you need more support, your doctor or nurse will recommend a different support surface.

Caregivers should know that pressure sores are often painful, and a hand check may increase pain. Caregivers should ask if it will be okay to do a hand check, which should be done as gently as possible.

Good body positions: Your position is important to relieving pressure on the sore and preventing new ones. You need to switch positions whether you are in a bed or a chair.

In bed. Follow these guidelines:

- Do not lie on the pressure sore. Use foam pads or pillows to relieve pressure on the sore.
- Change position at least every 2 hours.
- Do not rest directly on your hip bone when lying on your side. A 30-degree side-lying position is best.
- When lying on your back, keep your heels up off the bed by placing a thin foam pad or pillow under your legs from midcalf to ankle. The pad or pillow should raise the heels just enough so a piece of paper can be passed between them and the bed. Do not place the pad or pillow directly under the knee when on your back, because this could reduce blood flow to your lower leg.
- Do not use donut-shaped (ring) cushions—they reduce blood flow to tissue.
- Use pillows or small foam pads to keep knees and ankles from touching each other.
- Raise the head of the bed as little as possible. Raise it no more than 30 degrees from horizontal. If you have other health problems (such as respiratory ailments) that are improved by sitting up, ask your doctor or nurse which positions are best.
- Use the upright position during meals to prevent choking. The head of the bed can be moved back to a lying or semi-reclining position 1 hour after eating.

In a chair or wheelchair. When sitting, you should have good posture and be able to keep upright in the chair or wheelchair. A good position will allow you to move more easily and help prevent new sores.

For your specific needs, use cushions designed to relieve pressure on sitting surfaces. Even if pressure can be relieved with cushions, your position should be changed every hour. Remember to:

- Avoid sitting directly on the pressure sore.
- Keep the top of your thighs horizontal and your ankles in a comfortable, "neutral" position on the floor or footrest. Rest your elbows, forearms, and wrists on arm supports.
- If you cannot move yourself, have someone help you change your position at least every hour. If you can move yourself, shifting your weight every 15 minutes is even better.
- If your position in a chair cannot be changed, have someone help you back to bed so you can change position.
- Do not use donut-shaped or ring cushions, because they reduce blood flow to tissue.

Changing positions: Change your body position often—at least every hour while seated in a chair and at least every 2 hours while lying in bed. A written turning schedule or a turn clock (with positions written next to times) may help you and your caregiver remember turning times and positions. You may want to set a kitchen timer.

Be sure your plan works for you. It should consider your skin's condition, personal needs and preferences, and your comfort level.

Pressure Sore Care

The second principle of healing is proper care of the sore. The three aspects of care are: cleaning, removing dead tissue and debris (debridement), and dressing (bandaging) the pressure sore.

You should know about sore care even if only your caregiver is caring for the sore. Knowing about your care will help you make informed decisions about it.

Cleaning

Pressure sores heal best when they are clean. They should be free of dead tissue (which may look like a scab), excess fluid draining from the sore, and other debris. If not, healing can be slowed, and infection can result.

A health care professional will show you and your caregiver how to clean and/or rinse the pressure sore. Clean the sore each time dressings are changed.

Cleaning usually involves rinsing or "irrigating" the sore. Loose material may also be gently wiped away with a gauze pad. It is important to use the right equipment and methods for cleaning the sore. Tissue that is healing can be hurt if too much force is used when rinsing. Cleaning may be ineffective if too little force is used.

Use only cleaning solutions recommended by a health care professional. Usually saline is best for rinsing the pressure sore. Saline can be bought at a drugstore or made at home. Caution: Sometimes water supplies become contaminated. If the health department warns against drinking the water, use saline from the drugstore or use bottled water to make saline for cleaning sores.

Do not use antiseptics such as hydrogen peroxide or iodine. They can damage sensitive tissue and prevent healing.

Cleansing methods are usually effective in keeping sores clean. However, in some cases, other methods will be needed to remove dead tissue.

Removing Dead Tissue and Debris

Dead tissue in the pressure sore can delay healing and lead to infection. Removing dead tissue is often painful. You may want to take pain-relieving medicine 30 to 60 minutes before these procedures.

Under supervision of health care professionals, dead tissue and debris can be removed in several ways:

- Rinsing (to wash away loose debris).
- Wet-to-dry dressings. In this special method, wet dressings are put on and allowed to dry. Dead tissue and debris are pulled off when the dry dressing is taken off. This method is only used to remove dead tissue; it is never used on a clean wound.
- Enzyme medications to dissolve dead tissue only.
- Special dressings left in place for several days help the body's natural enzymes dissolve dead tissue slowly. This method should not be used if the sore is infected. With infected sores, a faster method for removing dead tissue and debris should be used.

Qualified health care professionals may use surgical instruments to cut away dead tissue. Based on the person's general health and the condition of the sore, the doctor or nurse will recommend the best method for removing dead tissue.

Choosing and Using Dressings

Choosing the right dressings is important to pressure sore care. The doctor or nurse will consider the location and condition of the pressure sore when recommending dressings.

The most common dressings are gauze (moistened with saline), film (see-through), and hydrocolloid (moisture- and oxygen-retaining) dressings. Gauze dressings must be moistened often with saline and changed at least daily. If they are not kept moist, new tissue will be pulled off when the dressing is removed.

Unless the sore is infected, film or hydrocolloid dressings can be left on for several days to keep in the sore's natural moisture.

The choice of dressing is based on:

- The type of material that will best aid healing.
- How often dressings will need to be changed.
- Whether the sore is infected.

In general, the dressing should keep the sore moist and the surrounding skin dry. As the sore heals, a different type of dressing may be needed.

Storing and Caring for Dressings

Clean (rather than sterile) dressings usually can be used, if they are kept clean and dry. There is no evidence that using sterile dressings is better than using clean dressings. However, contamination between patients can occur in hospitals and nursing homes. When clean dressings are used in institutions, procedures that prevent cross contamination should be followed carefully.

At home, clean dressings may also be used. Carefully follow the methods given below on how to store, care for, and change dressings.

To keep dressings clean and dry:

- Store dressings in their original packages (or in other protective, closed plastic packages) in a clean, dry place.
- Wash hands with soap and water before touching clean dressings.
- Take dressings from the box only when they will be used.

- Do not touch the packaged dressing once the sore has been touched.
- Discard the entire package if any dressings become wet or dirty.

Changing dressings. Ask your doctor or nurse to show how to remove dressings and put on new ones. If possible, he or she should watch you change the dressings at least once.

Ask for written instructions if you need them. Discuss any problems or questions about changing dressings with the doctor or nurse.

Wash your hands with soap and water before and after each dressing change. Use each dressing only once. You should check to be sure the dressing stays in place when changing positions. After the used dressing is removed, it must be disposed of safely to prevent spread of germs that may be on dressings.

Using plastic bags for removal. A small plastic bag (such as a sandwich bag) can be used to lift the dressing off the pressure sore. Seal the bag before throwing it away. If you use gloves, throw them away after each use.

Good Nutrition

Good nutrition is the third principle of healing. Eating a balanced diet will help your pressure sore heal and prevent new sores from forming.

You and your doctor, dietitian, or nurse should review any other medical conditions you have (such as diabetes or kidney problems) before designing a special diet.

Weigh yourself weekly. If you find you cannot eat enough food to maintain your weight or if you notice a sudden increase or decrease, you may need a special diet and vitamin supplements. You may need extra calories as part of a well-balanced diet.

Tell your doctor or nurse about any weight change. An unplanned weight gain or loss of 10 pounds or more in 6 months should be looked into.

Section 42.2

Treating Chronic Skin Sores

"Studies Offer Important Advances in Treating Chronic Skin Ulcers," National Institute of Arthritis and Musculoskeletal and Skin Diseases, March 2005. Available online at http://www.niams.nih.gov; accessed June 1, 2005.

Chronic skin wounds, like the one that contributed to the death of actor Christopher Reeve, are a far-too-common problem in people with diabetes, circulatory problems or, in Reeve's case, paralysis due to injuries or disease.

While new technologies—including grafts of bioengineered skin—exist to help promote the healing of chronic wounds, doctors have had no way to determine early on which wounds might require these advanced and expensive procedures. Furthermore, development of more effective and perhaps less expensive treatments have been hampered by the length and expense of clinical trials required to study them. New research supported by the National Institute of Arthritis and Musculoskeletal and Skin Diseases addresses both of these issues.

Focusing on prognostic models for leg ulcers caused by insufficient blood flow, David Margolis, M.D., at the University of Pennsylvania and his colleagues studied data on more than 20,000 people with the ulcers to try to determine which, if any, factors predicted complete healing of the wound by the 24th week. Among their findings: Wounds smaller than 10 square centimeters and less than a year old had about 70 percent chance of healing by the 24th week, while a wound older and larger than that had about an 80 percent chance of staying open after 24 weeks. Using information such as this concerning which wounds are unlikely to heal on their own, they say, doctors can better target technologies to the wounds likely to need them most.

In a separate NIAMS-supported study, Vincent Falanga, M.D., at the Roger Williams Medical Center in Providence, R.I., and his colleagues applied a classification system for both diabetic and venous ulcers to evaluate healing following the use of a bioengineered skin. The scoring system evaluated both the appearance of the natural skin and the appearance of the bioengineered skin 7 and 14 days after application in order to try to predict which wounds would heal and how quickly. The researchers say applying a system like this, once it is validated, would reduce the time and the expense it would take to conduct trials on treatments for skin ulcers, because scientists would not have to wait until wounds were completely healed to determine if a treatment was effective.

The researchers say both studies have the potential to help people with chronic skin wounds by determining which ones require special treatment and by facilitating the process by which those treatments are developed and studied and ultimately brought to market.

Margolis DJ, et al. The accuracy of venous leg ulcer prognostic models in a wound care system. *Wound Repair Regen* 2004; 12(2): 163-168.

Saap LJ, et al. Clinical classification of bioengineered skin use and its correlation with healing of diabetic and venous ulcers. *Dermatol Surg* 2004; 30(8): 1095-1100.

Chapter 43

Cutaneous Porphyria

Porphyria cutanea tarda (PCT) is the most common and also the most readily treated form of porphyria. Blisters and crusting of sun-exposed areas of skin are the most prominent features. PCT is caused by a deficiency of the enzyme uroporphyrinogen decarboxylase (UROD) in the liver. UROD is the fifth in the series of eight enzymes that are responsible for the synthesis of heme. PCT is somewhat more common in men than women. It usually develops in middle age, hence, the name *tarda*, which is Latin for late.

Causes of PCT

How a deficiency of UROD develops in the liver is not completely understood. Most of the time, this reduced level of activity of UROD is nevertheless sufficient to carry out heme synthesis normally. However, at other times, the activity is insufficient and results in a decreased synthesis of heme and an accumulation of the products of the early part of the heme biosynthetic pathway, which is still working normally. When this happens, porphyrins accumulate in the site of synthesis, which is mainly the liver, and spill out into the blood, from where they may be either excreted into the urine, or deposited in various tissues around the body. When these porphyrins are deposited in the skin, they can absorb light. Other porphyrins (for example,

---

chlorophyll, which is a heme-like molecule containing magnesium) are able to absorb light and store the energy in the form of carbohydrates, but the porphyrins which accumulate in PCT are unable to store the energy of the light. This energy is released into the skin in photochemical reactions that cause damage to the skin. Persistent exposure to light thus leads to skin damage, blistering, and scarring. Most of the known causative factors (listed below) are acquired and, therefore, can be avoided or treated. Not all of these factors are present in every patient with PCT.

Approximately 20% of PCT patients have an inherited (autosomal dominant) deficiency of UROD and are said to have familial (Type II) PCT. More than one case may occur in the same family (Type II). At birth UROD is approximately 50% normal in all tissues in these patients. However one or more of the additional causative factors listed below are important in these patients. Type II PCT becomes manifest when the enzyme activity in liver becomes much less than 50% of normal, due to one or more of these additional factors. Patients with familial PCT respond to the same treatments as those who do not have an inherited enzyme deficiency.

Iron has a central role in causing PCT. Liver iron is often increased in PCT. Removal of iron from the body always leads to a remission. Most PCT patients do not have a great excess of iron, because removal of only 5 to 6 pints of blood is needed for successful treatment in most cases. A serum ferritin measurement is often used to assess the degree of excess iron. The ferritin is usually normal to moderately increased. Marked increases in ferritin suggest that the patient has an iron overload condition called hemochromatosis, in addition to PCT. Because iron overload contributes to PCT and hemochromatosis is one of the most common genetic diseases (occurring in about 1 of 200 people in the population), it is not surprising that some patients have both conditions.

Excess alcohol intake is very common in PCT. How iron and alcohol lead to UROD deficiency in the liver is not known, but both can generate reactive and damaging forms of oxygen within liver cells.

Hepatitis C is common in PCT. In some areas where this viral infection is quite prevalent, especially in southern Europe and some parts of the United States, as many as 80% of PCT patients are infected with this virus. How this particular virus contributes to developing PCT is not known. Other hepatitis viruses are seldom implicated.

Estrogens are contributing factors, especially in women. PCT develops in some women taking estrogen containing oral contraceptive pills and in older women taking estrogens after menopause. Men have developed PCT after being treated with estrogens (for example, for cancer of the prostate). Other types of hormones do not appear to be important in causing PCT.

Other factors are important in some patients. High iron levels are known to inhibit the activity of UROD. Therefore, unusual diets which are very rich in iron, or iron supplementation of the diet with tablets, are contraindicated in PCT. Barbiturates and other drugs that increase porphyrin synthesis in the liver commonly exacerbate acute intermittent porphyria but are less important in PCT. Human immunodeficiency virus (HIV), the virus that causes AIDS, can be associated with PCT but much less often than hepatitis C. Industrial chemicals such as dioxin and hexachlorobenzene are sometimes implicated. Deficiencies in vitamin C and other nutrients may also contribute.

When UROD does become markedly deficient in the liver, porphyrins accumulate and spill out into the blood. They are then transported to other tissues such as the skin and are excreted in urine and feces. Porphyrins in the skin absorb light and release this absorbed energy in a manner that leads to generation of reactive forms of oxygen that damage the skin. Therefore, exposure to light leads to skin fragility, blistering, and scarring.

Symptoms

The most common symptoms are fragility and blistering of light-exposed areas of the skin—especially the backs of the hands, the lower arms, and the face. Patients often report that their skin is unusually fragile, so small bumps or knocks can scrape away the upper layer of the skin or cause a blister. The blisters contain fluid, rupture easily, crust over, and then heal slowly. Skin infections, scarring and changes in coloration may result. Small white spots called "milia" are commonly found on the hands and fingers.

Another feature which is often seen is excessive growth of facial hair. The reason for this is not at present understood, but once the disease is under control, the hair can usually be easily and effectively removed by conventional methods. Some patients develop severe scarring and thickening of the skin, which is referred to as pseudoscleroderma.

PCT is accompanied by some degree of liver damage. This is often mild or moderate. But over time there is a risk of developing cirrhosis and even liver cancer. Liver damage in PCT may be due in part to the excess porphyrins, which accumulate in very large amounts particularly in the liver. But other factors, such as alcohol, hepatitis C, and excess iron, can be important causes of liver damage.

Neurological symptoms, which are common in acute porphyrias, such as pain in the abdomen and extremities, are not features of PCT.

Diagnosis

The best screening test when PCT is suspected may be a plasma total porphyrin measurement. A normal result excludes active PCT. This test will also detect any other type of porphyria that is causing skin problems. Further testing is then needed to establish the type of porphyria. Urine porphyrins are commonly measured for screening for PCT and other porphyrias. But it must be remembered that increases in urinary porphyrins can occur in medical conditions other than porphyria, especially conditions that affect the liver and bone marrow.

The excess porphyrins in plasma and urine in PCT are mostly uroporphyrin (octacarboxylporphyrin) and heptacarboxylporphyrin. These porphyrins have 8 and 7 carboxyl groups, respectively, on the porphyrin molecule. Coproporphyrin (tetracarboxylporphyrin—with 4 carboxyl groups) is also increased in urine, but this is not a finding that is specific for PCT or even for porphyria. Fecal total porphyrins are usually only slightly increased, but a predominance of isocoproporphyrins, which are measured only in some specialty laboratories, is very specific for PCT.

UROD can be measured in red blood cells to establish whether or not a patient has inherited a deficiency of the enzyme. This is not essential in all cases, because the treatment of patients with familial PCT is not fundamentally different from those who do not have an inherited enzyme deficiency.

Some patients with “pseudoporphyria” have skin lesions that are essentially identical to those in PCT. These patients are most readily distinguished from PCT by finding normal levels of porphyrins in plasma. A photosensitizing drug is found to cause the sensitivity to light in some of these individuals.

Treatment

It is important to discontinue use of alcohol and, if possible, other contributing factors such as estrogens. Resumption of heavy alcohol intake is likely to lead to recurrence. However, in postmenopausal women who have been treated for PCT, there is seldom a recurrence when estrogens are restarted.

The most widely preferred treatment is repeated phlebotomy (venesection). The objective of the treatment is to decrease the amount of iron in the body to the lower limit of normal. Red blood cells contain large amounts of iron (in hemoglobin). When red blood cells are removed from the body, new cells and hemoglobin are made by the bone marrow. With repeated phlebotomy, the body's iron stores are gradually depleted. This process also removes iron from the liver, and the activity of the UROD is gradually restored. A pint of blood is removed every 1 to 2 weeks until the ferritin reaches the lower limit of normal.

The course of treatment is best followed by measuring the serum ferritin and plasma or serum porphyrin levels. Blood hematocrit or hemoglobin is also measured to avoid developing significant anemia. The plasma porphyrin levels also then gradually decrease, and the development of new skin lesions stops. Healing of damaged skin occurs more gradually. After the plasma porphyrin levels become normal, the patient is able to tolerate sunlight.

Low-dose chloroquine is a suitable alternative treatment, especially in patients who cannot tolerate phlebotomies. Chloroquine mobilizes excess porphyrins from the liver. Normal doses of chloroquine (as used for treating malaria or rheumatoid arthritis) can markedly worsen PCT and also cause liver damage before inducing a remission of PCT. If very small doses are used for treating PCT, these adverse effects are usually avoided. Only 125 milligrams of chloroquine or 100 milligrams of hydroxychloroquine should be given to patients twice weekly. Because tablets this small are not manufactured, the tablets must be cut by the patient or a pharmacist. Chloroquine and hydroxychloroquine rarely damage the retina of the eye.

PCT may be unusually severe in patients with advanced kidney diseases. Erythropoietin and phlebotomy, but not low-dose chloroquine, can be effective in these cases.

Treatment of hepatitis C with interferon alpha and ribavirin is available but is often not effective. Patients with PCT and hepatitis C should usually first undergo treatment of PCT. Treatment of hepatitis C can be considered later. There is some evidence that iron depletion may improve the results of treatment of hepatitis C.

The treatment of PCT is almost always successful, and the prognosis is usually excellent. The condition is not progressive and is seldom disabling. After treatment, periodic measurement of plasma porphyrins may be advised, especially if a contributing factor such as estrogen exposure is resumed. If a recurrence does occur, it can be detected early and retreated promptly.

Chapter 44

Epidermolysis Bullosa

What is epidermolysis bullosa (EB)?

EB is a group of blistering skin conditions. The skin is so fragile in people with EB that even minor rubbing may cause blistering. At times, the person with EB may not be aware of rubbing or injuring the skin even though blisters develop. In severe EB, blisters are not confined to the outer skin. They may develop inside the body, in such places as the linings of the mouth, esophagus, stomach, intestines, upper airway, bladder, and the genitals.

The skin has an outer layer called the epidermis and an underlying layer called the dermis. The place where the two layers meet is called the basement membrane zone. The main forms of EB are EB Simplex, Junctional EB, and Dystrophic EB. EB Simplex occurs in the outer layer of skin; Junctional EB and Dystrophic EB occur in the basement membrane zone. These major types of EB, which will be described throughout this text, also have many subtypes.

Who gets epidermolysis bullosa?

It is estimated that 2 to 4 out of every 100,000 people, or up to 12,000 people in the United States, have some form of EB. It occurs in all racial and ethnic groups and affects males and females equally.

Excerpted from "Questions and Answers about Epidermolysis Bullosa," National Institute of Arthritis and Musculoskeletal and Skin Diseases, June 2003. Available online at http://www.niams.nih.gov; accessed June 1, 2005.

The disease is not always evident at birth. Milder cases of EB may become apparent when a child crawls, walks, or runs, or when a young adult engages in vigorous physical activity.

What causes epidermolysis bullosa?

Most people with EB have inherited the condition through faulty genes they receive from one or both parents. Genes are located in the body's cells and determine inherited traits passed from parent to child. They also govern every body function, such as the formation of proteins in the skin. More than 10 genes are known to underlie the different forms of EB. Genes are located on chromosomes, which are structures in each cell's nucleus.

In an autosomal dominant form of EB, the disease gene is inherited from only one parent who has the disease, and there is a 50 percent (1 in 2) chance with each pregnancy that a baby will have EB. In the autosomal recessive form, the disease gene is inherited from both parents. Neither parent has to show signs of the disease; they simply need to "carry" the gene, and there is a 25 percent (1 in 4) chance with each pregnancy that a baby will have EB. EB can also be acquired through a mutation (abnormal change) in a gene that occurred during the formation of the egg or sperm reproductive cell in a parent. Neither the sex of the child nor the order of birth determines which child or how many children will develop EB in a family that has the faulty gene.

Although EB Simplex can occur when there is no evidence of the disease in the parents, it is usually inherited as an autosomal dominant disease. In EB Simplex, the faulty genes are those that provide instructions for producing keratin, a fibrous protein in the top layer of skin. As a result, the skin splits in the epidermis, producing a blister.

In Junctional EB, there is a defect in the genes inherited from both parents (autosomal recessive) that normally promote the formation of anchoring filaments (thread-like fibers) or hemidesmosomes (complex structures composed of many proteins). These structures anchor the epidermis to the underlying basement membrane. The defect leads to tissue separation and blistering in the upper part of the basement membrane.

There are both dominant and recessive forms of Dystrophic EB. In this condition, the filaments that anchor the epidermis to the underlying dermis are either absent or do not function. This is due to defects in the gene for type VII collagen, a fibrous protein that is the main component of the anchoring filaments.

Epidermolysis bullosa acquisita (EBA) is a rare autoimmune disorder where the body attacks its own anchoring fibrils with antibodies, the special proteins that help fight and destroy foreign substances that invade the body. In a few cases, it has occurred following drug therapy for another condition; in most cases, the cause is unknown.

How is epidermolysis bullosa diagnosed?

Dermatologists can identify where the skin is separating to form blisters and what kind of EB a person has by doing a skin biopsy (taking a small sample of skin that is examined under a microscope). One diagnostic test involves use of a microscope and reflected light to see if proteins needed for forming connecting fibrils, filaments, or hemidesmosomes are missing or reduced in number. Another test involves use of a high-power electron microscope, which can greatly magnify tissue images, to identify structural defects in the skin.

Recent techniques make it possible to identify defective genes in EB patients and their family members. Prenatal diagnosis can now be accomplished by amniocentesis (removing and examining a small amount of amniotic fluid surrounding the fetus in the womb of a pregnant woman) or sampling the chorionic villus (part of the outer membrane surrounding the fetus) as early as the tenth week of pregnancy.

What are the symptoms of epidermolysis bullosa?

The major sign of all forms of EB is fragile skin that blisters, which can lead to serious complications. For example, blistering areas may become infected, and blisters in the mouth or parts of the gastrointestinal tract may interfere with proper nutrition.

Following is a summary of some of the characteristic signs of various forms of EB.

- **EB Simplex (EBS):** A generalized form of EBS usually begins with blistering that is evident at birth or shortly afterward. In a localized, mild form called Weber-Cockayne, blisters rarely extend beyond the feet and hands. In some subtypes of EBS, the blisters occur over widespread areas of the body. Other signs may include thickened skin on the palms of the hands and soles of the feet; rough, thickened, or absent fingernails or toenails; and blistering of the soft tissues inside the mouth. Less common signs include growth retardation; blisters in the esophagus; anemia (a reduction in the red blood cells that carry oxygen to all parts of the body); scarring of the skin; and milia, which are small white skin cysts.

- **Junctional EB (JEB):** This disease is usually severe. In the most serious forms, large, ulcerated blisters on the face, trunk, and legs can be life threatening due to complicated infections and loss of body fluid that leads to severe dehydration. Survival is also threatened by blisters that affect the esophagus, upper airway, stomach, intestines, and the urogenital system. Other signs found in both severe and mild forms of JEB include rough and thickened or absent fingernails and toenails; a thin appearance to the skin (called atrophic scarring); blisters on the scalp or loss of hair with scarring (scarring alopecia); malnutrition and anemia; growth retardation; involvement of soft tissue inside the mouth and nose; and poorly formed tooth enamel.
- **Dystrophic EB (DEB):** The dominant and recessive inherited forms of DEB have slightly different symptoms. In some dominant and mild recessive forms, blisters may appear only on the hands, feet, elbows, and knees; nails usually are shaped differently; milia may appear on the skin of the trunk and limbs; and there may be involvement of the soft tissues, especially the esophagus. The more severe recessive form is characterized by blisters over large body surfaces, loss of nails or rough or thick nails, atrophic scarring, milia, itching, anemia, and growth retardation. Severe forms of recessive DEB also may lead to severe eye inflammation with erosion of the cornea (clear covering over the front of the eye), early loss of teeth due to tooth decay, and blistering and scarring inside the mouth and gastrointestinal tract. In most people with this form of EB, some or all the fingers or toes may fuse (pseudosyndactyly). Also, individuals with recessive DEB have a high risk of developing a form of skin cancer called squamous cell carcinoma. It primarily occurs on the hands and feet. The cancer may begin as early as the teenage years. It tends to grow and spread faster in people with EB than in those without the disease.

How is epidermolysis bullosa treated?

Persons with mild forms of EB may not require extensive treatment. However, they should attempt to keep blisters from forming and prevent infection when blisters occur. Individuals with moderate and severe forms may have many complications and require psychological support along with attention to the care and protection of the skin and soft tissues. Patients, parents, or other care providers should not feel that they must tackle all the complicated aspects of EB care alone. There are doctors, nurses, social workers, clergy members, psychologists, dietitians, and patient and parent support groups that can assist with care and provide information and emotional support.

Preventing Blisters: In many forms of EB, blisters will form with the slightest pressure or friction. This may make parents hesitant to pick up and cuddle young babies. However, a baby needs to feel a gentle human touch and affection, and can be picked up when placed on a soft material and supported under the buttocks (bottom) and behind the neck. A baby with EB should never be picked up under the arms.

A number of things can be done to protect the skin from injury. These include:

- avoiding overheating by keeping rooms at an even temperature.
- applying lubricants to the skin to reduce friction and keep the skin moist.
- using simple, soft clothing that requires minimal handling when dressing a child.
- using sheepskin on car seats and other hard surfaces.
- wearing mittens at bedtime to help prevent scratching.

Caring for Blistered Skin: When blisters appear, the objectives of care are to reduce pain or discomfort, prevent excessive loss of body fluid, promote healing, and prevent infection.

The doctor may prescribe a mild analgesic to prevent discomfort during changes of dressings (bandages). Dressings that are sticking to the skin may be removed by soaking them off in warm water. While daily cleansing may include a bath with mild soaps, it may be more comfortable to bathe in stages where small areas are cleaned at a time.

Blisters can become quite large and create a large wound when they break. Therefore, a medical professional will likely provide instructions on how to safely break a blister in its early stages while still leaving the top skin intact to cover the underlying reddened area. One technique is to pat the blister with an alcohol pad before popping it at the sides with a sterile needle or other sterile tool. The fluid can then drain into a sterile gauze that is used to dab the blister. After opening and draining, the doctor may suggest that an antibiotic ointment be applied to the area of the blister before covering it with a sterile, nonsticking bandage. To prevent irritation of the skin from tape, a bandage can be secured with a strip of gauze that is tied around it. In milder cases of EB or where areas are difficult to keep covered, the doctor may recommend leaving a punctured blister open to the air.

A moderately moist environment promotes healing, but heavy drainage from blister areas may further irritate the skin, and an absorbent or foam dressing may be needed. There are also contact layer dressings where a mesh layer through which drainage can pass is placed on the wound and is topped by an outer absorbent layer. The doctor or other health care professional may recommend gauze or bandages that are soaked with petroleum jelly, glycerin, or moisturizing substances, or may suggest more extensive wound care bandages or products.

Treating Infection: The chances of skin infection can be reduced by good nutrition, which builds the body's defenses and promotes healing, and by careful skin care with clean hands and use of sterile materials. For added protection, the doctor may recommend antibiotic ointments and soaks.

Even in the presence of good care, it is possible for infection to develop. Signs of infection are redness and heat around an open area of skin, pus or a yellow drainage, excessive crusting on the wound surface, a red line or streak under the skin that spreads away from the blistered area, a wound that does not heal, and/or fever or chills. The doctor may prescribe a specific soaking solution, an antibiotic ointment, or an oral antibiotic to reduce the growth of bacteria. Wounds that are not healing may be treated by a special wound covering or biologically developed skin.

Treating Nutritional Problems: Blisters that form in the mouth and esophagus in some people with EB are likely to cause difficulty in chewing and swallowing food and drinks. If breast or bottle feeding results in blisters, infants may be fed using a preemie nipple (a soft nipple with large holes), a cleft palate nipple, an eyedropper, or a syringe. When the baby is old enough to take in food, adding extra liquid to pureed (finely mashed) food makes it easier to swallow. Soups, milk drinks, mashed potatoes, custards, and puddings can be given to young children. However, food should never be served too hot.

Dietitians are important members of the health care team that assists people with EB. They can work with family members and older patients to find recipes and prepare food that is nutritious and easy to consume. For example, they can identify high-calorie and protein-fortified foods and beverages that help replace protein lost in the fluid from draining blisters. They can suggest vitamin and mineral nutritional supplements that may be needed, and show how to mix these into the food and drinks of young children. Dietitians can also recommend adjustments in the diet to prevent gastrointestinal problems, such as constipation, diarrhea, or painful elimination.

Surgical Treatment: Surgical treatment may be necessary in some forms of EB. Individuals with the severe forms of autosomal recessive Dystrophic EB whose esophagus has been narrowed by scarring may require dilation of their esophagus for food to travel from the mouth to the stomach. Other individuals who are not getting proper nutrition may need a feeding tube that permits delivery of food directly to the stomach. Also, patients whose fingers or toes are fused together may require surgery to rclease them.

Chapter 45

Pemphigus

What Is Pemphigus?

Pemphigus is a group of rare autoimmune blistering diseases of the skin and/or mucous membranes.

Our immune system produces antibodies that normally attack hostile viruses and bacteria in an effort to keep us healthy. In a person with pemphigus, however, the immune system mistakenly perceives the cells in skin and/or mucous membrane as foreign, and attacks them. Antibodies that attack one's own cells are called autoantibodies. The part of the cells that are attacked in pemphigus are proteins called desmogleins. Desmogleins form the glue that attaches adjacent skin cells, keeping the skin intact.

When autoantibodies attack desmogleins, the cells become separated from each other. The skin virtually becomes unglued. This causes burn-like lesions or blisters that do not heal. In some cases, these blisters can cover a significant area of the skin.

There are several types of pemphigus, and early diagnosis is important. Though there may be a genetic predisposition and some groups with a higher incidence of the disease, the disease appears to affect people across racial and cultural lines, so it's not possible to say who may get pemphigus.

Treatment is available, as is help for living with pemphigus, including information on nutrition and caregiving.

Who Gets Pemphigus?

To date, definitive statistics on the incidence and prevalence of pemphigus are not available, but estimates of the number of new cases diagnosed each year ranges from as high as 5 per 100,000 to as low as 1 per 1,000,000, depending upon the type of pemphigus and the ethnicity of the affected population. It is known to affect people across racial and cultural lines. However, there are certain groups of people (such as eastern European Jews and people of Mediterranean descent) who have a higher incidence of the disease. Men and women are equally affected. Research studies suggest a genetic predisposition to the disease. Although the onset usually occurs in middle-aged and older adults, PV [pemphigus vulgaris] and PF [pemphigus foliaceus] also occur in young adults and children.

Pemphigus is frequently the last disease considered during diagnosis. If you have any persistent skin or mouth lesions, consult your dermatologist. Early diagnosis may permit treatment with low levels of medication.

Types of Pemphigus

There are three main categories of pemphigus: pemphigus vulgaris, pemphigus foliaceus, and paraneoplastic pemphigus.

Pemphigus is not pemphigoid, cicatricial pemphigoid, or benign familial pemphigus, also known as Hailey-Hailey disease.

Pemphigus Vulgaris (PV)

The term "vulgar" means "common," and PV is the most frequently diagnosed form of pemphigus. Sores and blisters almost always start in the mouth.

Because the skin is an organ, PV is called a one-organ disease. It does not affect any of the internal organs. The blisters can go as far down as the vocal cords, but no further. PV does not cause permanent scars unless there is infection associated with the lesion.

In PV, autoantibodies attack the protein "glue," which holds skin cells together, called desmogleins. The lesions are painful. Sometimes there is the Nikolsky effect where just touching the skin can cause it to tear.

Before drug treatment, PV was 99% fatal, but today, with the current therapies, the mortality rate is only 5% to 15%.

Pemphigus Foliaceus (PF)

In pemphigus foliaceus, blisters and sores do not occur in the mouth. Crusted sores or fragile blisters usually first appear on the face and scalp and later involve the chest and back.

Autoantibodies are produced by the immune system but they bind only to desmoglein 1. The blisters are superficial and often itchy, but are not usually as painful as PV.

In PF, disfiguring skin lesions can occur, but the mortality rate from the disease is much lower than in PV.

Paraneoplastic Pemphigus (PNP)

PNP is the most serious form of pemphigus. It occurs most often in someone who has already been diagnosed with a malignancy (cancer). Fortunately, it is also the least common. Painful sores of the mouth, lips, and esophagus are almost always present; and skin lesions of different types occur. PNP can affect the lungs. In some cases, the diagnosis of the disease will prompt doctors to search for a hidden tumor. In some cases the tumor will be benign and the disease will improve if the tumor is surgically removed.

It is important to know that this condition is rare and looks different than the other forms of pemphigus. The antibodies in the blood are also different and the difference can be determined by laboratory tests.

Treatment of Pemphigus

Treatment for pemphigus vulgaris (PV) involves the use of one or more drugs. Initially, PV is treated with a corticosteroid. Other drugs are usually used in conjunction with corticosteroids.

Corticosteroids

Prompt and sufficient doses of corticosteroids, usually prednisone or prednisolone, are required to bring pemphigus under control. Once controlled, the steroid is reduced slowly to minimize side effects. Some patients then go into remission; however, many patients need a small maintenance dose to keep the disease under control.

Immunosuppressants

- Azathioprine (Imuran®)
- Mycophenolate mofetil (CellCept®)
- Cyclophosphamide (Cytoxan®)
- Cyclosporine

Additional Drugs

Other drugs that are used routinely with varying effects are:

- Dapsone®;
- Gold injections;
- Methotrexate;
- Tetracycline, minocycline, or doxycycline combined with niacinamide.

All of these medications can have serious side effects. Patients on these medications must have blood and urine monitored on a regular basis. There is some evidence suggesting that treatment is easier in the early stages of the disease.

Treatment should always be addressed according to the disease activity that is clinically apparent. An indirect immunofluorescence test (antibody titer count) will generally show a high count when the disease is more active, and will be low or undetectable when the disease is in remission.

However, this is not always true. The antibody titer test may be most useful with patients on maintenance doses of drugs. If a titer count is low, then it could be reassuring that the flare is controllable and short. A high titer might indicate the need for further treatment.

To date, no studies have shown that alternative, homeopathic, or any other nontraditional method has been successful in treating these diseases. For the best possible results, it is imperative that traditional treatments be administered.

However, once the disease is under control, alternative therapies may be useful to help reduce drug side effects.

Chapter 46

Lichenification Disorders

Chapter Contents

Section 46.1

Lichen Planus

Definition

Lichen planus is a disorder of the skin and mucous membranes resulting in inflammation, itching, and distinctive skin lesions.

Causes, Incidence, and Risk Factors

Lichen planus is an uncommon disorder involving a recurrent, itchy, inflammatory rash or lesion on the skin or in the mouth. The exact cause is unknown, but the disorder is likely to be related to an allergic or immune reaction.

The disorder has been known to develop after exposure to potential allergens such as medications, dyes, and other chemical substances. Symptoms are increased with emotional stress, possibly because of changes in immune system during stress.

Lichen planus generally occurs at or after middle age. It is less common in children. The initial attack may last for weeks to months, resolve, then recur for years.

Lichen planus may be associated with several other disorders, most notably hepatitis C.

Chemicals or medications associated with development of lichen planus include gold (used to treat rheumatoid arthritis), antibiotics, arsenic, iodides, chloroquine, quinacrine, quinidine, antimony, phenothiazines, diuretics such as chlorothiazide, and many others.

Symptoms

- Itching in the location of a lesion, mild to severe
- Skin lesion:
  - Usually located on the inner areas of the wrist, legs, torso, or genitals

    - Generalized, with symmetric appearance
    - Single lesion or clusters of lesions, often at sites of skin trauma
    - Papule of 2–4 cm in size
    - Papules clustered into a plaque or large, flat-topped lesion
    - Distinct, sharp borders to lesions
    - Possibly covered with fine white streaks or linear scratch marks called Wickham's striae
    - Shiny or scaly appearance
    - Color dark—reddish-purple (skin) or gray-white (mouth)
    - Possibility of developing blisters or ulcers
- Ridges in the nails (nail abnormalities)
- Dry mouth
- Metallic taste in the mouth
- Mouth lesions
    - Tender or painful (mild cases may have no discomfort)
    - Located on the sides of the tongue or the inside of the cheek
    - Occasionally located on the gums
    - Poorly defined area of blue-white spots or "pimples"
    - Linear lesions forming a lacy-appearing network of lesions
    - Gradual increase in size of affected area
    - Lesions occasionally erode to form painful ulcers
- Hair loss

Signs and Tests

Your physician will suspect lichen planus based on the distinctive appearance of the lesions. Your dentist may diagnose oral lichen planus based on the distinctive appearance of mouth lesions. A skin lesion biopsy or biopsy of a mouth lesion can confirm the diagnosis.

Treatment

The goal of treatment is to reduce your symptoms and speed healing of the skin lesions. If symptoms are mild, no treatment may be needed.

Treatments may include:

- Antihistamines
- If you have mouth lesions, lidocaine mouth washes may numb the area temporarily and make eating more comfortable.
- Topical corticosteroids (such as triamcinolone acetonide cream) or oral corticosteroids (such as prednisone) may be prescribed to reduce inflammation and suppress immune responses. Corticosteroids may be injected directly into a lesion.
- Topical retinoic acid cream (a form of vitamin A) and other ointments or creams may reduce itching and inflammation and may aid healing.
- Occlusive dressings may be placed over topical medications to protect the skin from scratching.
- Ultraviolet light therapy may be beneficial in some cases.

Expectations (Prognosis)

Lichen planus is generally not harmful and may resolve with treatment, but can persist for months to years. Oral lichen planus usually clears within 18 months.

Complications

Long-standing mouth ulcers may develop into oral cancer.

Calling Your Health Care Provider

Call your health care provider if symptoms persist, or if there are changes in the appearance of skin or oral lesions.

Call for an appointment with your health care provider if oral lichen planus persists or worsens despite treatment, or if your dentist recommends adjustment of medications or treatment of conditions that trigger the disorder.

Section 46.2

Lichen Sclerosus

Excerpted from "Questions and Answers About Lichen Sclerosus," National Institute of Arthritis and Musculoskeletal and Skin Diseases, June 2004. Available online at http://www.niams.nih.gov; accessed June 1, 2005.

What is lichen sclerosus?

Lichen sclerosus is a chronic inflammatory skin disorder that can affect men, women, or children, but is most common in women. It usually affects the vulva (the outer genitalia or sex organ) and the anal area. While lichen sclerosus appears predominantly in postmenopausal women, this skin condition is also known to develop on the head of the penis in men. Occasionally, lichen sclerosus is seen on other parts of the body, especially the upper body, breasts, and upper arms.

The symptoms are the same in children and adults. Early in the disease, small, subtle white spots appear. These areas are usually slightly shiny and smooth. As time goes on, the spots develop into bigger patches, and the skin surface becomes thinned and crinkled. As a result, the skin tears easily, and bright red or purple discoloration from bleeding inside the skin is common. More severe cases of lichen sclerosus produce scarring that may cause the inner lips of the vulva to shrink and disappear, the clitoris to become covered with scar tissue, and the opening of the vagina to narrow.

Lichen sclerosus of the penis occurs almost exclusively in uncircumcised men (those who have not had the foreskin removed). Affected foreskin can scar, tighten, and shrink over the head of the penis. Skin on other areas of the body affected by lichen sclerosus usually does not develop scarring.

How common is it?

Although definitive data are not available, lichen sclerosus is considered a rare disorder that can develop in people of all ages. It usually appears in postmenopausal women and primarily affects the vulva. It is uncommon for women who have vulvar lichen sclerosus to have the disease on other skin surfaces. The disease is much less common in childhood. In boys, it is a major cause of tightening of the foreskin, which requires circumcision. Otherwise, it is very uncommon in men.

What are the symptoms?

Symptoms vary depending on the area affected. Patients experience different degrees of discomfort. When lichen sclerosus occurs on parts of the body other than the genital area, most often there are no symptoms, other than itching. If the disease is severe, bleeding, tearing, and blistering caused by rubbing or bumping the skin can cause pain.

Very mild lichen sclerosus of the genital area often causes no symptoms at all. If the disease worsens, itching is the most common symptom. Rarely, lichen sclerosus of the vulva may cause extreme itching that interferes with sleep and daily activities. Rubbing or scratching to relieve the itching can create painful sores and bruising, so that many women must avoid sexual intercourse, tight clothing, tampons, riding bicycles, and other common activities that involve pressure or friction. Urination can be accompanied by burning or pain, and bleeding can occur, especially during intercourse. When lichen sclerosus develops around the anus, the discomfort can lead to constipation that is difficult to relieve. This is particularly common in children. It is important to note that the signs of lichen sclerosus in children may sometimes be confused with those of sexual abuse.

Most men with genital lichen sclerosus have not been circumcised. They sometimes experience difficulty pulling back the foreskin and have decreased sensation at the tip of the penis. Occasionally, erections are painful, and the urethra (the tube through which urine flows) can become narrow or obstructed.

What causes lichen sclerosus?

The cause is unknown, although an overactive immune system may play a role. Some people may have a genetic tendency toward the disease, and studies suggest that abnormal hormone levels may also play a role. Lichen sclerosus has also been shown to appear at sites of previous injury or trauma where the skin has already experienced scarring or damage.

Is it contagious?

No, lichen sclerosus is not contagious.

How is it diagnosed?

Doctors can diagnose an advanced case by looking at the skin. However, early or mild disease often requires a biopsy (removal and examination of a small sample of affected skin). Because other diseases of the genitalia can look like lichen sclerosus, a biopsy is advised whenever the appearance of the skin is not typical of lichen sclerosus.

How is it treated?

Patients with lichen sclerosus of nongenital skin often do not need treatment because the symptoms are very mild and usually go away over time. The amount of time involved varies from patient to patient.

However, lichen sclerosus of the genital skin should be treated, even when it is not causing itching or pain, because it can lead to scarring that may narrow openings in the genital area and interfere with either urination or sexual intercourse or both. There is also a very small chance that skin cancer may develop within the affected areas.

In uncircumcised men, circumcision is the most widely used therapy for lichen sclerosus. This procedure removes the affected skin, and the disease usually does not recur.

Prescription medications are required to treat vulvar lichen sclerosus, nongenital lichen sclerosus that is causing symptoms, and lichen sclerosus of the penis that is not cured by circumcision. The treatment of choice is an ultrapotent topical corticosteroid (a very strong cortisone cream or ointment). These creams or ointments may be applied daily for several weeks, which will be sufficient to stop the itching. However, long-term but less frequent applications (sometimes as infrequently as twice a week) will be needed to keep the lesions from reactivating and to help restore the skin's normal texture and strength. Treatment does not reverse the scarring that may have already occurred.

Because prolonged use of ultrapotent corticosteroid creams and ointments can cause thinning and redness of the skin, give rise to "stretch marks" around the area of application, and predispose individuals to vulvar yeast infections, periodic followup by a doctor is necessary.

Young girls may not require lifelong treatment, since lichen sclerosus can sometimes, but not always, disappear permanently at puberty. Scarring and changes in skin color, however, may remain even after the symptoms have disappeared.

Ultrapotent topical corticosteroids are so effective that other therapies are rarely prescribed. The previous standard therapy was testosterone cream or ointment, but this has been proven to produce no more benefit than a placebo (inactive) cream. Prolonged use of the testosterone cream or ointment can cause masculinization (low-pitched voice, increased coarse facial hairs). Another hormone cream, progesterone, was previously used to treat the disease, but has also been shown to be ineffective. Retinoids, or vitamin A-like medications, may be helpful for patients who cannot tolerate or are not helped by ultrapotent topical corticosteroids.

Tacrolimus (Protopic) ointment has been reported to benefit some patients, but more research is needed to confirm this. Tacrolimus is a steroid-free ointment; it is not a corticosteroid. Tacrolimus has no apparent side effects other than local irritation in some patients. [*Note:* Brand names included in this chapter are provided as examples only, and their inclusion does not mean that these products are endorsed by the National Institutes of Health or any other government agency. Also, if a particular brand name is not mentioned, this does not mean or imply that the product is unsatisfactory.]

There are some early indications that different forms of ultraviolet light treatments, with or without psoralens (pills that intensify the effect of ultraviolet A light), may be effective and well-tolerated treatments for some patients with lichen sclerosus on nongenital skin.

Patients who need medication should ask their doctor how the medication works, what its side effects might be, and why it is the best treatment for their lichen sclerosus.

For women and girls, surgery to remove the affected skin is not an acceptable option because lichen sclerosus comes back after removal. Surgery may be useful for scarring, but only after lichen sclerosus is controlled with medication.

Sometimes, people do not respond to the ultrapotent topical corticosteroid. Other factors, such as low estrogen levels, an infection, irritation, or allergy to the medication, can keep symptoms from clearing up. Your doctor may need to treat these as well. If you feel that you are not improving as you would expect, talk to your doctor.

Section 46.3

Prurigo Nodularis

Prurigo nodularis (PN) is a skin condition in which hard crusty lumps form on the skin that itches intensely. PN may itch constantly, mostly at night, or only when a light brush of clothing sets off a round of severe itch. For many, itching only ends when the PN is scratched to the point of bleeding or pain.

A PN sore is hard, and usually about a half inch across. The top is dry and rough and often scratched open. Old white scars are often found nearby from old sores. They tend to be in the areas most easily reached: arms, shoulders, and legs. There may be just a few or dozens.

PN, however, is actually the end result of scratching. Scratching causes the skin nerves to thicken, and when stimulated, they send unusually strong itch signals. Scratching is like "exercise" for the nerves; the more it is done, the stronger they become. What starts the scratching going at first can be different from one sufferer to the next. Once PN sets in full force the end is similar, and it may last years.

Factors triggering PN, and keeping it going include nervous and mental conditions, reduced function of the liver and kidneys, and skin diseases such as eczema, bullous pemphigoid, and dermatitis herpetiformis. In many patients, the true cause is never found.

Treatment is difficult. Due to the intensity of the itch patients often go from doctor to doctor looking for relief. No one treatment is always effective and several treatments may need to be tried. Initial treatment is often potent prescription steroid creams. If these help, a milder cream can be used for longer-term control. Antihistamine creams (Zonalon, Pramoxine) or pills (Atarax, Periactin) are often added for additional relief. Intralesional steroid injections, antidepressant pills, and non-prescription Zostrix cream helps many of those not improved with the usual treatment.

Severe and resistant cases can be controlled with cryotherapy (freezing the sores with liquid nitrogen spray), oral steroids, or PUVA [PUVA stands for psoralen and long-wave ultraviolet radiation]. Of course, try not to scratch the spots. In resistant cases blood tests and biopsy of the sores may be needed to look for a cause driving the PN.

Part Seven

Infectious, Inflammatory, and Other Skin Conditions

Chapter 47

Group A Streptococcal Skin Infections: Impetigo, Cellulitis, and Erysipelas

Overview

Group A streptococcal (strep) infections are caused by group A streptococcus, a bacterium responsible for a variety of health problems.

These infections can range from mild skin infection or sore throat to severe, life-threatening conditions such as toxic shock syndrome (multi-organ failures) and necrotizing fasciitis (soft tissue disease), commonly known as flesh-eating disease. Most people are familiar with strep throat, which along with minor skin infection, is the most common form of the disease. Health experts estimate that more than 10 million mild infections (throat and skin) like these occur every year.

In addition to strep throat and superficial skin infections, group A strep bacteria can cause infections in tissues at specific body sites, including lungs, bones, spinal cord, and abdomen.

Skin Infections: Impetigo, Cellulitis, Erysipelas

What is impetigo?

Impetigo is an infection of the top layers of the skin and is most common among children ages 2 to 6 years. It usually starts when the

---

Excerpted from "Group A Streptococcal Infections," National Institute of Allergy and Infectious Diseases, November 2004. Available online at http://www.niaid.nih.gov; accessed June 1, 2005.

bacteria get into a cut, scratch, or insect bite. Impetigo is usually caused by staphylococcus (staph), a different bacterium, but can be caused by group A streptococcus. Skin infections are usually caused by different types of strep bacteria than those that cause strep throat. Therefore, the types of strep germs that cause impetigo are usually different from those that cause strep throat.

What are the symptoms of impetigo?

Symptoms start with red or pimple-like lesions (sores) surrounded by reddened skin. These lesions can be anywhere on your body, but mostly on your face, arms, and legs. Lesions fill with pus, then break open after a few days and form a thick crust. Itching is common. Your health care provider can diagnose the infection by looking at the skin lesions.

How is impetigo spread?

The infection is spread by direct contact with wounds or sores or nasal discharge from an infected person. Scratching may spread the lesions. From the time of infection until you show symptoms is usually 1 to 3 days. Dried streptococci in the air are not infectious to skin with no breaks.

What is the treatment for impetigo?

Your health care provider will prescribe oral antibiotics, as with strep throat. This treatment may also include an antibiotic ointment to be used on the skin.

What are cellulitis and erysipelas?

Cellulitis is inflammation of the skin and deep underlying tissues. Erysipelas is an inflammatory disease of the upper layers of the skin. Group A strep germs are the most common cause of both conditions.

What are the symptoms of cellulitis and erysipelas?

Symptoms of cellulitis may include fever and chills and swollen glands or lymph nodes. Your skin will be painful, red, and tender. Your skin may blister and then scab over. You may also have perianal (around the anus) cellulitis with itching and painful bowel movements.

With erysipelas, a fiery red rash with raised borders may occur on your face, arms, or legs. Your skin will be hot, red, and have sharply defined raised areas. The infection may come back, causing chronic swelling of your arms or legs (lymphedema).

How does a person get cellulitis or erysipelas?

Both cellulitis and erysipelas begin with a minor incident, such as a bruise. They can also begin at the site of a burn, surgical cut, or wound, and usually affect your arm or leg. When the rash appears on your trunk, arms, or legs, however, it is usually at the site of a surgical cut or wound. Even if you have no symptoms, you carry the germs on your skin or in your nasal passages and can transmit the disease to others.

How are these skin infections diagnosed and what is the treatment?

A health care provider may take a sample or culture from your skin lesions to identify the bacteria causing infection. He or she may also recover the bacteria from your blood. Depending on how severe the infection is, treatment involves either oral or intravenous (through the vein) antibiotics.

Research

Through research, health experts have learned that there are more than 120 different strains of group A streptococci, each producing its own unique proteins. Some of these proteins are responsible for specific group A streptococcal diseases. With the support of the National Institute of Allergy and Infectious Diseases (NIAID), scientists have determined the genetic sequence, or DNA code, for three different strains of the group A streptococcus organism.

By studying an organism's genes, scientists learn which proteins are responsible for virulence, crucial information that will lead to new and improved drugs and vaccines. NIAID funds are supporting research for developing a group A streptococcus vaccine. As a result of NIAID-supported research, the first group A streptococci vaccine clinical trial in 30 years was conducted. The vaccine was well tolerated by patients and has led to further clinical evaluation of a similar vaccine candidate. An effective vaccine will prevent not only strep throat and impetigo, but more serious invasive disease and post-infectious complications like rheumatic fever.

Chapter 48

Staphylococcal Skin Infections: Boils

Alternative Names

Infection—hair follicle; hair follicle infection; boils

Definition

A furuncle is an infection of a hair follicle.

Causes, Incidence, and Risk Factors

A furuncle (boil) is a skin infection involving an entire hair follicle and the adjacent subcutaneous tissue.

Furuncles are very common. They are caused by staphylococcus bacteria, which are normally found on the skin surface. Damage to the hair follicle allows these bacteria to enter deeper into the tissues of the follicle and the subcutaneous tissue. Furuncles may occur in the hair follicles anywhere on the body, but they are most common on the face, neck, armpit, buttocks, and thighs.

Furuncles are generally caused by *Staphylococcus aureus*, but they may be caused by other bacteria or fungi. They may begin as a tender, red, subcutaneous nodule but ultimately become fluctuant (feel like a water-filled balloon). A furuncle may drain spontaneously, producing pus. More often the patient or someone else opens the furuncle.

Furuncles can be single or multiple. Some people have recurrent bouts with abscesses and little success at preventing them. Furuncles can be very painful if they occur in areas like the ear canal or nose. A health care provider should treat furuncles of the nose. Furuncles that develop close together may expand and join, causing a condition called carbunculosis.

Symptoms

The lesions themselves are the primary symptoms:

- Small firm tender red nodule in skin (early)
- Fluctuant nodule (later)
- Located with hair follicles
- Tender, mildly to moderately painful
- May be single or multiple
- Usually pea-sized, but may be as large as a golf ball
- Swollen
- Pink or red
- May grow rapidly
- May develop white or yellow centers (pustules)
- May weep, ooze, crust
- May join together or spread to other skin areas
- Increasing pain as pus and dead tissue fills the area
- Decreasing pain as the area drains
- Skin redness or inflammation around the lesion

Less common symptoms include the following:

- Fever
- Fatigue
- General discomfort, uneasiness, or malaise

Note: Itching (pruritus) of the skin may occur before the lesion develops.

Signs and Tests

Diagnosis is primarily based on the appearance of the skin. Skin or mucosal biopsy culture may show staphylococcus or other bacteria.

Treatment

Furuncles may heal on their own after an initial period of itching and mild pain. More often, they progress to pustules that increase in discomfort as pus collects. They finally burst, drain, and then heal spontaneously.

Furuncles usually must drain before they will heal. This most often occurs in less than 2 weeks. Boils that persist longer than 2 weeks, recur, are located on the spine or the middle of the face, or that are accompanied by fever or other symptoms require treatment by a health care provider because of the risk of complications from the spread of infection.

Warm moist compresses encourage furuncles to drain, which speeds healing. Gently soak the area with a warm, moist cloth several times each day. Deep or large lesions may need to be drained surgically by the health care provider. Never squeeze a boil or attempt to lance it at home because this can spread the infection and make it worse.

Meticulous hygiene is vital to prevent the spread of infection. Draining lesions should be cleaned frequently. The hands should be washed thoroughly after touching a boil. Do not reuse or share washcloths or towels. Clothing, washcloths, towels, and sheets or other items that contact infected areas should be washed in very hot (preferably boiling) water. Dressings should be changed frequently and discarded in a manner that contains the drainage, such as by placing them in a bag that can be closed tightly before discarding.

Antibacterial soaps and topical antibiotics are of little benefit once a furuncle has formed. Systemic antibiotics may help to control infection.

Drainage is the definitive treatment.

Expectations (Prognosis)

Full recovery is expected. Some people may experience many repeated episodes.

Complications

- Spread of infection to other parts of the body or skin surfaces

- Abscess formation
- Sepsis (general internal infection)
- Abscess of kidneys or other internal organs
- Osteomyelitis
- Endocarditis
- Brain infection
- Brain abscess
- Spinal cord infection
- Spinal cord abscess
- Permanent scarring

Calling Your Health Care Provider

Call for an appointment with your health care provider if furuncles develop and do not heal with home treatment within one week.

Call for an appointment with your provider if furuncles recur or are located on the face or spine.

Call for an appointment with your provider if boils are accompanied by fever, red streaks extending from the boil, large fluid collections around the boil, or other symptoms.

Prevention

- Good attention to hygiene
- Antibacterial soaps
- Antiseptic washes

Chapter 49

Warts

Many of us have had a wart somewhere on our bodies at some time. But other than being a nuisance, most warts are harmless.

More common in kids than in adults, warts are skin infections caused by viruses of the human papillomavirus (HPV) family. They can affect any area of the body, but are usually found on the fingers, hands, and feet. Warts are usually painless with the exception of the warts on the soles of the feet.

Types of warts include:

- **Common warts.** Usually found on fingers, hands, knees, and elbows, a common wart is a small, hard bump that's dome-shaped and usually grayish-brown. It has a rough surface that may look like the head of a cauliflower, with black dots inside.
- **Flat warts**, also called juvenile warts. These are about the size of a pinhead, are smoother than other kinds of warts, and have flat tops. Flat warts may be pink, light brown, or yellow. Most kids who get flat warts have them on their faces, but they can also grow on arms, knees, or hands and can appear in clusters.
- **Plantar warts.** Found on the bottom of the foot, plantar warts can be very uncomfortable—like walking on a small stone.

This information was provided by KidsHealth, one of the largest resources online for medically reviewed health information written for parents, kids, and teens. For more articles like this one, visit www.KidsHealth.org, or www.TeensHealth.org. Reviewed by Patrice Hyde, M.D., June 2004.

- **Filiform warts.** These have a finger-like shape, are usually flesh-colored, and often grow on or around the mouth, eyes, or nose.

Warts can also involve the genital area, but this article focuses on warts that appear on the rest of the body.

Are warts contagious?

Simply touching a wart on someone doesn't guarantee that you'll get one, too. But the viruses that cause warts are passed from person to person by close physical contact. (You can't, however, get a wart from holding a frog or toad, as your child might have wondered!)

A tiny cut or scratch can make any area of skin more vulnerable to warts. Also, if your child picks at a wart, it can spread to other parts of the body.

The length of time between when a person is exposed to the virus that causes warts and when a wart appears varies. However, warts can grow very slowly and may take weeks or longer, in some cases, to develop.

Can warts be prevented?

Although there's no way to prevent warts, it's always a good idea to encourage kids to wash their hands and skin regularly and well. If your child cuts or scratches his or her skin, be sure to use soap and water to clean the area because open wounds are more susceptible to warts and other infections.

It's also wise to have your child wear waterproof sandals or flip-flops in public showers, locker rooms, and around public pools (this can help protect against plantar warts and other infections, like athlete's foot, too).

How long do warts last?

About 25% of warts are gone in about 6 months without treatment, but most go away in 2 to 3 years. With treatment, warts may be removed more quickly, but can return if the virus isn't completely removed from the skin.

How are warts treated?

Warts don't generally cause any problems, so it's not always necessary to have them removed, unless you have concerns (see the section on When Should I Call My Child's Doctor?). Another reason to treat warts is to prevent them from spreading further.

Doctors have different ways of removing warts, including:

- using prescription medications to put on the wart
- burning the wart off (using a light electrical current)
- freezing the wart with liquid nitrogen (called cryosurgery)
- using laser treatment (which works very well for plantar warts or other warts that are more difficult to remove)

Within a few days after the doctor's treatment, the wart may fall off, but several treatments are sometimes necessary. Doctors don't usually cut off the wart, because it can cause scarring and the wart may return.

If your older child has a simple wart on the finger, talk to your child's doctor about using an over-the-counter wart remedy containing mild acids that help remove the wart. The medicine comes in either a liquid form that's painted on the skin or as a patch that sticks onto the wart. This treatment can take several weeks or months before you see results, but eventually, the wart should crumble away from the healthy skin.

However, wart medicines contain strong chemicals and should be used with care because they can also damage areas of healthy skin. Never use over-the-counter wart medicine on the face or genitals.

It's also important to make sure your child:

- soaks the wart in warm water and removes dead skin on the surface of the wart with an emery board before applying the medicine
- keeps the area of the wart covered while the medicine works
- knows not to rub, scratch, or pick at it to avoid spreading the virus to another part of the body or causing the wart to become infected

You may also have heard that you can use duct tape to remove a wart. Talk to your child's doctor about whether this type of home treatment is OK for your child.

When should I call my child's doctor?

Before you try to remove a wart with a store-bought remedy, call your child's doctor if:

- you have a young child or infant with a wart anywhere on the body.
- your child (of any age) has a wart on the face, genitals, or rectum.

Also call your child's doctor if a wart, that's treated or untreated, or surrounding skin is:

- painful;
- red;
- bleeding;
- swollen;
- oozing pus.

Although they may seem like a nuisance to your child, warts are common in childhood and usually cause no serious problems.

Chapter 50

Human Papillomavirus and Genital Warts

What is human papillomavirus?

Human papillomavirus (HPV) is one of the most common causes of sexually transmitted infection (STI) in the world. More than 100 different types of HPV exist, most of which are harmless. About 30 types are spread through sexual contact. Some types of HPV cause genital warts—single or multiple bumps that appear in the genital areas of men and women including the vagina, cervix, vulva (area outside of the vagina), penis, and rectum. Many people infected with HPV have no symptoms.

There are high-risk and low-risk types of HPV. High-risk HPV may cause abnormal Pap smear results, and could lead to cancers of the cervix, vulva, vagina, anus, or penis. Low-risk HPV also may cause abnormal Pap results or genital warts.

Health experts estimate there are more cases of genital HPV infection than any other STI in the United States. According to the American Social Health Association, approximately 5.5 million new cases of sexually transmitted HPV infections are reported every year. At least 20 million people in this country are already infected.

What are genital warts?

Genital warts (sometimes called condylomata acuminata or venereal warts) are the most easily recognized sign of genital HPV

"Human Papillomavirus and Genital Warts," National Institute of Allergy and Infectious Diseases, July 2004. Available online at http://www.niaid.nih.gov; accessed June 1, 2005.

infection. Many people, however, have a genital HPV infection without genital warts.

Genital warts are soft, moist, or flesh colored and appear in the genital area within weeks or months after infection. They sometimes appear in clusters that resemble cauliflower-like bumps, and are either raised or flat, small or large. Genital warts can show up in women on the vulva and cervix, and inside and surrounding the vagina and anus. In men, genital warts can appear on the scrotum or penis. There are cases where genital warts have been found on the thigh and groin.

Can HPV cause other kinds of warts?

Some types of HPV cause common skin warts, such as those found on the hands and soles of the feet. These types of HPV do not cause genital warts.

How are genital warts spread?

Genital warts are very contagious and are spread during oral, vaginal, or anal sex with an infected partner. They are transmitted by skin-to-skin contact during vaginal, anal, or (rarely) oral sex with someone who is infected. About two thirds of people who have sexual contact with a partner with genital warts will develop warts, usually within 3 months of contact.

In women, the warts occur on the outside and inside of the vagina, on the opening to the uterus (cervix), or around the anus.

In men, genital warts are less common. If present, they usually are seen on the tip of the penis. They also may be found on the shaft of the penis, on the scrotum, or around the anus.

Rarely, genital warts also can develop in your mouth or throat if you have oral sex with an infected person.

Like many STIs, genital HPV infections often do not have signs and symptoms that can be seen or felt. One study sponsored by the National Institute of Allergy and Infectious Diseases (NIAID) reported that almost half of women infected with HPV had no obvious symptoms. If you are infected but have no symptoms, you can still spread HPV to your sexual partner and/or develop complications from the virus.

How are HPV and genital warts diagnosed?

Your health care provider usually diagnoses genital warts by seeing them. If you are a woman with genital warts, you also should be examined for possible HPV infection of the cervix.

Your provider may be able to identify some otherwise invisible warts in your genital tissue by applying vinegar (acetic acid) to areas of your body that might be infected. This solution causes infected areas to whiten, which makes them more visible. In some cases, a health care provider will take a small piece of tissue from the cervix and examine it under the microscope.

If you have an abnormal Pap smear result, it may indicate the possible presence of cervical HPV infection. A laboratory worker will examine cells scraped from your cervix under a microscope to see if they are cancerous.

How are HPV and genital warts treated?

HPV has no known cure. There are treatments for genital warts, though they often disappear even without treatment. There is no way to predict whether the warts will grow or disappear. Therefore, if you suspect you have genital warts, you should be examined and treated, if necessary.

Depending on factors such as the size and location of your genital warts, your health care provider will offer you one of several ways to treat them.

- Imiquimod cream
- 20 percent podophyllin antimitotic solution
- 0.5 percent podofilox solution
- 5 percent 5-fluorouracil cream
- Trichloroacetic acid (TCA)

If you are pregnant, you should not use podophyllin or podofilox because they are absorbed by your skin and may cause birth defects in your baby. In addition, you should not use 5-fluorouracil cream if you are expecting.

If you have small warts, your health care provider can remove them by one of three methods.

- freezing (cryosurgery)
- burning (electrocautery)
- laser treatment

If you have large warts that have not responded to other treatment, you may have to have surgery to remove them.

Some health care providers use the antiviral drug alpha interferon, which they inject directly into the warts, to treat warts that have returned after removal by traditional means. The drug is expensive, however, and does not reduce the rate that the genital warts return.

Although treatments can get rid of the warts, none get rid of the virus. Because the virus is still present in your body, warts often come back after treatment.

How can HPV infection be prevented?

The only way you can prevent getting an HPV infection is to avoid direct contact with the virus, which is transmitted by skin-to-skin contact. If you or your sexual partner has warts that are visible in the genital area, you should avoid any sexual contact until the warts are treated.

Research studies have not confirmed that male latex condoms prevent transmission of HPV, but studies do suggest that using condoms may reduce your risk of developing diseases linked to HPV, such as genital warts and cervical cancer. Unfortunately, many people who don't have symptoms don't know that they can spread the virus to an uninfected partner.

What re the possible complications of HPV and genital warts?

Cancer: Some types of HPV can cause cervical cancer. Other types are associated with vulvar cancer, anal cancer, and cancer of the penis (a rare cancer).

Most HPV infections do not progress to cervical cancer. If you are a woman with abnormal cervical cells, a Pap test will detect them. If you have abnormal cervical cells, it is particularly important for you to have regular pelvic exams and Pap tests so you can be treated early, if necessary.

Pregnancy and Childbirth: Genital warts may cause a number of problems during pregnancy. Sometimes they get larger during pregnancy, making it difficult to urinate. If the warts are in the vagina, they can make the vagina less elastic and cause obstruction during delivery.

Rarely, infants born to women with genital warts develop warts in their throats (laryngeal papillomatosis). Although uncommon, it is a potentially life-threatening condition for the child, requiring frequent laser surgery to prevent obstruction of the breathing passages. Research on the use of interferon therapy with laser surgery indicates that this drug may show promise in slowing the course of the disease.

What research is underway?

Scientists are doing research on two types of HPV vaccines. One type would be used to prevent infection or disease (warts or precancerous tissue changes). The other type would be used to treat cervical cancers. Researchers are testing both types of vaccines in people.

Chapter 51

Cold Sores and Genital Herpes

What is herpes?

Herpes is a common and usually mild infection. It can cause cold sores or fever blisters on the mouth or face (known as oral herpes) and similar symptoms in the genital area (genital herpes).

What causes herpes?

Either of two viruses can cause herpes: herpes simplex type 1 (HSV-1) and herpes simplex type 2 (HSV-2). Both are part of a larger family of herpesviruses that includes varicella zoster virus, the cause of chicken pox and shingles; and Epstein Barr virus, the cause of mononucleosis.

Herpes simplex is different from many other common viral infections in several ways. Most importantly, herpes sets up a lifelong presence in the body. The virus can travel the nerve pathways in a particular part of the body and hide away in the nerve roots for long periods of time.

This means that even though HSV may not be causing cold sores or genital symptoms at a given time, it can still cause symptoms later when HSV wakes up (reactivates) and travels back to the skin.

Excerpted from the "Herpevac Trial for Women," National Institute of Allergy and Infectious Diseases, 2003. Available online at http://www.niaid.nih.gov; accessed June 3, 2005.

What are the symptoms of oral herpes?

The majority of oral herpes infections are caused by HSV-1, and most people contract oral herpes when they are young. This may occur when a child receives a kiss from a person who has a cold sore or from other childhood physical contact (at daycare, for example).

Many people with oral HSV do not have cold sores or other symptoms. It's estimated that only 20% to 40% of people with oral herpes have recurrent cold sores as adults.

Classic symptoms of oral herpes can appear as a single blister or cluster of blisters (cold sores) on the lips but may also occur on other areas around the face such as the cheeks, chin, or nose. Subtle oral HSV symptoms can be easily mistaken for another infection or condition such as a small crack or cut in the skin, chapped lips, bug bite, or a pimple, to name a few examples.

What are the symptoms of genital herpes?

Most often caused by HSV-2, symptoms of genital herpes vary greatly from one person to the next. The majority of people have such mild symptoms that they may not recognize the infection for many years. Out of the one in five adults (males and females) in the United States who have genital herpes, more than 80% have not been diagnosed and are unaware they have it.

The most noticeable symptoms tend to occur shortly after a person contracts the virus, when her or his immune response to herpes is not fully developed (this is called the first episode). Later symptoms tend to be milder because the immune response recognizes the virus and can quickly respond to it.

For some, symptoms during a first episode can be severe, appearing as small fluid-filled blisters that crust over and scab like a small cut, sometimes taking more than two weeks to fully heal. Symptoms of a first episode may also include flu-like symptoms, such as fever and swollen glands, particularly in the groin. On the other hand, most people have first episode symptoms so mild they don't even notice them. It may be another episode, or reactivation, that is first noticed months or even years later.

Right before an outbreak, many people experience an itching, tingling, or burning feeling in the area where their herpes symptoms will develop.

This sort of warning symptom is called a prodrome and often precedes visible signs of infection by a day or two. In some people, prodrome will involve pain in the buttocks, the back of the legs, or even lower back.

How is it that herpes symptoms can go unrecognized?

Many people have very subtle forms of recurrent herpes that can heal in a matter of days. While recurrences of herpes may cause the classic blisters, other symptoms caused by HSV can easily be mistaken for insect bites, ingrown hairs, abrasions, yeast infections, jock itch, hemorrhoids, and other conditions.

Can herpes be active without causing symptoms?

It was once thought that all of HSV's active times were marked by outbreaks—a sore, blister, bump, rash, or some other kind of symptom like an itch. However, researchers have learned that there are days when HSV can become active without causing symptoms. This is often called asymptomatic viral shedding. And during these times, because there are no recognizable signs that the virus has made its way to the skin, there is no way of knowing when asymptomatic shedding is occurring.

How is herpes transmitted?

Herpes is spread most efficiently by direct skin-to-skin contact. More specifically, the soft moist tissue of the mouth and genitals are most vulnerable to HSV if these areas come into contact with the virus.

The following scenarios illustrate how HSV is most often transmitted:

- If a person has a cold sore and kisses someone, the virus can be passed to the other person's mouth.
- If a person has active genital herpes and engages in direct genital-to-genital contact, the virus can be transmitted from her or his genitals to a partner's.
- If someone with a cold sore places his or her mouth on a partner's genitals (oral sex), the partner can contract genital herpes.

Herpes can be transmitted through sexual contact during asymptomatic viral shedding or times when there are no obvious symptoms. Herpes is often passed by people who do not know they have herpes, or by people who simply don't recognize that their herpes infection is in an active phase.

Can herpes be prevented?

Preventing herpes can be a difficult challenge. First, HSV is widespread, with more than two out of three adults infected with HSV-1 or HSV-2. Second, most people who have HSV are unaware that they have the infection. And third, even among those who are aware of their infection, there are times of asymptomatic viral shedding when HSV becomes active without symptoms and can be transmitted.

While there are vaccines in development to prevent herpes, currently the only 100% effective method of preventing genital herpes infection is to abstain from any form of genital-to-genital contact or oral-to-genital contact.

However, given that most adults will have a sexual relationship at some point in their lives, it is important to understand how herpes is transmitted along with other ways to reduce the risk of contracting the virus.

How can one reduce the risk of getting herpes?

In a sexual relationship, there are ways to reduce the risk of contracting herpes:

- **Talk.** Talk with a partner about herpes, other sexually transmitted diseases, and birth control before engaging in sexual contact. Finding out if a partner has herpes or other sexually transmitted diseases (STD)s can help both individuals decide which precautions are right for them.
- **Avoid skin-to-skin contact with herpes lesions.** If your partner has a cold sore or a genital lesion, avoid kissing, oral-genital, or genital-to-genital contact. Symptoms of prodrome and outbreaks indicate viral activity and pose the greatest risk of passing the virus to another person.
- **Use condoms between outbreaks as a guard against unrecognized herpes.** Consistent and correct use of condoms effectively reduces (but does not eliminate) the risk of contracting herpes. Condoms are not recommended as protection during herpes outbreaks because a lesion may be in a place the condom doesn't cover. But they decrease the risk of genital herpes during asymptomatic shedding, especially if used consistently.

- **Antiviral medication may help.** For individuals with genital herpes, taking a 500-milligram dose of valacyclovir each day has been shown to decrease the risk of a partner developing genital herpes symptoms by 77% and the overall risk of HSV infection by 50%.

What about testing for herpes?

There are several tests for herpes. If signs and symptoms are present, a health care provider can look at the area, take a sample (culture) from the symptomatic area, and test to see if the herpes virus is present.

From this culture test, a second test can be run to tell whether the virus present is HSV-1 or HSV-2. A culture test will not work if the lesions have healed, and might not work if they're more than a few days old.

Blood tests are also available to test to see if a person has herpes. Type-specific blood tests can accurately determine if a person has HSV-1 and/or HSV-2 by looking for an immune response (antibodies) to the virus. Some older blood tests for herpes are not type-specific and can give false results. Therefore, if a blood test is performed, it is important to ensure that it can accurately identify HSV antibodies.

Chapter 52

Varicella Disease (Chickenpox)

What is varicella (chickenpox)?

Chickenpox is an infectious disease caused by the varicella zoster virus, which results in a blister-like rash, itching, tiredness, and fever.

The rash appears first on the trunk and face, but can spread over the entire body causing between 250 to 500 itchy blisters. Most cases of chickenpox occur in persons less than 15 years old. Prior to the use of varicella vaccine, the disease had annual cycles, peaking in the spring of each year.

How do you get chickenpox?

Chickenpox is highly infectious and spreads from person to person by direct contact or through the air from an infected person's coughing or sneezing. A person with chickenpox is contagious 1 to 2 days before the rash appears and until all blisters have formed scabs. It takes from 10–21 days after contact with an infected person for someone to develop chickenpox.

What is the chickenpox illness like?

In children, chickenpox most commonly causes an illness that lasts about 5 to 10 days. Children usually miss 5 or 6 days of school or child

---

"Varicella Disease (Chickenpox)," Centers for Disease Control and Prevention, December 20, 2001. Available online at http://www.cdc.gov; accessed June 1, 2005.

care due to their chickenpox. About half of all children with chickenpox visit a health care provider due to symptoms of their illness such as high fever, severe itching, an uncomfortable rash, dehydration, or headache. In addition, about 1 child in 10 has a complication from chickenpox serious enough to visit a health care provider including infected skin lesions, other infections, dehydration from vomiting or diarrhea, exacerbation of asthma or more serious complications such as pneumonia.

Certain groups of persons are more likely to have more serious illness with complications. These include adults, infants, adolescents, and people with weak immune systems from either illnesses or from medications such a long-term steroids.

What are the serious complications from chickenpox?

Serious complications from chickenpox include bacterial infections, which can involve many sites of the body including the skin, tissues under the skin, bone, lungs (pneumonia), joints, and the blood. Other serious complications are due directly to the virus infection and include viral pneumonia, bleeding problems, and infection of the brain (encephalitis). Many people are not aware that, before a vaccine was available, there were approximately 11,000 hospitalizations and 100 deaths from chickenpox in the United States every year. One child and one adult died each week.

Can a healthy person with varicella die from the disease?

Yes, many of the deaths and complications from chickenpox occur in previously healthy children and adults. From 1990 to 1994, before there was a vaccine available, there were about 50 chickenpox deaths in children and 50 chickenpox deaths in adults every year; most of these persons were healthy or did not have a medical illness (such as cancer) that placed them at higher risk of getting severe chickenpox.

Since 1999, states have been encouraged to report chickenpox deaths to the Centers for Disease Control and Prevention (CDC). In 1999 and 2000, CDC received reports that showed that deaths from chickenpox continue to occur in healthy, unvaccinated children and adults. Most of the healthy adults who died from chickenpox contracted the disease from their unvaccinated children.

Can chickenpox be prevented?

Yes, chickenpox can now be prevented by vaccination.

Can you get chickenpox more than once?

Yes, but it is uncommon to do so. For most people, one infection is thought to confer lifelong immunity.

Chickenpox in children is usually not serious. Why not let children get the disease?

It is never possible to predict who will have a mild case of chickenpox and who will have a serious or even deadly case of disease. Now that there is a safe and effective vaccine available, it is not worth taking this chance.

Chapter 53

Shingles

In Italy, shingles also is called St. Anthony's fire, a fitting name for a disease that has bedeviled saints and sinners throughout the ages. Caused by the same varicella-zoster virus that causes chickenpox, shingles (also called herpes zoster) most commonly occurs in older people. Treatment was once limited to wet compresses and aspirin. Today's treatments provide a variety of ways to shorten the duration of a shingles outbreak and to control the associated pain. Sometimes, however, shingles leads to a chronic painful condition called postherpetic neuralgia (PHN) that can be difficult to treat.

Initial Symptoms

After an attack of chickenpox, the varicella-zoster virus retreats to nerve cells in the body, where it may lie dormant for decades. But under certain conditions, usually related to aging or disease, the virus can reactivate and begin to reproduce. Once activated, the virus travels along the path of a nerve to the skin's surface, where it causes shingles.

Shingles' symptoms may be vague and nonspecific at first. People with shingles may experience numbness, tingling, itching, or pain before the classic rash appears. In the pre-eruption stage, diagnosis may be difficult, and the pain can be so severe that it may be mistaken

---

Excerpted from "Shingles: An Unwelcome Encore," by Evelyn Zamula, U.S. Food and Drug Administration, *FDA Consumer* Magazine, May-June 2001. Available online at http://www.fda.gov; accessed June 3, 2005.

for pleurisy, kidney stones, gallstones, appendicitis, or even a heart attack, depending on the location of the affected nerve.

The Outbreak

Pain may come first, but when the migrating virus finally reaches the skin—usually the second to the fifth day after the first symptoms—the rash tells all. The virus infects the skin cells and creates a painful, red rash that resembles chickenpox.

Doctors can distinguish shingles from chickenpox (or dermatitis or poison ivy) by the way the spots are distributed. Since shingles occurs in an area of the skin that is supplied by sensory fibers of a single nerve—called a dermatome—the rash usually appears in a well-defined band on one side of the body, typically the torso; or on one side of the face, around the nose and eyes. (Shingles' peculiar name derives from the Latin *cingulum*, which means girdle or belt.) If a diagnosis is in doubt, lab tests can confirm the presence of the virus.

The rash usually begins as clusters of small bumps that soon develop into fluid-filled blisters (vesicles). In turn, the blisters fill with pus (pustules), break open, and form crusty scabs. In about four or five weeks, the disease runs its course, the scabs drop off, the skin heals, and the pain fades. Most healthy individuals make an uneventful, if not particularly pleasant, recovery.

Not everyone sails through without incident, however. Although it's difficult to resist scratching the itchy rash, it's better to keep hands off, as the damaged skin may develop a bacterial infection requiring antibiotic treatment. After such an infection, the skin may be left with significant scarring, some of it serious enough to require plastic surgery.

Another complication called the Ramsay Hunt syndrome occurs when the varicella-zoster virus spreads to the facial nerve, causing intense ear pain. The rash can appear on the outer ear, inside the ear canal, on the soft palate (part of the roof of the mouth), around the mouth, and on the face, neck and scalp. The hearing loss, vertigo, and facial paralysis that may result are usually, but not always, temporary.

Occasionally, the rash will appear as a single spot or cluster of spots on the tip of the nose, called Hutchinson's sign. This is not good news. It means that the ophthalmic nerve is probably involved and the eye may become affected, possibly causing temporary or permanent blindness.

"My husband was undergoing chemotherapy treatment for prostate cancer," says Julia Hershfield, of Kensington, Maryland, "when he developed shingles in his right eye. The pain was so bad, that he lost all will to live. Shingles finished him." In people whose immune systems are extremely weakened, the shingles virus can also spread to the internal organs and affect the lungs, central nervous system, and the brain, sometimes causing death.

Chickenpox Redux

Like other members of the herpes family (such as the herpes simplex viruses that cause cold sores and genital herpes), the varicella-zoster virus that causes chickenpox never completely leaves the body. Most people don't get chickenpox a second time. However, anyone who has had chickenpox has the potential to develop shingles, because after recovery from chickenpox, the virus settles in the nerve roots.

Researchers are not sure exactly what triggers the virus to spontaneously start reproducing in nerve cells later in life and reappear as shingles. However, they do know the virus may reactivate when the immune system is weak.

Certain factors can cause the immune system to let down its guard. Age is one of them. Immunity declines with aging, so susceptibility to disease increases. The incidence of shingles and of resulting PHN rises with increasing age. More than 50 percent of cases occur in people over 60. Older people may also lack exposure to children with chickenpox, thereby losing an opportunity to boost immunity and prevent virus reactivation. Although most people have only one attack of shingles, about 4 percent will have further attacks.

People who have had chickenpox cannot "catch" shingles from someone who has it. However, people who've never had chickenpox can be infected with chickenpox if exposed to someone with an active case of shingles. The rash sheds the varicella-zoster virus and can be contagious. A caregiver or other person who lacks immunity developed from a prior case of chickenpox or the vaccine must avoid coming into contact with the rash or contaminated materials.

Also at risk for shingles are people with leukemia, lymphoma, or Hodgkin's disease, and those whose immune systems have been weakened because they are HIV positive, or have undergone chemotherapy, radiation, transplant surgery with immunosuppression, or treatment with corticosteroids. Moreover, about 5 percent of people with shingles are found to have an underlying cancer, about twice the number of people in the population expected to have undiagnosed cancer.

It pays to be vigilant when unexplained symptoms occur. "New development of a rash or pain, especially when it occurs on only one side of the chest or face, should prompt a visit to the health-care provider," says Therese A. Cvetkovich, M.D., a medical officer in the Food and Drug Administration's Center for Drug Evaluation and Research (CDER).

Controlling the Outbreak

Although viral diseases can't be cured, doctors can prescribe oral antiviral medications, such as Zovirax (acyclovir), Famvir (famciclovir), and Valtrex (valacyclovir), that help control the infection by hindering reproduction of the virus in the nerve cells. "Antiviral therapy may shorten the course of an episode of shingles," says Cvetkovich. "However, therapy must be started as early as possible after symptoms develop—within 48 hours—in order to have an effect."

To relieve pain, the doctor may recommend over-the-counter analgesics (pain-relieving drugs), such as ibuprofen and naproxen, or prescription drugs, such as indomethacin, all members of a class of medications known as nonsteroidal anti-inflammatory drugs. Acetaminophen is also commonly used to relieve the pain. If pain is severe, doctors may add stronger analgesics, such as codeine or oxycodone.

When the Pain Persists

In some patients, the misery continues long after the rash has healed. Many of the 1 million people who develop shingles each year experience a complication called post-herpetic neuralgia (PHN). This term refers to pain that is present in the affected area for months, or even years, afterward. Although the acute pain of shingles and the chronic pain of PHN (called neuropathic pain) both originate in the nerve cells, their duration and the reaction to treatment is different.

Pain that occurs with the initial outbreak responds to treatment and is limited in duration. In contrast, PHN lasts longer, is difficult to treat and can be incapacitating. Furthermore, for unknown reasons, older people suffer more from this debilitating pain than younger people. In many individuals, the skin is so sensitive that clothing or even a passing breeze cannot be tolerated on the affected area. Described by PHN sufferers as agonizing, excruciating, and burning, the pain can result in an inability to perform daily tasks of living, and lead to loss of independence and, ultimately, depression and isolation.

"I would rather have ten babies than the pain I've endured for the past ten years," says 87-year-old Etta Watson Zukerman of Bethesda, Maryland, who has lost partial use of her right arm and hand due to nerve damage from PHN. "Nothing my doctor prescribed helped. I even went to a sports medicine specialist who recommended exercises. They didn't help either." Many PHN sufferers receive no relief at all, no matter what medications or therapies they use. And what works for one doesn't necessarily work for another.

Treating the Pain

Doctors use other methods to alleviate pain with varying degrees of success. "One of the relatively new medications that I'm enthusiastic about is the Lidoderm patch," says Veronica Mitchell, M.D., director of the pain management center and inpatient pain service at Georgetown University Hospital, Washington, D.C. "It's the transdermal form of lidocaine and it's been studied in the PHN population with very good results," adds Mitchell. "We prescribed the Lidoderm patch for a patient who had intolerable side effects with oral medications—and no relief—and she's had about a 50 percent-plus improvement in pain relief. It's one of my first-line therapies." The medication contained in this soft, pliable patch penetrates the skin, reaching the damaged nerves just under the skin without being absorbed significantly into the bloodstream. This means that the patch can be used for long periods of time without serious side effects.

Yet another method used to treat PHN is transcutaneous electrical nerve stimulation, or TENS. A device that generates low-level pulses of electrical current is applied to the skin's surface, causing tingling sensations and offering some people pain relief. One theory as to how TENS works is that the electrical current stimulates production of endorphins, the body's natural painkillers.

TENS is not for everyone. "TENS didn't help at all," says Einar Raysor of Rockville, Maryland. "I found there was a problem in fine-tuning the administration of the electrical current. Low doses of the electrical current didn't do anything for me. When the technician increased the current, it gave me a painful response. After this happened a couple of times, we dropped the treatment."

As a last resort, invasive procedures called nerve blocks may be used to provide temporary relief. These procedures usually entail the injection of a local anesthetic into the area of the affected nerves. "We have controversial results in the terms of the efficacy of nerve blocks," says Mitchell. "I do consider nerve blocks in treating PHN and I would perform them because there's some evidence that they work, but the real efficacy is to catch and treat the patient in the acute shingles phase. As PHN presents mostly in the elderly, and the older patient often is unable to tolerate some of the medications we use, I find nerve blocks useful in these cases."

Injection directly into the spine is another option for relief of pain that is not easily treated. A Japanese clinical study published in the *New England Journal of Medicine* found that an injection of the steroid methylprednisolone combined with the anesthetic lidocaine reduced pain by more than 70 percent in one patient group compared with groups that received lidocaine alone or an inactive substance.

Prevention, Almost Perfect

Before the FDA approved the chickenpox vaccine in 1995, about 95 percent of the U.S. population developed chickenpox before age 18. Since then, more than 60 percent of American youngsters have been vaccinated against chickenpox.

"The vaccine is a live attenuated strain of the chickenpox virus," says Philip R. Krause, M.D., lead research investigator in the FDA's Center for Biologics Evaluation and Research. "However, it's a weaker form so it gives rise to a milder infection. But in the course of giving rise to this milder infection, it induces enough immunity to prevent people from getting the natural infection." It is estimated that the vaccine is between 75 and 85 percent effective in preventing chickenpox. "But the important thing," says Krause, "is that it is almost completely effective in preventing severe cases of chickenpox."

Now that we have a chickenpox vaccine, are shingles and PHN on their way out? Although the FDA hasn't evaluated the effects of the vaccine on shingles, Krause believes that "in the long term, if you can prevent enough people from getting the wild (natural) type of chickenpox, you're likely to see a beneficial effect on the incidence of shingles and post-herpetic neuralgia. But it may take several generations for this to happen."

—by Evelyn Zamula, freelance writer in Potomac, Maryland

Chapter 54

Molluscum Contagiosum

What is molluscum contagiosum?

A skin disease caused by the molluscum contagiosum virus (MCV) usually causing one or more small lesions/bumps. MCV is generally a benign infection and symptoms may self-resolve. MCV was once a disease primarily of children, but it has evolved to become a sexually transmitted disease in adults. It is believed to be a member of the pox virus family.

How is molluscum contagiosum transmitted?

- Molluscum contagiosum may be sexually transmitted by skin-to-skin contact (does not have to be mucous membranes) and/or lesions. Transmission through sexual contact is the most common form of transmission for adults.
- MCV may be transmitted from inanimate objects such as towels and clothing that come in contact with the lesions. MCV transmission has been associated with swimming pools and sharing baths with an infected person.

 For additional information, contact the American Social Health Association (ASHA) at P.O. Box 13827, Research Triangle Park, NC 27709, (919) 361-8400, or visit the ASHA website at http://www.ashastd.org.

- MCV also may be transmitted by autoinoculation, such as touching a lesion and touching another part of the body.

What is the incubation period for molluscum contagiosum?

The incubation period averages 2 to 3 months and may range from 1 week to 6 months.

How long are you infectious?

This is not known for certain, but researchers assume that if the virus is present it may be transmitted.

What are the symptoms of molluscum contagiosum?

- Lesions are usually present on the thighs, buttocks, groin and lower abdomen of adults, and may occasionally appear on the external genital and anal region.
- Children typically develop lesions on the face, trunk, legs, and arms.
- The lesions may begin as small bumps which can develop over a period of several weeks into larger sores/bumps. The lesions can be flesh-colored, gray-white, yellow, or pink. They can cause itching or tenderness in the area, but in most cases the lesions cause few problems. Lesions can last from 2 weeks to 4 years—the average is 2 years.
- People with AIDS or others with compromised immune systems may develop extensive outbreaks.

How is molluscum contagiosum diagnosed?

Diagnosis is usually made by the characteristic appearance of the lesion. MCV may be diagnosed by collecting a specimen from the lesion, placing it onto a slide and staining with a Gram stain which shows changes in infected cells. Diagnosis may be made by collecting a specimen from the lesion and viewing it under an electron microscope.

How is molluscum contagiosum treated?

- Most symptoms are self-resolving, but generally lesions are removed. Removal of lesions reduces autoinoculation and transmission to others.

- Lesions can be removed surgically and/or treated with a chemical agent such as podophyllin, cantharidin, phenol, silver nitrate, trichloroacetic acid, or iodine.
- Cryotherapy is an alternative method of removal.

Lesions may recur, but it is not clear whether this is due to reinfection, exacerbation of subclinical infection, or reactivation of latent infection.

How can I keep from getting molluscum contagiosum?

- Because transmission through sexual contact is the most common form of transmission for adults, preventing skin-to-skin contact with an infected partner will be most effective in preventing MCV.
- Latex condoms or other moisture barriers for vaginal, oral, and anal sex may help to prevent such contact. Limitations of such barriers must be recognized as MCV does not require mucous membrane contact to be passed.
- Using water-based spermicide for vaginal intercourse. Spermicide is not recommended for oral sex, and has not been found safe or effective for anal intercourse.
- Using condoms may protect the penis or vagina from infection, but do not protect from contact with other areas such as the scrotum or anal area.
- Mutual monogamy (sex with only one uninfected partner).

If you do get molluscum contagiosum, avoid touching the lesion and then touching another part of the body without washing your hands to prevent chance of autoinoculation.

What about complications from molluscum contagiosum?

In people with HIV infection, molluscum contagiosum is often a progressive disease.

Chapter 55

Tinea Infections

Chapter Contents

Section 55.1

Athlete's Foot, Jock Itch, and Ringworm

If your kids are active, chances are that locker-room showers and heaps of sweaty clothing are part of their everyday lives. It's important to take the proper precautions so that your child doesn't develop fungal skin infections that can be itchy and uncomfortable.

Jock itch, athlete's foot, and ringworm are all types of fungal skin infections known collectively as tinea. They are caused by fungi called dermatophytes that live on skin, hair, and nails and thrive in warm, moist areas.

Symptoms of these infections can vary depending on where they are on the body. The source of the fungus is usually the soil, an animal (usually a cat, dog, or rodent), or most often, another person. Minor trauma to the skin (for instance, scratches) and poor skin hygiene increase the potential for infection.

It's important to learn some of the signs and symptoms of these infections so that you can get the proper treatment for your child. Many of these infections can be treated with over-the-counter medication, but some of them may require treatment from your child's doctor.

Ringworm

Ringworm isn't a worm, but a fungal infection of the scalp or skin that got its name from the ring or series of rings that it can produce. Ringworm may first appear on your child as a red, scaly patch or bump on the skin that becomes very itchy. It may cause your child to experience dandruff-like scaling and hair loss (with broken stubbles of hair).

Symptoms of Ringworm

Ringworm of the scalp may start as a small sore that resembles a pimple before becoming patchy, flaky, or scaly. These flakes may be confused with dandruff. It may cause some hair to fall out or break into stubbles. It can also cause the scalp to become swollen, tender, and red.

Sometimes, there may be a swollen, inflamed mass known as a kerion, which oozes fluid. These symptoms can be confused with impetigo or cellulitis. The distinctive features of ringworm are itching, redness on the skin, and a circular patchy lesion that spreads along its borders and clears at the center.

Ringworm of the nails may affect one or more nails on your child's hands or feet. The nails may become thick, white or yellowish, and brittle.

If you suspect that your child has ringworm, you may want to call your child's doctor.

Treating Ringworm

Ringworm is fairly easy to diagnose and treat. Most of the time, the doctor can diagnose it by looking at it or by scraping off a small sample of the flaky infected skin to test for the fungus. The doctor may recommend an antifungal ointment for ringworm of the skin or an oral medication for ringworm of the scalp and nails.

Preventing Ringworm

A child usually gets ringworm from another infected person, so it's important to encourage your child to avoid sharing combs, brushes, pillows, and hats with others.

Jock Itch

Jock itch, an infection of the groin and upper thighs, got its name because cases are commonly seen in active kids who sweat a lot while playing sports. But the fungus that causes the jock itch infection can thrive on the skin of any kids who spend time in hot and humid weather, wear tight clothing like bathing suits that cause friction, share towels and clothing, and don't completely dry off their skin. It can last for weeks or months if it goes untreated.

Symptoms of Jock Itch

The symptoms of jock itch may include:

- itching, chafing, or burning in the groin, thigh, or anal area
- skin redness in the groin, thigh, or anal area
- flaking, peeling, or cracking skin

Treating Jock Itch

Jock itch can usually be treated with over-the-counter antifungal creams and sprays. If you are using one of these substances, make sure that your child takes the following steps so that the treatment is as effective as possible:

- Wash and then dry the area using a clean towel.
- Apply the antifungal cream, powder, or spray as directed on the label.
- Change clothing, especially the underwear, every day.
- Continue this treatment for 2 weeks, even if symptoms disappear, to prevent the infection from recurring.

If the ointment or spray is not effective, you may want to call your child's doctor, who can prescribe other treatment.

Preventing Jock Itch

Jock itch can be prevented by keeping the groin area clean and dry, particularly after showering, swimming, and performing sweaty activities.

Athlete's Foot

Athlete's foot typically affects the soles of the feet, the areas between the toes, and sometimes the toenails. It can also spread to the palms of the hands, the groin, or the underarms if your child touches the affected foot and then touches another body part. The condition got its name because it affects people whose feet tend to be damp and sweaty, which is often the case with athletes.

Symptoms of Athlete's Foot

The symptoms of athlete's foot may include itching, burning, redness, and stinging on the soles of the feet. The skin may flake, peel, blister, or crack.

Treating Athlete's Foot

A doctor can often diagnose athlete's foot simply by examining your child's foot or by taking a small scraping of the affected skin to detect the presence of the fungus that causes athlete's foot.

Over-the-counter antifungal creams and sprays may effectively treat mild cases of athlete's foot within a few weeks. Athlete's foot can recur or be more serious. If that's the case, you may want to call your child's doctor who may prescribe a stronger treatment.

Preventing Athlete's Foot

Because the fungus that causes athlete's foot thrives in warm, moist areas, infections can be prevented by keeping your child's feet and the space between the toes clean and dry.

Athlete's foot is contagious and can be spread in damp areas, such as public showers or pool areas, so you may want take some extra precautions with the feet. You may want to encourage your child to:

- wear waterproof shoes or flip-flops in public showers, like those in locker rooms
- alternate shoes or sneakers to prevent moisture buildup and fungus growth
- avoid socks that trap moisture or make the feet sweat and instead choose cotton or wool socks or socks made of fabric that wicks away the moisture
- choose sneakers that are well ventilated with small holes to keep the feet dry

By taking the proper precautions and teaching them to your child, you can prevent these uncomfortable skin infections from putting a crimp in your active child's lifestyle.

Section 55.2

Tinea Versicolor

Reprinted with permission from the American Osteopathic College of Dermatology (AOCD), © 2005. All rights reserved. For additional information, visit the AOCD website at www.aocd.org.

Tinea versicolor is caused by a yeast type of skin fungus, which is present on normal skin. If the skin is oily enough, warm enough, and moist enough, it starts to grow into small "colonies" on the surface of the skin. In these colonies the yeast grows like crazy and leaks out an acidic bleach. This changes the skin color. The patches are light reddish brown on very pale skin but they don't tan. Because of lack of any tanning, they look like white spots on darker or tanned skin. This is most often seen on the neck, upper chest, upper arms, and back. There may be a fine, dry scale on it.

Usually the infection produces few symptoms, but some people get itching, especially when sweating. The warmer the weather, the worse this condition gets. Tanning booths are warm places, so avoid them. The reasons why some get this problem and others do not are not known.

A dermatologist can easily recognize this infection, but occasionally it can be mistaken for other skin conditions. If there is any doubt a KOH prep, a test done quickly in the office, will confirm the diagnosis.

The infection is treated with either topical or oral medications. In very mild cases, nonprescription antifungal creams will work. Prescription antifungal lotions and sprays may work better. The most economical effective treatment is to apply an antifungal shampoo (Nizoral, Loprox) to the body as if it were soap, but leave it on for some minutes before rinsing.

For severe, extensive, or recurrent cases, a few tablets of Nizoral pills will clear things up. A newer pill, Sporanox, may replace Nizoral for this problem. These will eliminate the fungus and relive any itch and scale. The uneven color of the skin will remain several months, perhaps until one gets a tan again the next summer.

Remember, since we all have some of this fungus, no treatment can prevent one from picking it up again. In many people, the rash reappears for the next few years. To prevent recurrence, preventative retreatment with the same medication may be advised. This condition is not seen beyond midlife, so rest assured it won't keep coming back forever.

Chapter 56

Sporotrichosis and Yeast Skin Infections

Chapter Contents

Section 56.1

Sporotrichosis

From the Centers for Disease Control and Prevention (CDC), February 17, 2004. Available online at http://www.cdc.gov; accessed June 1, 2005.

What is sporotrichosis?

Sporotrichosis is a fungal infection caused by a fungus called *Sporothrix schenckii*. It usually infects the skin.

Who gets sporotrichosis?

Persons handling thorny plants, sphagnum moss, or baled hay are at increased risk of getting sporotrichosis. Outbreaks have occurred among nursery workers handling sphagnum moss, rose gardeners, children playing on baled hay, and greenhouse workers handling bayberry thorns contaminated by the fungus. A number of cases have recently occurred among nursery workers, especially workers handling sphagnum moss topiaries.

How is the fungus spread?

The fungus can be found in sphagnum moss, in hay, in other plant materials, and in the soil. It enters the skin through small cuts or punctures from thorns, barbs, pine needles, or wires. It is not spread from person to person.

What are the symptoms of sporotrichosis?

The first symptom is usually a small painless bump resembling an insect bite. It can be red, pink, or purple in color. The bump (nodule) usually appears on the finger, hand, or arm where the fungus first enters through a break on the skin. This is followed by one or more additional bumps or nodules, which open and may resemble boils. Eventually lesions look like open sores (ulcerations) and are very slow to heal. The infection can spread to other areas of the body.

Does sporotrichosis involve any other organs besides the skin?

The majority of infections are limited to the skin. Cases of joint, lung, and central nervous system infection have occurred but are very rare. Usually they occur only in persons with previous disorders of the immune system.

How soon do symptoms appear?

The first nodule may appear any time from 1 to 12 weeks after exposure to the fungus. Usually the nodules are visible within 3 weeks after the fungus enters the skin.

How is sporotrichosis diagnosed?

Sporotrichosis can be confirmed when a doctor obtains a swab or a biopsy of a freshly opened skin nodule and submits it to a laboratory for fungal culture.

If I have symptoms should I see my doctor?

Yes. It is important for the diagnosis to be confirmed by a doctor so that proper treatment can be provided.

How is sporotrichosis treated?

Sporotrichosis is generally treated with potassium iodide, taken by mouth in droplet form. A new drug, called itraconazole (Sporanox), is available for treatment, but experience with this drug is still limited. Treatment is often extended over a number of weeks, until the skin lesions are completely healed.

How can sporotrichosis be prevented?

Control measures include wearing gloves and long sleeves when handling wires, rose bushes, hay bales, conifer (pine) seedlings, or other materials that may cause minor skin breaks. It is also advisable to avoid skin contact with sphagnum moss. Moss has been implicated as a source of the fungus in a number of outbreaks.

Section 56.2

Cutaneous Candidiasis (Yeast Skin Infection)

Definition

Cutaneous candidiasis is an infection of the skin caused by the fungus candida.

Causes, Incidence, and Risk Factors

The body normally hosts a variety of microorganisms including bacteria and fungi. Some of these are useful to the body, some produce no harm or benefits, while others may cause harmful infections.

Fungal infections are caused by microscopic organisms (fungi) that can live on the skin. They can live on the dead tissues of the hair, nails and outer skin layers. Fungal infections include mold-like fungi (dermatophytes, which cause tinea infections) and yeast-like fungi (such as candida).

Cutaneous candidiasis involves infection of the skin with candida. It may involve almost any skin surface on the body, but usually occurs in warm, moist, creased areas (such as armpits and groins). Cutaneous candidiasis is fairly common.

Candida is the most common cause of diaper rash in infants, where it takes advantage of the warm moist conditions inside the diaper. The most common fungus to cause these infections is *Candida albicans*.

Candida infection is particularly common in individuals with diabetes and in people who are obese. Antibiotics and oral contraceptives increase the risk of cutaneous candidiasis. Candida can also cause infections of the nail, referred to as onychomycosis, and infections around the corners of the mouth, called angular cheilitis.

Oral thrush, a form of candida infection found on the mucous membranes of the mouth, may be a sign of HIV infection or other immunodeficiency disorders when it occurs in adults. Infected individuals are not usually considered infectious to others, though in some settings transmission to immunocompromised people can occur.

Candida is also the most frequent cause of vaginal yeast infections, which are extremely common.

Symptoms

- itching (may be intense)
- skin lesion or rash
    - skin redness or inflammation
    - enlarging patch
    - macule or papule
    - may have satellite lesions
    - located on the skin folds, genitals, trunk, buttocks, under the breasts or other skin areas
    - infection of hair follicles ("folliculitis") may have a pimple-like appearance

Signs and Tests

Diagnosis is primarily based on the appearance of the skin, particularly if risk factors are present. A skin scraping can show typical yeast forms, suggestive of candida.

Treatment

General hygiene is vital to the treatment of cutaneous candidiasis; keeping the skin dry and exposed to air is helpful. Weight loss may eliminate the problem in obese people, and good sugar control in diabetics may also be helpful. Topical antifungal medications may be used to treat infection of the skin; systemic antifungal medications may be necessary for folliculitis or nail infection.

Expectations (Prognosis)

Cutaneous candidiasis is usually treatable, but occasionally is difficult to eradicate. Recurrence is common.

Complications

- Recurrence of candida skin infection
- Infection of nails may cause nails to become oddly shaped and may cause paronychia (infection around the nail)

- Disseminated candidiasis may occur in immunocompromised individuals

Calling Your Health Care Provider

Call for an appointment with your health care provider if symptoms indicate cutaneous candidiasis.

Prevention

Good general health and hygiene help prevent candida infections. Keep the skin clean and dry. Drying powders may help prevent fungal infections in people who are susceptible to them. Weight loss and good sugar control in diabetics may help prevent these infections.

Chapter 57

Scabies

What is scabies?

Scabies is an infestation of the skin with the microscopic mite *Sarcoptes scabei*. Infestation is common, found worldwide, and affects people of all races and social classes. Scabies spreads rapidly under crowded conditions where there is frequent skin-to-skin contact between people, such as in hospitals, institutions, child-care facilities, and nursing homes.

What are the signs and symptoms of scabies infestation?

- Pimple-like irritations, burrows or rash of the skin, especially the webbing between the fingers; the skin folds on the wrist, elbow, or knee; the penis, the breast, or shoulder blades.
- Intense itching, especially at night and over most of the body.
- Sores on the body caused by scratching. These sores can sometimes become infected with bacteria.

How did I get scabies?

By direct, prolonged, skin-to-skin contact with a person already infested with scabies. Contact must be prolonged (a quick handshake

---

From the Centers for Disease Control and Prevention (CDC), February 10, 2005. Available online at http://www.cdc.gov; accessed June 2, 2005.

or hug will usually not spread infestation). Infestation is easily spread to sexual partners and household members. Infestation may also occur by sharing clothing, towels, and bedding.

Who is at risk for severe infestation?

People with weakened immune systems and the elderly are at risk for a more severe form of scabies, called Norwegian or crusted scabies.

How long will mites live?

Once away from the human body, mites do not survive more than 48 to 72 hours. When living on a person, an adult female mite can live up to a month.

Did my pet spread scabies to me?

No. Pets become infested with a different kind of scabies mite. If your pet is infested with scabies, (also called mange) and they have close contact with you, the mite can get under your skin and cause itching and skin irritation. However, the mite dies in a couple of days and does not reproduce. The mites may cause you to itch for several days, but you do not need to be treated with special medication to kill the mites. Until your pet is successfully treated, mites can continue to burrow into your skin and cause you to have symptoms.

How soon after infestation will symptoms begin?

For a person who has never been infested with scabies, symptoms may take 4 to 6 weeks to begin. For a person who has had scabies, symptoms appear within several days. You do not become immune to an infestation.

How is scabies infestation diagnosed?

Diagnosis is most commonly made by looking at the burrows or rash. A skin scraping may be taken to look for mites, eggs, or mite fecal matter to confirm the diagnosis. If a skin scraping or biopsy is taken and returns negative, it is possible that you may still be infested. Typically, there are fewer than 10 mites on the entire body of an infested person; this makes it easy for an infestation to be missed.

Can scabies be treated?

Yes. Several lotions are available to treat scabies. Always follow the directions provided by your physician or the directions on the package insert. Apply lotion to a clean body from the neck down to the toes and left overnight (8 hours). After 8 hours, take a bath or shower to wash off the lotion. Put on clean clothes. All clothes, bedding, and towels used by the infested person 2 days before treatment should be washed in hot water; dry in a hot dryer. A second treatment of the body with the same lotion may be necessary 7 to 10 days later. Pregnant women and children are often treated with milder scabies medications.

Who should be treated for scabies?

Anyone who is diagnosed with scabies, as well as his or her sexual partners and persons who have close, prolonged contact to the infested person should also be treated. If your health care provider has instructed family members to be treated, everyone should receive treatment at the same time to prevent reinfestation.

How soon after treatment will I feel better?

Itching may continue for 2 to 3 weeks, and does not mean that you are still infested. Your health care provider may prescribe additional medication to relieve itching if it is severe. No new burrows or rashes should appear 24 to 48 hours after effective treatment.

Chapter 58

Lice (Pediculosis)

Chapter Contents

Section 58.1

Head Lice

"Head Lice Infestation" is from the Centers for Disease Control and Prevention (CDC), October 19, 2004. Available online at http://www.cdc.gov; accessed June 2, 2005.

What are head lice?

Also called *Pediculus humanus capitis*, head lice are parasitic insects found on the heads of people. Having head lice is very common. However, there are no reliable data on how many people get head lice in the United States each year.

Who is at risk for getting head lice?

Anyone who comes in close contact with someone who already has head lice, or contact with clothing or other personal items (such as brushes or towels) that belong to an infested person. Preschool and elementary-age children, 3 to 10, and their families are infested most often. Girls get head lice more often than boys, women more than men. In the United States, African Americans rarely get head lice.

What do head lice look like?

There are three forms of lice: the nit, the nymph, and the adult.

- **Nit:** Nits are head lice eggs. They are hard to see and are often confused for dandruff or hair spray droplets. Nits are found firmly attached to the hair shaft. They are oval and usually yellow to white in color. Nits take about 1 week to hatch.
- **Nymph:** The nit hatches into a baby louse called a nymph. It looks like an adult head louse, but is smaller. Nymphs mature into adults about 7 days after hatching. To live, the nymph must feed on blood.
- **Adult:** The adult louse is about the size of a sesame seed, has six legs, and is tan to grayish-white. In persons with dark hair,

the adult louse will look darker. Females lay nits; they are usually larger than males. Adult lice can live up to 30 days on a person's head. To live, adult lice need to feed on blood. If the louse falls off a person, it dies within 2 days.

Where are head lice most commonly found?

They are most commonly found on the scalp, behind the ears, and near the neckline at the back of the neck. Head lice hold on to hair with hook-like claws found at the end of each of their six legs. Head lice are rarely found on the body, eyelashes, or eyebrows.

What are the signs and symptoms of head lice infestation?

- Tickling feeling of something moving in the hair.
- Itching, caused by an allergic reaction to the bites.
- Irritability.
- Sores on the head caused by scratching. These sores can sometimes become infected.

How did my child get head lice?

- Contact with an already infested person. Contact is common during play at school and at home (slumber parties, sports activities, at camp, on a playground).
- Wearing infested clothing, such as hats, scarves, coats, sports uniforms, or hair ribbons.
- Using infested combs, brushes, or towels.
- Lying on a bed, couch, pillow, carpet, or stuffed animal that has recently been in contact with an infested person.

How is head lice infestation diagnosed?

An infestation is diagnosed by looking closely through the hair and scalp for nits, nymphs, or adults. Finding a nymph or adult may be difficult; there are usually few of them and they can move quickly from searching fingers. If crawling lice are not seen, finding nits within a 1/4 inch of the scalp confirms that a person is infested and should be treated. If you only find nits more than 1/4 inch from the scalp, the infestation is probably an old one and does not need to be treated. If you are not sure if a person has head lice, the diagnosis should be made by a health care provider, school nurse, or a professional from the local health department or agricultural extension service.

Section 58.2

Pubic Lice

"Pubic Lice Infestation" is from the Centers for Disease Control and Prevention (CDC), October 19, 2004. Available online at http://www.cdc.gov; accessed June 2, 2005.

What are pubic lice?

Also called crabs, pubic lice are parasitic insects found in the genital area of humans. Infection is common and found worldwide.

How did I get pubic lice?

Pubic lice are usually spread through sexual contact. Rarely, infestation can be spread through contact with an infested person's bed linens, towels, or clothes. A common misunderstanding is that infestation can be spread by sitting on a toilet seat. This isn't likely, since lice cannot live long away from a warm human body. Also, lice do not have feet designed to walk or hold onto smooth surfaces such as toilet seats.

Infection in a young child or teenager may indicate sexual activity or sexual abuse.

Where are pubic lice found?

Pubic lice are generally found in the genital area on pubic hair; but may occasionally be found on other coarse body hair, such as hair on the legs, armpits, mustache, beard, eyebrows, or eyelashes. Infestations of young children are usually on the eyebrows or eyelashes. Lice found on the head are not pubic lice; they are head lice.

Animals do not get or spread pubic lice.

What are the signs and symptoms of pubic lice?

Signs and symptoms of pubic lice include:

- Itching in the genital area
- Visible nits (lice eggs) or crawling lice

What do pubic lice look like?

There are three stages in the life of a pubic louse: the nit, the nymph, and the adult.

- **Nit:** Nits are pubic lice eggs. They are hard to see and are found firmly attached to the hair shaft. They are oval and usually yellow to white. Nits take about 1 week to hatch.
- **Nymph:** The nit hatches into a baby louse called a nymph. It looks like an adult pubic louse, but it is smaller. Nymphs mature into adults about 7 days after hatching. To live, the nymph must feed on blood.
- **Adult:** The adult pubic louse resembles a miniature crab when viewed through a strong magnifying glass.

Pubic lice have six legs, but their two front legs are very large and look like the pincher claws of a crab; this is how they got the nickname "crabs." Pubic lice are tan to grayish-white in color. Females lay nits and are usually larger than males. To live, adult lice must feed on blood.

If the louse falls off a person, it dies within 1 to 2 days.

How is a pubic lice infestation diagnosed?

A lice infestation is diagnosed by looking closely through pubic hair for nits, nymphs, or adults. It may be difficult to find nymph or adult lice; there are usually few of them and they can move quickly away from light. If crawling lice are not seen, finding nits confirms that a person is infested and should be treated. If you are unsure about infestation or if treatment is not successful, see a health care provider for a diagnosis.

How is a pubic lice infestation treated?

A lice-killing shampoo (also called a pediculicide) made of 1% permethrin or pyrethrin is recommended to treat pubic lice. These products are available without a prescription at your local drugstore. Medication is generally very effective; apply the medication exactly as directed on the bottle. A prescription medication, called Lindane (1%) is available through your health care provider. Lindane is not recommended for pregnant or nursing women, or for children less than 2 years old.

Malathion lotion 0.5% (Ovide) is another prescription medication that is effective against pubic lice.

How to treat pubic lice infestations: (Note: see section below for treatment of eyelashes or eyebrows. The lice medications described in this section should not be used near the eyes.)

1. Wash the infested area; towel dry.
2. Thoroughly saturate hair with lice medication. If using permethrin or pyrethrin, leave medication on for 10 minutes; if using Lindane, only leave on for 4 minutes. Thoroughly rinse off medication with water. Dry off with a clean towel.
3. Following treatment, most nits will still be attached to hair shafts. Nits may be removed with fingernails.
4. Put on clean underwear and clothing after treatment.
5. To kill any lice or nits (attached to hairs) that may be left on clothing or bedding, machine wash those washable items that the infested person used during the 2 to 3 days before treatment. Use the hot water cycle (130 degrees Fahrenheit). Use the hot dryer cycle for at least 20 minutes.
6. Dry clean clothing that is not washable.
7. Inform any sexual partners that they are at risk for infestation.
8. Do not have sex until treatment is complete.
9. Do not have sex with infected partners until partners have been treated and infestation has been cured.
10. Repeat treatment in 7 to 10 days if lice are still found.

To treat nits and lice found on eyebrows or eyelashes:

- If only a few nits are found, it may be possible to remove live lice and nits with your fingernails or a nit comb.
- If additional treatment is needed for pubic lice nits found on the eyelashes, applying an ophthalmic-grade petrolatum ointment (only available by prescription) to the eyelids twice a day for 10 days is effective. Vaseline is a kind of petrolatum, but is likely to irritate the eyes if applied.

Chapter 59

Pilonidal Disease

Pilonidal disease was first reported in 1833. Sacrococcygeal pilonidal sinus is a common disorder among young adults. It is observed most commonly in people aged 15 to 30 years, occurring after puberty when sex hormones are known to affect the pilosebaceous gland and change healthy body hair growth. The onset of pilonidal disease in people older than 40 years is rare.

History

In the 1950s, pilonidal sinus disease was thought to be of congenital origin rather than an acquired disorder. The pilonidal sinus and abscess were thought to be secondary to a congenital remnant of an epithelial-lined tract from postcoccygeal epidermal cell rests or vestigial scent cells. Sinuses to the neural canal can occasionally extend to the dura, but these are rare and are located in the lumbar region rather than the sacral region. Pilonidal disease is now widely accepted as an acquired disorder based on the observations that congenital tracts do not contain hair and are lined by cuboidal epithelium. The recurrence of the disorder after complete excision of the disease tissue down to the sacrococcygeal fascia and the high incidence of chronic pilonidal sinus disease in patients who are hirsute further support an acquired theory of pathogenesis.

Problem

In a recent census and survey of patients admitted to England hospitals in 1985 for treatment of pilonidal sinus disease, 7000 patients required hospitalization for an average of 5 days. The hospitalization of these patients for the treatment of pilonidal disease resulted in a loss of productivity, a loss of earnings, and a disruption of education because patients recovered in the hospital.

Treatment options are now available that provide a rapid rate of cure, a lower recurrence rate, and a minimized number of hospital admissions. Although numerous randomized clinical studies have evaluated different treatments, no clear consensus has been reached as to the optimal medical or surgical treatment.

Frequency

The incidence rate of pilonidal disease is approximately 0.7%. Men are affected 2.2 to 4 times more frequently than women. During a population study involving college students, the incidence rate was found to be 1.1% (365 of 31,497 people) in males and 0.11% (24 of 21,367 people) in females. The onset of the disease is earlier in women, which may be due to earlier puberty in women.

Etiology

The incidence is also affected by hair characteristics such as kinking, medullation, coarseness, and growth rate. White persons are affected more frequently than African or Asian persons. Other factors affecting the incidence are increased sweating activity associated with sitting and buttock friction, poor personal hygiene, obesity, and local trauma, which help to explain why pilonidal sinus disease is common in army recruits. In an article examining pilonidal sinus in Turkish soldiers, the incidence was found to be 8.8%, with the correlation factors known to be family history, obesity, being the driver of a vehicle, and the presence of folliculitis or a furuncle at another site on the body.

Pathophysiology

After the onset of puberty, sex hormones affect the pilosebaceous glands, and, subsequently, the hair follicle becomes distended with keratin. As a result, a folliculitis is created, which produces edema and follicle occlusion. The infected follicle extends and ruptures into the subcutaneous tissue, forming a pilonidal abscess. This results in a sinus tract that leads to a deep subcutaneous cavity. The direction of the sinus tract is cephalad in 90% of the cases, which coincides with the directional growth of the hair follicle. This usually places the tracking follicle approximately 5 to 8 cm from the anus. In the more rare instance that the sinus is located caudally, it is usually found 4 to 5 cm from the anus. The laterally communicating sinus overlying the sacrum is created as the pilonidal abscess spontaneously drains to the skin surface. The original sinus tract from the natal cleft becomes an epithelialized tube. The laterally draining tract becomes a granulating sinus tract opening.

Loose hairs are drilled, propelled, and sucked into the pilonidal sinus by friction and movement of the buttocks whenever a patient stands or sits. Hair enters tip first, and the barbs on the hair prevent it from being expelled so that the hair becomes entrapped. Physical examination occasionally may reveal a tuft of hair emerging from the midline opening in the natal cleft. This trapped hair stimulates a foreign body reaction and infection. Rarely, foreign bodies other than human hair can cause this disease process. Rare case reports exist in which the hair did not come from the patient but, instead, from a bird's feather, the type used to stuff feather bedding.

Diagnosis

Although pilonidal disease may manifest as an abscess, pilonidal sinus, recurrent or chronic pilonidal sinus, or a perianal pilonidal sinus, the most common manifestation of pilonidal disease is a painful fluctuant mass in the sacrococcygeal region. Initially, 50% of patients first present with a pilonidal abscess that is cephalad to the hair follicle and sinus infection. Pain and purulent discharge from the sinus tract are present 70% to 80% of the time and are the 2 most frequently described symptoms. In the early stages prior to the development of an abscess, only a cellulitis or folliculitis is present. The abscess is formed when a folliculitis expands into the subcutaneous tissue or when a preexisting foreign body granuloma becomes infected. The subcutaneous cavity and laterally oriented secondary sinus tract openings are lined with granulation tissue, whereas only the midline natal cleft pit sinus is lined by epithelium.

The diagnosis of a pilonidal sinus can be made by identifying the epithelialized follicle opening, which can be palpated as an area of deep induration beneath the skin in the sacral region. These tracts most commonly run in the cephalad direction. When the tract runs in the caudal direction, perianal sepsis may be present. The distinctions among pilonidal disease, fistula-in-ano, and hidradenitis can be difficult to discern. In the differential diagnosis, also include skin furuncle, syphilitic granuloma, tubercular granuloma, and osteomyelitis of the underlying sacrum with a draining sinus.

Recurrent pilonidal disease is observed most commonly after the incision and drainage of a pilonidal abscess. In this setting, the pilonidal sinus has not been excised and is still present after the abscess cavity heals, only to precipitate a recurrence. After surgical excision, the hair follicle has been removed and is no longer the pathogenic precipitating cause of the chronic pilonidal sinus. Instead, the base of the unhealed surgical wound is believed to become filled with granulation tissue, hair, and skin debris, which is a nidus for the ongoing foreign body reaction that takes place to create the chronic disease. This theory, coupled with the known predisposing intergluteal anatomy that draws hair into the pilonidal sinus cavity or surgical wound, is thought to precipitate the extensive recurrent and chronic disease.

Endoanal pilonidal sinus is a rare variety of pilonidal disease that affects the perianal skin directly or may occur circumferentially around the anus, involving the skin of the anal verge. Three causes of perianal pilonidal disease have been described. First, the pilonidal sinus may tract down caudally, creating a perianal fissure or fistula communicating with the anal canal. Second, hair may enter the healing wound of a surgically managed fistula-in-ano. Third, hair may be propelled and penetrate the normal anoderm and produce a similar foreign body reaction, which is usually observed in the sacrococcygeal region.

Treatment

Medical Therapy

Phenol injections used as treatment of the pilonidal sinus are more common in Europe than in the United States. Both chronic pilonidal disease and acute pilonidal abscess (after drainage) may be managed by phenol injection. Eighty percent phenol is injected into the sinus, left there for 1 minute, and then expressed out of the cavity. The sinus is then curetted. This may be repeated as many as 3 times for a total of 3 minutes of phenol exposure at one treatment. The treatments may be repeated every 4 to 6 weeks as necessary as wound healing progresses. Paraffin jelly may be used to protect the skin from the phenol, which destroys the epithelium.

Phenol sterilizes the sinus tract and removes embedded hair. Phenol injections may be combined with local excision of the sinus. Wound healing usually requires 4 to 8 weeks. The incidence of recurrence is reported to be approximately 9% to 27%, which is similar to the incidence following simple excision and packing open the wound. Because of the intense local inflammatory response after the phenol injection, patients usually stay in the hospital overnight. Thereafter, the patient is allowed to return home with instructions to bathe daily and keep the area shaved. Dressings are used for comfort.

Surgical Therapy

Pilonidal disease is divided into 3 categories to better determine the most appropriate surgical management. These 3 categories are (1) acute pilonidal abscess, (2) chronic pilonidal disease, and (3) complex or recurrent pilonidal disease.

Chapter 60

Psoriasis

Chapter Contents

Section 60.1

Understanding Psoriasis

"Psoriasis: More Than Cosmetic," by Linda Bren, U.S. Food and Drug Administration, *FDA Consumer* magazine, September-October 2004. Available online at http://www.fda.gov; accessed June 12, 2005.

It's not easy living in Leah Bird's skin. "The worst thing is when people just stare," says Bird. "I almost like it better if someone comes up to me and asks me what it is."

Then she'll tell them, "I have psoriasis. It's not contagious."

Bird, 51, of suburban Boston, has had flare-ups of this chronic skin disease since she was a teenager. The dry, red, scaly patches of skin that characterize psoriasis have covered as much as 85 percent of her body, she says. "It alarms people. It looks very scary to people who don't know what it is."

But psoriasis is more than cosmetic. "This disease is common, chronic, and costly, both in monetary terms and in quality of life," says Jonathan Wilkin, M.D., director of the Food and Drug Administration's Division of Dermatologic and Dental Drug Products.

More than 5 million Americans have psoriasis, and they spend between $1.6 billion and $3.2 billion each year to treat the disease, according to the National Psoriasis Foundation (NPF). Between 150,000 and 260,000 new cases are diagnosed each year, including 20,000 in children younger than 10.

"Psoriasis can be painful and can be profoundly disruptive to a person's life," says Jill Lindstrom, M.D., an FDA dermatologist. "People who don't have it don't understand how burdensome the disease can be. There is constant shedding of scales. There can be functional impairment, itching, and pain." And health complications, such as arthritis, accompany some cases.

There is no cure for psoriasis, but a broad range of treatments is available to reduce the symptoms, clear up the skin, and send the disease into remission. FDA-approved treatments range from creams rubbed into the skin, to lasers that aim ultraviolet rays at the skin, to the newest treatments—injectable drugs made from living cells.

What Is Psoriasis?

Psoriasis is an inflammatory skin disease in which skin cells replicate at an extremely rapid rate. New skin cells are produced about eight times faster than normal—over several days instead of a month—but the rate at which old cells slough off is unchanged. This causes cells to build up on the skin's surface, forming thick patches, or plaques, of red sores (lesions) covered with flaky, silvery-white dead skin cells (scales).

Rarely life threatening, at its mildest, psoriasis can be itchy and sore. At its worst, it's painful, disfiguring, and debilitating. About two-thirds of the people with psoriasis have a mild form of the disease, says the NPF. About one-third have moderate or severe psoriasis. Psoriasis can affect people at any age, but it most often strikes those between the ages of 15 and 35.

There are five forms of psoriasis. Plaque psoriasis is the most common—affecting 4 out of 5 people who have psoriasis, says the NPF. Plaque psoriasis may start with small red bumps and progress to larger lesions.

The plaques of psoriasis occur most frequently on the elbows, knees, other parts of the legs, scalp, back, face, palms, and soles of the feet.

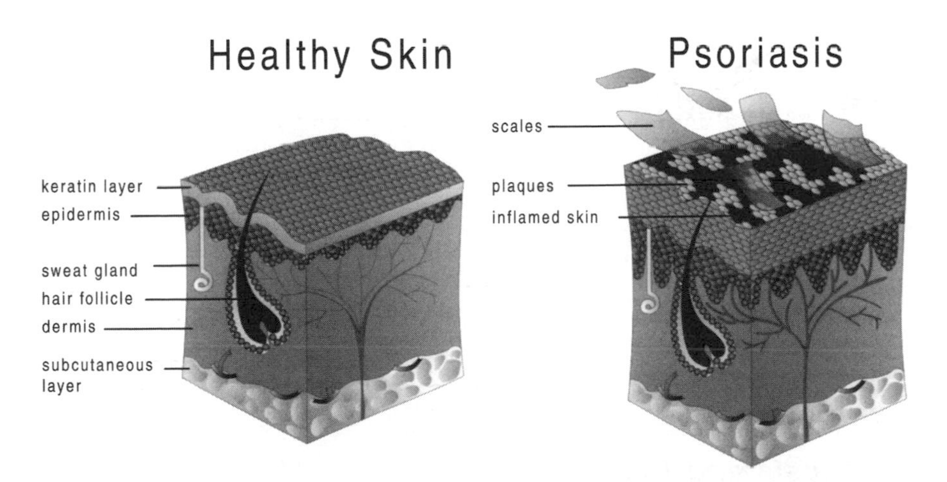

Figure 60.1. *In psoriasis, an activated immune system triggers the skin to reproduce every three to four days, building up on the outer layers (epidermis and keratin). The epidermis thickens, blood flow increases and reddens the skin, and silver-gray scales cover it.*

Psoriasis can also affect the fingernails and toenails, causing pitting, discoloration, or tissue buildup around the nails. According to the National Institute of Arthritis and Musculoskeletal and Skin Diseases, about 15 percent of people with psoriasis also get psoriatic arthritis, which can be progressively disabling if untreated.

Wayward White Blood Cells

Scientists believe that certain white blood cells called T lymphocytes (T cells) play an important role in psoriasis. "And the disease has a genetic component," says Lindstrom. In about one-third of psoriasis cases, there is a family history of the disease.

T cells circulate throughout the body, orchestrating the immune system's response to foreign invaders like bacteria or viruses. In people with psoriasis, the defective T cells are overactive and migrate to the skin as if to heal a wound or ward off an infection. This process leads to the rapid growth of skin cells, triggering inflammation and the development of lesions.

Both the environment and genetics may play a role in the development of psoriasis. "In genetically predisposed children, psoriasis can be triggered by a strep or other infection," says Lindstrom. That's what happened to author John Updike. After an attack of measles at the age of 6, Updike developed psoriasis "in all its flaming scabbiness from head to toe," as he later described it in his memoir, *Self-Consciousness*.

Remission and Reactivation

While the disease never goes away, the symptoms of psoriasis subside for a while (remission) and then return (flare-up, or reactivation). Remission can last for years in some people; in others, flare-ups occur every few weeks. Certain triggers, such as stress and seasonal changes, can reactivate psoriasis. "Certain drugs may also exacerbate it," says Lindstrom, including lithium, prescribed for bipolar disorder (also called manic-depressive illness), beta-blockers used to treat high blood pressure, and antimalarial drugs.

Diagnosis and Treatment

No single test exists to diagnose psoriasis, but a dermatologist can usually determine it by the appearance of the skin and by looking at an individual's personal and family medical history. In some cases, a specialist will confirm the diagnosis by examining a small piece of skin (biopsy) under a microscope.

Psoriasis treatments fall into three categories: medications externally applied to the skin (topical), ultraviolet light applied to the skin (phototherapy), and medications taken by mouth or injected (systemic).

Topical Treatments

Topical lotions, ointments, creams, gels, and shampoos for the skin and scalp are prescribed for mild-to-moderate cases of psoriasis or in combination with other treatments for more severe cases. FDA-approved prescription topicals to treat psoriasis include corticosteroids, retinoids, calcipotriene, and coal tar products. These drugs slow down skin cell production and reduce inflammation.

Corticosteroids are synthetic drugs that resemble naturally occurring hormones. Side effects may include thinning of the skin and stretch marks at the area where the topical is applied. Corticosteroids may also suppress the adrenal glands' production of natural steroids, which could leave the body susceptible to disease.

Retinoids are derivatives of vitamin A and calcipotriene is a synthetic form of vitamin D. Retinoids and calcipotriene are not the same as over-the-counter vitamin A and D supplements, which have no value for treating psoriasis, says Wilkin. "These topical creams on the skin deliver the vitamin-like chemicals right to where you want them," he says. Skin irritation where the topical is applied may be a side effect. Retinoids are also available by prescription as oral systemic drugs.

Coal tar products can help with scaling, itching, and inflammation but are not used as commonly as some other topicals, says Lindstrom. They are messy, can stain, and have a strong odor.

Carol Bentson of Washington, D.C., has had plaque psoriasis for more than 30 years, causing "major itching" all over and pain along the scalp line. She has treated it with topical corticosteroids, ultraviolet light, and cortisone injected into her scalp, elbows, toes, and legs. At times, "ointment wouldn't penetrate the areas of heavy plaque buildup, no matter how much I put on," she says.

Bentson has accumulated "sacks of lotions" to treat psoriasis. She would find a topical treatment that worked for a while but then quit working, forcing her to switch to another one.

"With a potent topical steroid, there is a phenomenon called tachyphylaxis," says Craig Leonardi, M.D., associate clinical professor of dermatology at the Saint Louis University Medical School. "Prolonged use can cause down-regulation [decrease] of steroid receptors in cells.

The net effect is that the skin becomes less responsive to steroids over time."

Wilkin adds that this unresponsiveness may be a temporary effect. "A patient may need to be off the steroid for a few days or a week and when put back on it, the responsiveness could come back."

Light Therapy

Exposing the skin to ultraviolet (UV) light—either from the sun or an artificial source—sets off a biological process that kills T cells, which slows the buildup of skin cells and reduces inflammation.

Light boxes that emit UV light to treat moderate-to-severe psoriasis and other skin diseases are medical devices that require licensing by the FDA. A person steps into the light box, which is about the size of a telephone booth, while lamps direct the light onto the body.

"Treatment with these devices is complex," says Richard Felten, an FDA chemist and senior medical device reviewer. The physician must determine an individual's sensitivity to UV and adjust the light emissions for the most effective treatment with the least risk of side effects, he says. Side effects may include burning, darkened skin, premature aging, and skin cancer. Three to five treatments per week for several weeks or months may be needed to get the psoriasis under control, followed by weekly maintenance treatments.

Light therapy, or phototherapy, is usually done in the physician's office or a medical facility that has the devices, says Felten. "The FDA has cleared some devices for home use under certain conditions and with a doctor's prescription," he says. Home devices include handheld devices for scalp psoriasis and stand-alone light boxes for other areas of the body.

Light therapy usually involves a short wavelength of ultraviolet light, called UVB. For people with resistant moderate-to-severe psoriasis, a combination of an oral or topical drug called psoralen and a longer wavelength ultraviolet A (UVA) light is used. This treatment is called "psoralen plus UVA" (PUVA).

"Psoralen makes the patient more sensitive to the UVA," says Lindstrom, "so once they've taken a dose of psoralen, a smaller dose of UVA is needed to treat them." Patients must be very careful to protect both skin and eyes for 24 hours after psoralen use to prevent damage, she says.

The FDA has also approved a special type of laser, an excimer laser, as a phototherapy device to treat mild-to-moderate psoriasis. "These lasers can deliver a much more controlled beam of light to small areas of the affected skin," says Felten.

Systemic Treatments

The FDA has approved oral and injected drugs that circulate throughout the body to treat psoriasis that is moderate, severe, or disabling. These systemic drugs are very powerful, and while some may be used continuously, others can only be used for a limited time because of their severe side effects. Once a drug is discontinued, the psoriasis may reactivate. The risk of birth defects prevents many systemics from being taken by pregnant women or women planning to become pregnant.

Systemic drugs that may be prescribed for psoriasis include acitretin, methotrexate, cyclosporine, and biologics, which are drugs made from proteins of living cells. Methotrexate, cyclosporine, and the biologic drugs are immunosuppressants, meaning they lower the body's normal immune response. "These drugs suppress the immune cells that cause psoriasis, but they don't distinguish these cells from the immune cells that protect our body from infections," says Elektra Papadopoulos, M.D., an FDA dermatologist.

Acitretin, a retinoid that is given orally for severe psoriasis, helps normalize the growth of skin cells. One of the side effects is raised fat (lipid) levels in the blood, and people taking this drug must get regular blood tests to monitor their cholesterol and triglyceride levels.

Methotrexate and cyclosporine slow the growth of skin cells. Methotrexate, taken orally or by injection, is also a chemotherapy drug for cancer patients. Cyclosporine, taken orally, was first approved to prevent organ rejection in transplant recipients. People using either of these drugs must be closely monitored and should use them only for short periods of time because of serious, potentially fatal, side effects.

Biologics are the newest systemic psoriasis treatments. Since 2003, the FDA has licensed three biologics to treat moderate-to-severe plaque psoriasis: Amevive (alefacept), manufactured by Biogen Inc.; Raptiva (efalizumab), made by Genentech Inc.; and Enbrel (etanercept), marketed by Amgen Inc. and Wyeth Pharmaceuticals. Enbrel was first licensed in 2002 to treat the arthritis associated with psoriasis, and in 2004 to treat psoriasis itself.

"All are immunosuppressive and have different proposed mechanisms," says Papadopoulos. Amevive simultaneously reduces the number of immune cells, including T cells, and inhibits T-cell activation. Raptiva inhibits the activation of T cells and the migration of those cells across blood vessels and into tissues, including the skin.

Enbrel inhibits the action of an inflammatory chemical messenger in the immune system called tumor necrosis factor-alpha (TNF-alpha), which is believed to play a role in both the skin and the joint symptoms of psoriasis.

All three biologics are injected. The FDA has licensed Amevive to be given in a physician's office, either injected into the muscle or into a vein (intravenously). It's a once-a-week treatment for 12 weeks; further treatments may be given after a waiting period.

The FDA has licensed Raptiva and Enbrel for home treatment. People can inject themselves with Raptiva under the skin once a week or with Enbrel once or twice a week. Both drugs are recommended for continuous use to maintain results.

Since biologic drugs are immunosuppressants, they may carry an increased risk of infection and cancer. Rare but serious effects have also included blood abnormalities and autoimmune diseases such as lupus. Other side effects are flu-like symptoms and pain and inflammation at the injection site.

Some dermatologists prescribe biologics alone for psoriasis or in combination with topical treatments. Leonardi says when he prescribes biologics, "I don't have to resort to adding other systemic therapies such as methotrexate, cyclosporine, acitretin, or phototherapy."

"Biologics are an alternative treatment to some of the traditional therapies," says Papadopoulos.

"Now we need to get the expense down," says Leonardi, who has patients who pay $30,000 per year on drugs to treat psoriasis.

Bird feels fortunate that her insurance company covers most of the expense of Enbrel, which is prescribed for both her psoriasis and psoriatic arthritis. Because of the arthritis pain, she has used a cane to help her walk and has had surgery on her wrist to correct some of the arthritis damage. Although Enbrel has been less effective over time for the psoriasis, she says, it's reduced her arthritic pain by about 95 percent. "I can jog down to the corner to chase after the dog," she says. "And last summer, I went hiking with my children in Colorado."

Reducing Treatment Risks

Biologics, other systemic drugs, and phototherapy are powerful treatments with increased risks, says Lindstrom.

Biologics may raise the risk for developing cancer and serious bacterial or fungal infections that spread throughout the body (sepsis).

Cyclosporine can damage the kidneys, methotrexate puts the liver and lungs at risk, and phototherapy can cause skin cancer. To reduce these risks, doctors often put patients on "rotational therapy." "The thought is by moving from one therapy to another therapy over time, the risk to any individual organ is reduced," says Lindstrom.

"We also try to choose a drug with an appropriate benefit-risk ratio," she says. For mild psoriasis, a topical steroid may be appropriate. For more severe disease, where it becomes impractical to apply topicals over a large surface area several times a day, a patient may need a systemic treatment.

Most of the highly effective treatments for psoriasis affect the immune system in some way. For steroid drugs, which have been around for more than 50 years, the risks are well known. But less is known about the long-term side effects of newer drugs, such as the biologics. The safety and side effects of biologics and other immune-suppressing drugs to treat psoriasis continue to be monitored by drug manufacturers and the FDA.

Emotional Impact

For many people, dealing with the emotional impact of psoriasis can be as challenging as treating the disease.

Bird says that mothers have pulled their children away from her on the subway, and some people, horrified by her skin lesions, have asked her if she has AIDS. As her disease has evolved over 30 years, so has Bird's way of dealing with these reactions. In her teens, she'd tell people she had leprosy just for the shock value, she says. Today, Bird is open about the disease but still relies on her defiant attitude to "steel myself for the experience" of going to the beach. "I love to swim," she says. But Bird knows that without covering herself up in a public place, she "runs the risk of people just rubbernecking."

"When I'm feeling forgiving, I try to ignore them," she says, "but when I'm angry, I think 'didn't your mother teach you not to stare?'"

Bird advises others with psoriasis to find out what works best for them to cope with the emotional effects of the disease. Going to therapy has helped her, she says. So has leading a support group for psoriasis sufferers. "It's important for people to work on their emotional well-being," says Bird, "however they choose—whether it's meditation, yoga, or putting on long pants and going out dancing."

The Future of Psoriasis Treatment

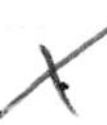

Researchers continue to look for reasons why immune cells overreact and what genes may be responsible for psoriasis, hoping to find better treatments, and eventually a cure. Psoriasis research is aided by the visibility of the symptoms on the skin.

"You can see the disease," says Leonardi. "You don't have to do invasive testing to see the effects of therapy." Psoriasis research has a "tremendous spillover into other fields besides dermatology," he adds. "There is a huge need for drugs to suppress the immune system without the side effects."

Multiple sclerosis, Crohn disease, rheumatoid arthritis, and type 1 diabetes are just a few of the diseases that may also benefit from psoriasis research.

Section 60.2

Biologic Advances in the Treatment of Psoriasis

Recently approved and investigational biologic therapies are changing the way dermatologists treat psoriasis, a chronic disease that physically and emotionally challenges 4.5 million Americans. As more research is conducted into the effectiveness of these biologics, they are showing great promise for improving the health and well-being of patients with psoriasis.

Dermatologist Jeffrey M. Weinberg, M.D., assistant clinical professor in the department of dermatology at Columbia University, New York, N.Y., discussed the aims of biologics for the treatment of psoriasis and psoriatic arthritis.

"Biologics are designed to provide select, immunologically directed intervention within the body to target psoriasis-causing reactions, controlling the condition and helping to prevent flare-ups," said Dr. Weinberg. "Biologics also are proving to have fewer side effects than traditional psoriasis therapies, meaning patients can find relief for longer periods of time without having to switch treatments."

Caused by the unusually rapid growth of skin cells due to faulty signals from the body's immune system, psoriasis is characterized by thick, red, white or scaly patches on the skin's surface. The extra cells build up on the skin's surface and form plaques—usually around the knees, elbows, scalp, hands, feet or lower back—causing itching and severe discomfort.

Research has shown that the activation of T-cells, a type of white blood cell, is the key immune system trigger in the development of psoriasis. Once activated, these cells release cytokines—chemicals used by the immune system to communicate messages. In psoriasis patients, these cytokines signal skin cells to reproduce and mature at an accelerated rate, thereby setting off other reactions that lead to psoriatic lesions forming on the skin.

Two biologics—alefacept and efalizumab—are approved by the U.S. Food and Drug Administration (FDA) for treating psoriasis and a third biologic—etanercept—is FDA-approved for the treatment of both psoriasis and psoriatic arthritis. These three biologics are approved for treating adults with moderate to severe psoriasis.

Alefacept

Alefacept is a biologic that is given by intramuscular injection at a dermatologist's office once a week for 12 weeks and works by directly reducing the number of activated T-cells in the skin, thereby stopping the cycle of psoriasis.

In a recent study, patients underwent two alefacept treatment courses, each with a 12-week treatment and 12-week follow-up phase, that did not include biologic treatment, only monitoring. During the first course of treatment, patients' Psoriasis Activity and Severity Index (PASI) scores were recorded. The PASI is the standard measurement tool to determine what percentage of the body is affected by psoriasis and how severe a patient's psoriasis is at any given time. Nearly 14 percent of patients achieved a 75 percent reduction from their baseline PASI around week 14. After the 12-week follow-up phase, patients from this same trial were randomly selected to receive a second course of alefacept and they showed additional improvement, with 40 percent achieving between 50 and 75 percent PASI improvement almost immediately upon beginning the second course of treatment.

"Alefacept provides a long period of remission for patients, in many cases from seven months to one year," stated Dr. Weinberg. "Once remission lapses, a repeat 12-week course of therapy can be administered if 12 weeks have passed since the last shot was given, making alefacept a viable long-term treatment option."

Efalizumab

The biologic efalizumab prevents the migration of activated T-cells into the skin from the lymph nodes. Injected into the skin by patients at home, efalizumab is taken on a weekly basis.

Clinical trials of various strengths of efalizumab as compared to placebo showed nearly 30 percent of patients achieved a 75 percent or more improvement from their baseline PASI as compared to only 3.4 percent of patients treated with the placebo who achieved that same PASI score. "What is proving most effective about efalizumab is that it works rapidly to treat psoriasis, allowing almost immediate relief in most cases," stated Dr. Weinberg. "However, once efalizumab is stopped, signs and symptoms of psoriasis usually reappear."

Etanercept

Etanercept is a biologic approved for the treatment of both psoriasis and psoriatic arthritis, a condition that can affect joints in the hands, feet, knees, hips, shoulders, lower back and ankles, making them painfully swollen, red, and stiff. Etanercept is injected by the patient once or twice a week at home and can provide long-term therapy.

"Because etanercept works by neutralizing a cytokine that is primary to immune response, when taken continually it can greatly benefit patients who experience severe psoriasis flare-ups," said Dr. Weinberg. "It also is advantageous because it treats not only psoriasis but psoriatic arthritis, which affects more than 25 percent of patients with psoriasis."

In clinical trials evaluating etanercept, the biologic was injected in 25 milligrams and 50 milligrams doses twice weekly by patients. After 12 weeks at the 25 milligram dose, nearly 34 percent of patients achieved a 75 percent or more improvement from their baseline PASI. At the higher dose, 49 percent of patients achieved a 75 percent or more PASI improvement at 12 weeks, and at 24 weeks, nearly 59 percent of patients achieved that PASI improvement.

Biologics on the Horizon

Another biologic currently in phase III testing with the FDA is infliximab. This biologic blocks TNF-a, tumor necrosis factor-alpha, one of the main cytokines that signals the psoriasis cycle to begin. Infliximab can be given intravenously in the dermatologist's office over a course of several weeks to reduce the severity of psoriasis.

"Biologics are a positive step forward in finding innovative ways to treat psoriasis," stated Dr. Weinberg. "As more and more research is being conducted in this area, I'm confident that dermatologists can help more patients with psoriasis find the best therapy available for their condition."

Chapter 61

Scleroderma

What Is Scleroderma?

Derived from the Greek words "sklerosis," meaning hardness, and "derma," meaning skin, scleroderma literally means hard skin. Though it is often referred to as if it were a single disease, scleroderma is really a symptom of a group of diseases that involve the abnormal growth of connective tissue, which supports the skin and internal organs. It is sometimes used, therefore, as an umbrella term for these disorders. In some forms of scleroderma, hard, tight skin is the extent of this abnormal process. In other forms, however, the problem goes much deeper, affecting blood vessels and internal organs, such as the heart, lungs, and kidneys.

Scleroderma is called both a rheumatic disease and a connective tissue disease. The term rheumatic disease refers to a group of conditions characterized by inflammation and/or pain in the muscles, joints, or fibrous tissue. A connective tissue disease is one that affects the major substances in the skin, tendons, and bones.

Different Types of Scleroderma

The group of diseases we call scleroderma falls into two main classes: localized scleroderma and systemic sclerosis. (Localized diseases

---

Excerpted from "Handout on Health: Scleroderma," National Institute of Arthritis and Musculoskeletal and Skin Diseases, May 2001. Available online at http://www.niams.nih.gov; accessed May 17, 2005.

affect only certain parts of the body; systemic diseases can affect the whole body.) Both groups include subgroups. Although there are different ways these groups and subgroups may be broken down or referred to (and your doctor may use different terms from what you see here), the following is a common way of classifying these diseases.

Localized Scleroderma

Localized types of scleroderma are those limited to the skin and related tissues and, in some cases, the muscle below. Internal organs are not affected by localized scleroderma, and localized scleroderma can never progress to the systemic form of the disease. Often, localized conditions improve or go away on their own over time, but the skin changes and damage that occur when the disease is active can be permanent. For some people, localized scleroderma is serious and disabling.

There are two generally recognized types of localized scleroderma:

Morphea: Morphea comes from a Greek word that means "form" or "structure." The word refers to local patches of scleroderma. The first signs of the disease are reddish patches of skin that thicken into firm, oval-shaped areas. The center of each patch becomes ivory colored with violet borders. These patches sweat very little and have little hair growth. Patches appear most often on the chest, stomach, and back. Sometimes they appear on the face, arms, and legs.

Morphea can be either localized or generalized. Localized morphea limits itself to one or several patches, ranging in size from a half-inch to 12 inches in diameter. The condition sometimes appears on areas treated by radiation therapy. Some people have both morphea and linear scleroderma. The disease is referred to as generalized morphea when the skin patches become very hard and dark and spread over larger areas of the body.

Regardless of the type, morphea generally fades out in 3 to 5 years; however, people are often left with darkened skin patches and, in rare cases, muscle weakness.

Linear scleroderma: As suggested by its name, the disease has a single line or band of thickened and/or abnormally colored skin. Usually, the line runs down an arm or leg, but in some people it runs down the forehead. People sometimes use the French term *en coup de sabre*, or "sword stroke," to describe this highly visible line.

Systemic Scleroderma (also known as Systemic Sclerosis)

Systemic scleroderma, or systemic sclerosis, is the term for the disease that not only includes the skin, but also involves the tissues beneath to the blood vessels and major organs. Systemic sclerosis is typically broken down into diffuse and limited disease. People with systemic sclerosis often have all or some of the symptoms that some doctors call CREST, which stands for the following:

- **Calcinosis:** the formation of calcium deposits in the connective tissues, which can be detected by x ray. They are typically found on the fingers, hands, face, and trunk and on the skin above elbows and knees. When the deposits break through the skin, painful ulcers can result.
- **Raynaud phenomenon:** a condition in which the small blood vessels of the hands and/or feet contract in response to cold or anxiety. As the vessels contract, the hands or feet turn white and cold, then blue. As blood flow returns, they become red. Fingertip tissues may suffer damage, leading to ulcers, scars, or gangrene.
- **Esophageal dysfunction:** impaired function of the esophagus (the tube connecting the throat and the stomach) that occurs when smooth muscles in the esophagus lose normal movement. In the upper esophagus, the result can be swallowing difficulties; in the lower esophagus, the problem can cause chronic heartburn or inflammation.
- **Sclerodactyly:** thick and tight skin on the fingers, resulting from deposits of excess collagen within skin layers. The condition makes it harder to bend or straighten the fingers. The skin may also appear shiny and darkened, with hair loss.
- **Telangiectasias:** small red spots on the hands and face that are caused by the swelling of tiny blood vessels. While not painful, these red spots can create cosmetic problems.

Limited scleroderma: Limited scleroderma typically comes on gradually and affects the skin only in certain areas: the fingers, hands, face, lower arms, and legs. Many people with limited disease have Raynaud phenomenon for years before skin thickening starts. Others start out with skin problems over much of the body, which improves over time, leaving only the face and hands with tight, thickened skin. Telangiectasias and calcinosis often follow. Because of the predominance of CREST in people with limited disease, some doctors refer to limited disease as the CREST syndrome.

Diffuse scleroderma: Diffuse scleroderma typically comes on suddenly. Skin thickening occurs quickly and over much of the body, affecting the hands, face, upper arms, upper legs, chest, and stomach in a symmetrical fashion (for example, if one arm or one side of the trunk is affected, the other is also affected). Some people may have more area of their skin affected than others. Internally, it can damage key organs such as the heart, lungs, and kidneys.

People with diffuse disease are often tired, lose appetite and weight, and have joint swelling and/or pain. Skin changes can cause the skin to swell, appear shiny, and feel tight and itchy.

The damage of diffuse scleroderma typically occurs over a few years. After the first 3 to 5 years, people with diffuse disease often enter a stable phase lasting for varying lengths of time. During this phase, skin thickness and appearance stay about the same. Damage to internal organs progresses little, if at all. Symptoms also subside: joint pain eases, fatigue lessens, and appetite returns.

Gradually, however, the skin starts to change again. Less collagen is made and the body seems to get rid of the excess collagen. This process, called "softening," tends to occur in reverse order of the thickening process: the last areas thickened are the first to begin softening. Some patients' skin returns to a somewhat normal state, while other patients are left with thin, fragile skin without hair or sweat glands. More serious damage to heart, lungs, or kidneys is unlikely to occur unless previous damage leads to more advanced deterioration.

People with diffuse scleroderma face the most serious long-term outlook if they develop severe kidney, lung, digestive, or heart problems. Fortunately, less than one-third of patients with diffuse disease develop these problems. Early diagnosis and continual and careful monitoring are important.

Sine scleroderma: Some doctors break systemic sclerosis down into a third subset called systemic sclerosis sine (Latin for "without") scleroderma. Sine may resemble either limited or diffuse systemic sclerosis, causing changes in the lungs, kidneys, and blood vessels. However, there is one key difference between sine and other forms of systemic sclerosis: it does not affect the skin.

Causes of Scleroderma

Although scientists don't know exactly what causes scleroderma, they are certain that people cannot catch it from or transmit it to others. Studies of twins suggest it is also not inherited. Scientists suspect that scleroderma comes from several factors that may include the following.

Abnormal immune or inflammatory activity: Like many other rheumatic disorders, scleroderma is believed to be an autoimmune disease. An autoimmune disease is one in which the immune system, for unknown reasons, turns against one's own body.

In scleroderma, the immune system is thought to stimulate cells called fibroblasts to produce too much collagen. In scleroderma, collagen forms thick connective tissue that builds up around the cells of the skin and internal organs. In milder forms, the effects of this buildup are limited to the skin and blood vessels. In more serious forms, it also can interfere with normal functioning of skin, blood vessels, joints, and internal organs.

Genetic makeup: While genes seem to put certain people at risk for scleroderma and play a role in its course, the disease is not passed from parent to child like some genetic diseases.

However, some research suggests that having children may increase a woman's risk of scleroderma. Scientists have learned that when a woman is pregnant, cells from her baby can pass through the placenta, enter her bloodstream, and linger in her body—in some cases, for many years after the child's birth. Recently, scientists have found fetal cells from pregnancies of years past in the skin lesions of some women with scleroderma. They think that these cells, which are different from the woman's own cells, may either begin an immune reaction to the woman's own tissues or trigger a response by the woman's immune system to rid her body of those cells. Either way, the woman's healthy tissues may be damaged in the process. Further studies are needed to find out if fetal cells play a role in the disease.

Environmental triggers: Research suggests that exposure to some environmental factors may trigger the disease in people who are genetically predisposed to it. Suspected triggers include viral infections, certain adhesive and coating materials, and organic solvents such as vinyl chloride or trichloroethylene. In the past, some people believed that silicone breast implants might have been a factor in developing connective tissue diseases such as scleroderma. But several studies have not shown evidence of a connection.

Hormones: By the middle to late childbearing years (ages 30 to 55), women develop scleroderma at a rate 7 to 12 times higher than men. Because of female predominance at this and all ages, scientists suspect that something distinctly feminine, such as the hormone estrogen, plays a role in the disease. So far, the role of estrogen or other female hormones has not been proven.

People at Risk

Although scleroderma is more common in women, the disease also occurs in men and children. It affects people of all races and ethnic groups. However, there are some patterns by disease type. For example:

- Localized forms of scleroderma are more common in people of European descent than in African Americans.
- Morphea usually appears between the ages of 20 and 40.
- Linear scleroderma usually occurs in children or teenagers.
- Systemic scleroderma, whether limited or diffuse, typically occurs in people from 30 to 50 years old. It affects more women of African American than European descent.

Because scleroderma can be hard to diagnose and it overlaps with or resembles other diseases, scientists can only estimate how many cases there actually are. Estimates for the number of people in the United States with systemic sclerosis range from 40,000 to 165,000. By contrast, a survey that included all scleroderma-related disorders, including Raynaud phenomenon, suggested a number between 250,000 and 992,500.

For some people, scleroderma (particularly the localized forms) is fairly mild and resolves with time. But for others, living with the disease and its effects day to day has a significant impact on their quality of life.

Scleroderma's Impact

Having a chronic disease can affect almost every aspect of your life, from family relationships to holding a job. For people with scleroderma, there may be other concerns about appearance or even the ability to dress, bathe, or handle the most basic daily tasks. Here are some areas in which scleroderma could intrude.

Appearance and self-esteem: Aside from the initial concerns about health and longevity, one of the first fears people with scleroderma have is how the disease will affect their appearance. Thick, hardened skin can be difficult to accept, particularly on the face. Systemic scleroderma may result in facial changes that eventually cause the opening to the mouth to become smaller and the upper lip to virtually disappear. Linear scleroderma may leave its mark on the forehead. Although these problems can't always be prevented, their effects may be minimized with proper treatment and skin care. Special cosmetics—and in some cases, plastic surgery—can help conceal scleroderma's damage.

Caring for yourself: Tight, hard connective tissue in the hands can make it difficult to do what were once simple tasks, such as brushing your teeth and hair, pouring a cup of coffee, using a knife and fork, unlocking a door, or buttoning a jacket. If you have trouble using your hands, consult an occupational therapist, who can recommend new ways of doing things or devices to make tasks easier. Devices as simple as Velcro fasteners and built-up brush handles can help you be more independent. [*Note:* Brand names included in this chapter are provided as examples only, and their inclusion does not mean that these products are endorsed by the National Institutes of Health or any other Government agency. Also, if a particular brand name is not mentioned, this does not mean or imply that the product is unsatisfactory.]

Family relationships: Spouses, children, parents, and siblings may have trouble understanding why you don't have the energy to keep house, drive to soccer practice, prepare meals, and hold a job the way you used to. If your condition isn't that visible, they may even suggest you are just being lazy. On the other hand, they may be overly concerned and eager to help you, not allowing you to do the things you are able to do or giving up their own interests and activities to be with you. It's important to learn as much about your form of the disease as you can and share any information you have with your family. Involving them in counseling or a support group may also help them better understand the disease and how they can help you.

Sexual relations: Sexual relationships can be affected when systemic scleroderma enters the picture. For men, the disease's effects on the blood vessels can lead to problems achieving an erection. In women, damage to the moisture-producing glands can cause vaginal dryness that makes intercourse painful. People of either sex may find they have difficulty moving the way they once did. They may be self-conscious about their appearance or afraid that their sexual partner will no longer find them attractive. With communication between partners, good medical care, and perhaps counseling, many of these changes can be overcome or at least worked around.

Pregnancy and childbearing: In the past, women with systemic scleroderma were often advised not to have children. But thanks to better medical treatments and a better understanding of the disease itself, that advice is changing. (Pregnancy, for example, is not likely to be a problem for women with localized scleroderma.) Although blood vessel involvement in the placenta may cause babies of women with systemic scleroderma to be born early, many women with the disease can have safe pregnancies and healthy babies if they follow some precautions.

One of the most important pieces of advice is to wait a few years after the disease starts before attempting a pregnancy. During the first 3 years you are at the highest risk of developing severe problems of the heart, lungs, or kidneys that could be harmful to you and your unborn baby.

If you haven't developed organ problems within 3 years of the disease's onset, chances are you won't, and pregnancy should be safe. But it is important to have both your disease and your pregnancy monitored regularly. You'll probably need to stay in close touch with the doctor you typically see for your scleroderma as well as an obstetrician experienced in guiding high-risk pregnancies.

Diagnosing Scleroderma

Depending on your particular symptoms, a diagnosis of scleroderma may be made by a general internist, a dermatologist (a doctor who specializes in treating diseases of the skin, hair, and nails), an orthopaedist (a doctor who treats bone and joint disorders), a pulmonologist (lung specialist), or a rheumatologist (a doctor specializing in treatment of rheumatic diseases). A diagnosis of scleroderma is based largely on the medical history and findings from the physical exam. To make a diagnosis, your doctor will ask you a lot of questions about what has happened to you over time and about any symptoms you may be experiencing. Are you having a problem with heartburn or swallowing? Are you often tired or achy? Do your hands turn white in response to anxiety or cold temperatures?

Once your doctor has taken a thorough medical history, he or she will perform a physical exam. Finding one or more of the following factors can help the doctor diagnose a certain form of scleroderma:

- Changed skin appearance and texture, including swollen fingers and hands and tight skin around the hands, face, mouth, or elsewhere.
- Calcium deposits developing under the skin.
- Changes in the tiny blood vessels (capillaries) at the base of the fingernails.
- Thickened skin patches.

Finally, your doctor may order lab tests to help confirm a suspected diagnosis. At least two proteins, called antibodies, are commonly found in the blood of people with scleroderma:

- Anti-topoisomerase-1 or Anti-Scl-70 antibodies appear in the blood of up to 40 percent of people with diffuse systemic sclerosis.
- Anticentromere antibodies are found in the blood of as many as 90 percent of people with limited systemic sclerosis.

A number of other scleroderma-specific antibodies can occur in people with scleroderma, although less frequently. When present, however, they are helpful in clinical diagnosis.

Because not all people with scleroderma have these antibodies and because not all people with the antibodies have scleroderma, lab test results alone cannot confirm the diagnosis.

In some cases, your doctor may order a skin biopsy (the surgical removal of a small sample of skin for microscopic examination) to aid in or help confirm a diagnosis. However, skin biopsies, too, have their limitations: biopsy results cannot distinguish between localized and systemic disease, for example.

Diagnosing scleroderma is easiest when a person has typical symptoms and rapid skin thickening. In other cases, a diagnosis may take months, or even years, as the disease unfolds and reveals itself and as the doctor is able to rule out some other potential causes of the symptoms. In some cases, a diagnosis is never made, because the symptoms that prompted the visit to the doctor go away on their own.

Treating Scleroderma

Because scleroderma can affect many different organs and organ systems, you may have several different doctors involved in your care. Typically, care will be managed by a rheumatologist, a specialist who treats people with diseases of the joints, bones, muscles, and immune system. Your rheumatologist may refer you to other specialists, depending on the specific problems you are having: for example, a dermatologist for the treatment of skin symptoms, a nephrologist for kidney complications, a cardiologist for heart complications, a gastroenterologist for problems of the digestive tract, and a pulmonary specialist for lung involvement.

In addition to doctors, professionals like nurse practitioners, physician assistants, physical or occupational therapists, psychologists, and social workers may play a role in your care. Dentists, orthodontists, and even speech therapists can treat oral complications that arise from thickening of tissues in and around the mouth and on the face.

Currently, there is no treatment that controls or stops the underlying problem—the overproduction of collagen—in all forms of scleroderma. Thus, treatment and management focus on relieving symptoms and limiting damage. Your treatment will depend on the particular problems you are having. Some treatments will be prescribed or given by your physician. Others are things you can do on your own.

Here are some of the potential problems that can occur in systemic scleroderma and the medical and nonmedical treatments for them. These problems do not occur as a result or complication of localized scleroderma. [*Note:* This is not a complete listing of problems or their treatments. Different people experience different problems with scleroderma and not all treatments work equally well for all people. Work with your doctor to find the best treatment for your specific symptoms.]

Raynaud Phenomenon

One of the most common problems associated with scleroderma, Raynaud phenomenon can be uncomfortable and can lead to painful skin ulcers on the fingertips. Smoking makes the condition worse. The following measures may make you more comfortable and help prevent problems:

- Don't smoke! Smoking narrows the blood vessels even more and makes Raynaud phenomenon worse.
- Dress warmly, with special attention to hands and feet. Dress in layers and try to stay indoors during cold weather.

- Use biofeedback (to control various body processes that are not normally thought of as being under conscious control) and relaxation exercises.
- For severe cases, speak to your doctor about prescribing drugs called calcium channel blockers, such as nifedipine (Procardia), which can open up small blood vessels and improve circulation. Other drugs are in development and may become available in the future.
- If Raynaud leads to skin sores or ulcers, increasing your dose of calcium channel blockers (under the direction of your doctor ONLY) may help. You can also protect skin ulcers from further injury or infection by applying nitroglycerin paste or antibiotic cream. Severe ulcerations on the fingertips can be treated with bioengineered skin.

Stiff, Painful Joints

In diffuse systemic sclerosis, hand joints can stiffen because of hardened skin around the joints or inflammation of the joints themselves. Other joints can also become stiff and swollen. The following may help:

- Exercise regularly. Ask your doctor or physical therapist about an exercise plan that will help you increase and maintain range of motion in affected joints. Swimming can help maintain muscle strength, flexibility, and joint mobility.
- Use acetaminophen or an over-the-counter or prescription nonsteroidal anti-inflammatory drug, as recommended by your doctor, to help relieve joint or muscle pain. If pain is severe, speak to a rheumatologist about the possibility of prescription-strength drugs to ease pain and inflammation.
- Learn to do things in a new way. A physical or occupational therapist can help you learn to perform daily tasks, such as lifting and carrying objects or opening doors, in ways that will put less stress on tender joints.

Skin Problems

When too much collagen builds up in the skin, it crowds out sweat and oil glands, causing the skin to become dry and stiff. If your skin is affected, you may need to see a dermatologist. To ease dry skin, try the following:

- Apply oil-based creams and lotions frequently, and always right after bathing.
- Apply sunscreen before you venture outdoors, to protect against further damage by the sun's rays.
- Use humidifiers to moisten the air in your home in colder winter climates. (Clean humidifiers often to stop bacteria from growing in the water.)
- Avoid very hot baths and showers, as hot water dries the skin.
- Avoid harsh soaps, household cleaners, and caustic chemicals, if at all possible. If that's not possible, be sure to wear rubber gloves when you use such products.
- Exercise regularly. Exercise, especially swimming, stimulates blood circulation to affected areas.

Dry Mouth and Dental Problems

Dental problems are common in people with scleroderma for a number of reasons: tightening facial skin can make the mouth opening smaller and narrower, which makes it hard to care for teeth; dry mouth due to salivary gland damage speeds up tooth decay; and damage to connective tissues in the mouth can lead to loose teeth. You can avoid tooth and gum problems in several ways:

- Brush and floss your teeth regularly. (If hand pain and stiffness make this difficult, consult your doctor or an occupational therapist about specially made toothbrush handles and devices to make flossing easier.)
- Have regular dental checkups. Contact your dentist immediately if you experience mouth sores, mouth pain, or loose teeth.
- If decay is a problem, ask your dentist about fluoride rinses or prescription toothpastes that remineralize and harden tooth enamel.
- Consult a physical therapist about facial exercises to help keep your mouth and face more flexible.
- Keep your mouth moist by drinking plenty of water, sucking ice chips, using sugarless gum and hard candy, and avoiding mouthwashes with alcohol. If dry mouth still bothers you, ask your doctor about a saliva substitute or a prescription medication called

pilocarpine hydrochloride (Salagen) that can stimulate the flow of saliva.

Gastrointestinal (GI) Problems

Systemic sclerosis can affect any part of the digestive system. As a result, you may experience problems such as heartburn, difficulty swallowing, early satiety (the feeling of being full after you've barely started eating), or intestinal complaints such as diarrhea, constipation, and gas. In cases where the intestines are damaged, your body may have difficulty absorbing nutrients from food. Although GI problems are diverse, here are some things that might help at least some of the problems you have:

- Eat small, frequent meals.
- Raise the head of your bed with blocks, and stand or sit for at least an hour (preferably two or three) after eating to keep stomach contents from backing up into the esophagus.
- Avoid late-night meals, spicy or fatty foods, and alcohol and caffeine, which can aggravate GI distress.
- Chew foods well and eat moist, soft foods. If you have difficulty swallowing or if your body doesn't absorb nutrients properly, your doctor may prescribe a special diet.
- Ask your doctor about prescription medications for problems such as diarrhea, constipation, and heartburn. Some drugs called proton pump inhibitors are highly effective against heartburn. Oral antibiotics may stop bacterial overgrowth in the bowel that can be a cause of diarrhea in some people with systemic sclerosis.

Lung Damage

About 10 to 15 percent of people with systemic sclerosis develop severe lung disease, which comes in two forms: pulmonary fibrosis (hardening or scarring of lung tissue because of excess collagen) and pulmonary hypertension (high blood pressure in the artery that carries blood from the heart to the lungs). Treatment for the two conditions is different.

- Pulmonary fibrosis may be treated with drugs that suppress the immune system such as cyclophosphamide (Cytoxan) or azathioprine (Imuran), along with low doses of corticosteroids.

- Pulmonary hypertension may be treated with drugs that dilate the blood vessels such as prostacyclin (Iloprost).

Regardless of the problem or its treatment, your role in the treatment process is essentially the same. To minimize lung complications, work closely with your medical team. Do the following:

- Watch for signs of lung disease, including fatigue, shortness of breath or difficulty breathing, and swollen feet. Report these symptoms to your doctor.
- Have your lungs closely checked, using standard lung-function tests, during the early stages of skin thickening. These tests, which can find problems at the earliest and most treatable stages, are needed because lung damage can occur even before you notice any symptoms.
- Get regular flu and pneumonia vaccines as recommended by your doctor. Contracting either illness could be dangerous for a person with lung disease.

Heart Problems

About 15 to 20 percent of people with systemic sclerosis develop heart problems, including scarring and weakening of the heart (cardiomyopathy), inflamed heart muscle (myocarditis), and abnormal heartbeat (arrhythmia). All of these problems can be treated. Treatment ranges from drugs to surgery, and varies depending on the nature of the condition.

Kidney Problems

About 15 to 20 percent of people with diffuse systemic sclerosis develop severe kidney problems, including loss of kidney function. Because uncontrolled high blood pressure can quickly lead to kidney failure, it's important that you take measures to minimize the problem. Things you can do:

- Check your blood pressure regularly and, if you find it to be high, call your doctor right away.
- If you have kidney problems, take your prescribed medications faithfully. In the past two decades, drugs known as ACE (angiotensin-converting enzyme) inhibitors, including captopril

(Capoten), enalapril (Vasotec), and quinapril (Accupril), have made scleroderma-related kidney failure a less-threatening problem than it was in the past. But for these drugs to work, you must take them.

Cosmetic Problems

Even if scleroderma doesn't cause any lasting physical disability, its effects on the skin's appearance—particularly on the face—can take their toll on your self-esteem. Fortunately, there are procedures to correct some of the cosmetic problems scleroderma causes.

- The appearance of telangiectasias, small red spots on the hands and face caused by swelling of tiny blood vessels beneath the skin, may be lessened or even eliminated with the use of guided lasers.
- Facial changes of localized scleroderma, such as the *en coup de sabre* that may run down the forehead in people with linear scleroderma, may be corrected through cosmetic surgery. (However, such surgery is not appropriate for areas of the skin where the disease is active.)

Scleroderma Research

No one can say for sure when—or if—a cure will be found. But research is providing the next best thing: better ways to treat symptoms, prevent organ damage, and improve the quality of life for people with scleroderma. In the past two decades, multidisciplinary research has also provided new clues to understanding the disease, which is an important step toward prevention or cure.

Leading the way in funding for this research is the National Institute of Arthritis and Musculoskeletal and Skin Diseases (NIAMS), a part of the National Institutes of Health (NIH). Other sources of funding for scleroderma research include pharmaceutical companies and organizations such as the Scleroderma Foundation, the Scleroderma Research Foundation, and the Arthritis Foundation. Scientists at universities and medical centers throughout the United States conduct much of this research.

Studies of the immune system, genetics, cell biology, and molecular biology have helped reveal the causes of scleroderma, improve existing treatment, and create entirely new treatment approaches. Research advances in recent years that have led to a better understanding of and/or treatment for the diseases include:

- The use of a hormone produced in pregnancy to soften skin lesions. Early studies suggest relaxin, a hormone that helps a woman's body to stretch to meet the demands of a growing pregnancy and delivery, may soften the connective tissues of women with scleroderma. The hormone is believed to work by blocking fibrosis, or the development of fibrous tissue between the body's cells.
- Finding a gene associated with scleroderma in Oklahoma Choctaw Native Americans. Scientists believe the gene, which codes for a protein called fibrillin-1, may put people at risk for the disease.
- The use of the drug Iloprost for pulmonary hypertension. This drug has increased the quality of life and life expectancy for people with this dangerous form of lung damage.
- The use of the drug cyclophosphamide (Cytoxan) for lung fibrosis. One recent study suggested that treating lung problems early with this immunosuppressive drug may help prevent further damage and increase chances of survival.
- The increased use of ACE inhibitors for scleroderma-related kidney problems. For the past two decades, ACE inhibitors have greatly reduced the risk of kidney failure in people with scleroderma. Now there is evidence that use of ACE inhibitors can actually heal the kidneys of people on dialysis for scleroderma-related kidney failure. As many as half of people who continue ACE inhibitors while on dialysis may be able to go off dialysis in 12 to 18 months.

Other studies are examining the following:

- Changes in the tiny blood vessels of people with scleroderma. By studying these changes, scientists hope to find the cause of cold sensitivity in Raynaud phenomenon and how to control the problem.
- Immune system changes (and particularly how those changes affect the lungs) in people with early diffuse systemic sclerosis.
- The role of blood vessel malfunction, cell death, and autoimmunity in scleroderma.
- Skin changes in laboratory mice in which a genetic defect prevents the breakdown of collagen, leading to thick skin and patchy hair loss. Scientists hope that by studying these mice,

they can answer many questions about skin changes in scleroderma.

- The effectiveness of various treatments, including (1) methotrexate, a drug commonly used for rheumatoid arthritis and some other inflammatory forms of arthritis; (2) collagen peptides administered orally; (3) halofuginone, a drug that inhibits the synthesis of type I collagen, which is the primary component of connective tissue; (4) ultraviolet light therapy for localized forms of scleroderma; and (5) stem cell transfusions, a form of bone marrow transplant that uses a patient's own cells, for early diffuse systemic sclerosis.

Scleroderma research continues to advance as scientists and doctors learn more about how the disease develops and its underlying mechanisms.

Part Eight

Hair and Nail Disorders

Chapter 62

Hair Disorders

Chapter Contents

Section 62.1

Hair Loss in Men

Definition

Male pattern baldness is the most common type of hair loss in men. It usually follows a typical pattern of receding hairline and hair thinning on the crown, and is caused by hormones and genetic predisposition.

Causes, Incidence, and Risk Factors

Hair grows about an inch every couple of months. Each hair grows for 2 to 6 years, remains at that length for a short period, then falls out. A new hair soon begins growing in its place. At any one time, about 85% of the hair on your head is in the growing phase and 15% is not.

Each hair sits in a cavity in the skin called a follicle. Baldness in men occurs when the follicle shrinks over time, resulting in shorter and finer hair. The end result is a very small follicle with no hair inside. Ordinarily, hair should grow back. However, in men who are balding, the follicle fails to grow a new hair. Why this occurs is not well understood, but it is related to your genes and male sex hormones. Even though the follicles are small, they remain alive, suggesting the possibility of new growth.

Symptoms

The typical pattern of male baldness begins at the hairline. The hairline gradually recedes to form an "M" shape. The existing hair may become finer and shorter. The hair at the crown also begins to thin. Eventually the top of the hairline meets the thinned crown, leaving a horseshoe pattern of hair around the sides of the head.

Hair loss in patches, diffuse shedding of hair, breaking of hair shafts, or hair loss associated with redness, scaling, pain, or rapid progression could be caused by other conditions.

Signs and Tests

Classic male pattern baldness is usually diagnosed based on the appearance and pattern of the hair loss. Any atypical hair loss may be caused by other medical disorders. A skin biopsy or other procedures may be needed to diagnose other disorders that cause loss of hair.

Hair analysis is not accurate for diagnosing nutritional or similar causes of hair loss. However, it may reveal substances such as arsenic or lead.

Treatment

Treatment is not necessary if you are comfortable with your appearance. Hair weaving, hairpieces, or change of hairstyle may disguise the hair loss. This is usually the least expensive and safest approach for male baldness.

There are two main drugs used to treat male pattern baldness:

- Minoxidil (Rogaine): A solution that you apply directly to the scalp to stimulate the hair follicles. It slows hair loss for many men, and some men grow new hair. The previous degree of hair loss returns when you stop applying the solution.
- Finasteride (Propecia, Proscar): A prescription pill that inhibits the production of the male hormone dihydrotestosterone. Like minoxidil, you are more likely to have slower hair loss than actual new hair growth. In general, it is somewhat more effective than minoxidil. The previous degree of hair loss returns when you stop taking the drug.

Hair transplants consist of removing tiny plugs of hair from areas where the hair is continuing to grow and placing them in areas that are balding. This can cause minor scarring in the donor areas and carries a modest risk for skin infection. The procedure usually requires multiple transplantation sessions and may be expensive. Results, however, are often excellent and permanent.

Suturing hairpieces to the scalp is not recommended. It can result in scars, infections, and abscess of the scalp. The use of hair implants made of artificial fibers was banned by the FDA because of the high rate of infection.

Expectations (Prognosis)

Male pattern baldness does not indicate a medical disorder, but it may affect self-esteem or cause anxiety. The hair loss is usually permanent.

Complications

- Psychological stress
- Loss of self-esteem due to change in appearance

Calling Your Health Care Provider

Call your doctor if:

- Your hair loss occurs in an atypical pattern—rapid hair loss, diffuse shedding, hair loss in patches, or breaking of hair shafts.
- Your hair loss is accompanied by itching, skin irritation, redness, scaling, pain, or other symptoms.
- Your hair loss begins after starting a medication.
- You want to attempt to treat your hair loss.

Prevention

There is no known prevention for male pattern baldness.

Section 62.2

Hair Loss in Women

Definition

Female pattern baldness involves a typical pattern of loss of hair in women, caused by hormones, aging, and genetic predisposition.

Causes, Incidence, and Risk Factors

Hair grows from its follicle at an average rate of about 1/2 inch per month. Each hair grows for 2 to 6 years, then rests, and then falls out. A new hair soon begins growing in its place. At any one time, about 85% of the hair is growing and 15% is resting.

Baldness occurs when hair falls out but new hair does not grow in its place. The cause of the failure to grow new hair in female pattern baldness is not well understood, but it is associated with genetic predisposition, aging, and levels of endocrine hormones (particularly androgens, the male sex hormones).

Changes in the levels of androgens can affect hair production. For example, after the hormonal changes of menopause, many women find that the hair on the head is thinned, while facial hair is coarser. Although new hair is not produced, follicles remain alive, suggesting the possibility of new hair growth.

The typical pattern of female pattern baldness is different from that of male pattern baldness. The hair thins all over the head, but the frontal hairline is maintained. There may be a moderate loss of hair on the crown, but this rarely progresses to total or near baldness as it may in men.

Hair loss can occur in women for reasons other than female pattern baldness, including the following:

- Temporary shedding of hair (telogen effluvium)
- Breaking of hair (from such things as styling treatments and twisting or pulling of hair)

- Patchy areas of total hair loss (alopecia areata—an immune disorder causing temporary hair loss)
- Medications
- Certain skin diseases

Symptoms

- Thinning of hair over the entire head
- Hair loss at the crown or hairline, mild to moderate

Signs and Tests

Female pattern baldness is usually diagnosed based on the appearance and pattern of hair loss and by ruling out other causes of hair loss.

A skin biopsy or other procedures may be used to diagnose medical disorders that cause loss of hair.

Hair analysis is not accurate for diagnosing nutritional or similar causes of hair loss, although it may reveal substances such as arsenic or lead.

Treatment

The hair loss of female pattern baldness is permanent. In most cases, it is mild to moderate. No treatment is required if the person is comfortable with her appearance.

The only drug or medication approved by the United States Food and Drug Administration (FDA) to treat female pattern baldness is minoxidil, used topically on the scalp. For women, the 2% concentration is recommended. Minoxidil may help hair to grow in 20% to 25% of the female population, and in the majority it may slow or stop the loss of hair. Treatment is expensive, however. Hair loss recurs when minoxidil's use is stopped.

Hair transplants consist of removal of tiny plugs of hair from areas where the hair is continuing to grow and placing them in areas that are balding. This can cause minor scarring in the donor areas and carries a modest risk for skin infection. The procedure usually requires multiple transplantation sessions and may be expensive. Results, however, are often excellent and permanent.

Suturing of hairpieces to the scalp is not recommended as it can result in scars, infections, and abscess of the scalp. The use of hair implants made of artificial fibers was banned by the FDA because of the high rate of infection.

Hair weaving, hairpieces, or change of hairstyle may disguise hair loss and improve cosmetic appearance. This is often the least expensive and safest method of treating female pattern baldness.

Expectations (Prognosis)

Female pattern baldness is of cosmetic importance only and does not indicate a medical disorder, but it may affect self-esteem or cause anxiety. The hair loss is usually permanent.

Complications

Complications are psychological stress and a loss of self-esteem due to change in appearance.

Calling Your Health Care Provider

Call your health care provider if hair loss occurs and persists. There might be a treatable medical cause for the loss of hair.

Also call your health care provider if female pattern baldness is present and you want to treat the hair loss; or if hair loss is accompanied by itching, skin irritation, or other symptoms.

Prevention

There is no known prevention for female pattern baldness.

Section 62.3

Excess Hair Growth in Women

"Coping with Hirsutism," by Drs. Maria I. New and Heino F. L. Meyer-Bahlburg. This article is available on the website of the Congenital Adrenal Hyperplasia Research, Education and Support (CARES) Foundation, Inc., www.caresfoundation.org. Reprinted by permission of the authors. Material is undated but was reviewed by author in April 2005.

Hair Basics

Hair is really just an outgrowth of the skin layer called the epidermis. In fact, hair and skin are composed of the same protein (keratin). The hair shaft is produced by the hair follicle within the skin. The hair follicle has two regions: the hair bulb and the mid-follicle region. The hair bulb contains actively growing cells and pigment (melanin) producing cells. In the mid-follicle region the actively growing cells die and harden into what we call hair.

The follicle can produce two types of hair: (1) vellus hairs, which are pale, fine, and silky; (2) terminal hairs, which are darker, coarser and larger. During its lifespan, hair goes through three distinct phases: anagen, catagen, and telogen. In the anagen phase, protein and keratin are continuously made to promote development and active growth of the hair shaft. At any point in time, 85% to 90% of hair is in the anagen phase, which can last from a few months up to six years. Hair then enters a transitional, or catagen, phase, when chemical and structural changes cause the follicle to regress and stop growing. In the final part of the cycle, the telogen phase, the hair follicle shuts down and goes into resting mode. In this stage hair can shed so that new hair growth can begin. The telogen phase can last up to 100 days.

Hair growth in humans is asynchronous, meaning that growth and shedding of each follicle is independent of surrounding follicles. The number of hair follicles throughout the body is genetically determined. Men and women typically have the same number of hairs. However, in men, high androgen levels cause hair follicles in the androgen-sensitive areas of the body to produce terminal, coarser hair. In women, in whom androgen levels are typically low, those same hair follicles produce less visible, vellus hair.

Excess Hair

When the delicate hormonal balance of the body is disturbed, hair production, among other things, can be affected. In the case of CAH [congenital adrenal hyperplasia], excess androgen (e.g., testosterone) production causes excess "terminal" hair to grow in the androgen-sensitive areas of the body. Excess hair can be categorized as either "hirsutism" or "hypertrichosis." Hirsutism indicates the presence of excess terminal hair growth in areas of the body that are androgen-sensitive. Androgen-sensitive areas of the body are the face, chest, areola, lower back, buttock, inner thigh, and external genitalia. Hypertrichosis indicates excess terminal hair growth in areas of the body that are not androgen sensitive. Androgen-insensitive areas of the body include forehead, forearms, and tops of the hands. In women with hirsutism, the hair follicles that would normally produce pale, fine vellus hairs have switched to producing the darker, coarser terminal hairs. On the scalp the effect is the opposite, with hair follicles switching to production of vellus hairs in the presence of high androgen levels. This is why temporal balding is seen in untreated women with CAH. In general, hypertrichosis is not a problem in CAH since it does not depend on high androgen levels.

Endocrinologists use the Ferriman-Gallwey (FG) scale to assess the degree of hirsutism in CAH patients. Measuring the degree of hirsutism in eleven areas of the body, the FG scale can range from 0 to 44 (the higher the score, the more severe the hirsutism). A typical score for someone with hirsutism is between 8 and 29. While this scale is somewhat subjective, it does allow the physician to monitor the improvement in hair growth.

Treatment for Hirsutism

In CAH patients, excess androgen levels can cause an increase in terminal hair production. Therefore, the first step doctors take to treat hirsutism is to ensure that the patient is adequately controlled with replacement cortisol (Cortef, prednisone, or dexamethasone).

Medications

Even with optimal replacement of cortisol, however, there are certain times during the day when androgen levels rise, and, therefore, replacement cortisol alone is often not sufficient to combat hirsutism once it has begun. Elevated androgen levels can trigger a condition called polycystic ovarian syndrome, or PCO. In PCO, the ovaries become enlarged with multiple cysts and begin to produce androgens. For this reason, if replacement therapy alone is not sufficient to combat hirsutism, you may be tested for PCO and, if found, oral contraceptives would be prescribed.

If hirsutism persists even with adequate replacement therapy and oral contraceptives, drugs that block androgen action may be tried. By blocking androgen action, terminal hair growth decreases with each passing cycle. However significant improvement can take several months to two years because of the cyclical nature of hair growth. If the androgen blocker is discontinued, hair growth will recur.

Spironolactone is an androgen blocker, which is also a weak diuretic (a drug that causes excess urination). While taking spironolactone, electrolytes should be monitored periodically. Cyproterone acetate is another androgen blocker, which is used in Europe and Australia but not approved in the United States. Cyproterone acetate also counteracts androgen action and is often combined with ethinyl estradiol (a type of estrogen), which counteracts the androgens produced by polycystic ovaries.

The combination of cyproterone acetate and ethinylestradiol is found in Diane and Dianette. These drugs therefore operate as both an oral contraceptive and an androgen blocker at the same time. Contraindications for cyproterone acetate (mainly due to the estrogen action) are varicose veins, uterine fibroids, smoking, and cardiovascular disease. Side effects for both spironolactone and cyproterone acetate can include breast tenderness, decreased libido (sex drive), fatigue, headaches, depression, weight gain, and irregular periods. In high doses, anti-androgens have been linked to liver toxicity. However, this is usually not a problem at the doses used to treat hirsutism. It is also extremely important that a woman does not become pregnant while on these medications as they will interfere with the normal development of a male fetus.

Flutamide, another anti-androgen medication, is no longer used by some medical centers because of two reported deaths tentatively associated with its use.

Hair Removal Methods

Bleaching: Many women use hydrogen peroxide to bleach their facial hair so that it is less noticeable. The only downside to this method is that sometimes the hair develops a yellow hue.

Shaving: This method offers temporary benefits and can sometimes cause skin irritation and infections. Many women have the mistaken belief that repeated shaving will cause the hair to grow in darker and coarser. After shaving, the only hairs that immediately regrow are the ones in the anagen phase.

Plucking: Plucking stimulates hairs that were in the telogen phase to begin their anagen phase. This means that plucking a hair that happens to be in the telogen phase actually speeds up the regrowth of that hair. Facial hair has a long telogen phase, so it is best to shave before plucking so that the only hairs plucked are already in the anagen phase.

Depilatory Creams: The most often used depilatory preparations contain thioglycolates, which target the keratin in hair. Since skin also contains keratin, depilatory creams often irritate the skin, sometimes causing dermatitis.

Vaniqa: A new cream called Vaniqa has been getting good reviews. Vaniqa is an enzyme inhibitor used topically to slow the growth of unwanted facial hair in women. Vaniqa must be prescribed by a physician.

Waxing: Waxing involves the application of warmed wax to hair-bearing skin. Upon cooling of the wax, hairs are imbedded within the wax and when the wax is pulled away in a quick motion, the trapped hairs are pulled away with it.

Waxing can be painful and may cause hyperpigmentation, folliculitis, scarring and, if performed improperly, thermal burns.

Electrolysis: Electrolysis has been an option for over a century and is considered the only permanent form of hair removal. It uses an electrical current to disrupt individual hair follicles in the anagen (actively growing) phase. Since only a percentage of hair follicles are in the anagen phase at any given time, electrolysis must be done over several visits to steadily destroy all follicles in a given area. For instance, removing excess hair from the upper lip and chin could take approximately 18 monthly treatments, with the initial visits lasting longer than subsequent visits. Most patients find it mildly uncomfortable, and some take anti-pain medication (e.g., Tylenol) before their appointment. For the minority of patients who experience electrolysis as painful there is the option of EMLA® cream (for which you need a prescription from an M.D.) or ELA-Max cream (an over-the-counter medication, but more expensive).

Some states require that electrologists be licensed. In these states we advise that you only use those who have a license. However, many states, including New York, do not require electrologists to obtain a license. In these states it is recommended that that an electrologist be accredited by the American Electrology Association (AEA) and be a Certified Professional Electrologist (CPE). The AEA hosts a website at www.electrology.com with information about electrolysis and with a search engine to find AEA members in a given area. Questions to ask of an electrologist when choosing one are:

- Are you a CPE?
- Do you use disposable probes and do you sterilize your forceps?
- Is your equipment new (at least within the last 10 years)?

In unskilled hands, electrolysis can cause folliculitis (a painful, red swelling of the hair follicle) and scarring. Typical complications include a mild redness that lasts for about 1 hour afterward, occasional breakouts, and minor temporary scabbing. Many electrologists will require a doctor's note if you have diabetes, are a pregnant woman, are on blood thinners, or have mitral valve prolapse (a common heart condition, which usually causes no symptoms and doesn't need to be treated). Electrologists should offer a free consultation (where you can ask all these questions). They have variable fees, and, while electrolysis is not usually reimbursed by insurance, some people have successfully lobbied their insurance companies for reimbursement.

Laser Treatment

Laser treatment is the newest method of hair removal. There is less data on safety. Laser uses light waves to target the melanin (pigment) in the hair follicle and disrupt the follicle bulb. Because skin also contains melanin, light-skinned dark-haired individuals usually have the best outcomes with laser therapy. Like electrolysis, laser only destroys hairs in the anagen phase so multiple treatments are required to achieve hair removal in a given area. Approximately 50% to 70% of the excess hair can be removed. With this method follicles do not need to be treated one at a time, and therefore each treatment is relatively quick and usually only mildly uncomfortable.

There are several kinds of lasers used in treating hirsutism. The type of laser is chosen based on skin type. Laser treatment does not cause permanent hair loss since with time, hair tends to regrow to a variable extent. This is why touch-ups are required on a yearly basis. Complications could include permanent scarring and hypopigmentation (loss of normal skin color); however, based on very short-term data, these risks appear to be low if the procedure is done by a trained dermatological surgeon.

At the moment there are no regulations governing the use of laser technology, and in fact it is offered in any number of settings from local spas to beauty parlors. We strongly recommend that laser treatment be done only by a dermatological surgeon. Surgeons should be a member of the American Society for Dermatologic Surgery (ASDS) and have had specific medical training in the use of lasers. The ASDS hosts a website (www.asds-net.org) that contains information about laser hair removal and it provides a search engine that enables the user to find local ASDS-approved dermatological surgeons.

Hair Loss

Women with untreated CAH often experience temporal balding due to the action of androgens on the hair follicles of the scalp. Unlike the other androgen sensitive areas of the body, the hair follicles of the scalp respond to high androgen levels by making vellus (soft, pale, and fine) hair instead of the usual terminal hair found on the scalp. Usually, when the underlying hormonal imbalance is treated with replacement cortisol (i.e., Cortef, prednisone, or dexamethasone), women have a fairly rapid improvement in scalp hair regrowth.

In Summary

In summary, there are many ways to battle hirsutism or hair loss. The first and most important step is to consult your endocrinologist and make sure that the replacement medication you are taking is adequate. Then, if hirsutism is the problem, discuss the various options presented here with your endocrinologist and/or dermatologist and find a treatment plan that you are comfortable with. If you chose electrolysis or laser therapy, your doctor may be able to recommend a well-trained local professional. If you see something on a message board or the Internet, discuss it with your doctor before jumping right in. What works for one woman, may not be the treatment of choice for someone else.

Section 62.4

Questions and Answers about Alopecia Areata

Excerpted from "Questions and Answers About Alopecia Areata," National Institute of Arthritis and Musculoskeletal and Skin Diseases, February 2003. Available online at http://www.niams.nih.gov; accessed June 1, 2005.

What is alopecia areata?

Alopecia areata is considered an autoimmune disease, in which the immune system, which is designed to protect the body from foreign invaders such as viruses and bacteria, mistakenly attacks the hair follicles, the tiny cup-shaped structures from which hairs grow. This can lead to hair loss on the scalp and elsewhere.

In most cases, hair falls out in small, round patches about the size of a quarter. In many cases, the disease does not extend beyond a few bare patches. In some people, hair loss is more extensive. Although uncommon, the disease can progress to cause total loss of hair on the head (referred to as alopecia areata totalis) or complete loss of hair on the head, face, and body (alopecia areata universalis).

What causes it?

In alopecia areata, immune system cells called white blood cells attack the rapidly growing cells in the hair follicles that make the hair. The affected hair follicles become small and drastically slow down hair production. Fortunately, the stem cells that continually supply the follicle with new cells do not seem to be targeted. So the follicle always has the potential to regrow hair.

Scientists do not know exactly why the hair follicles undergo these changes, but they suspect that a combination of genes may predispose some people to the disease. In those who are genetically predisposed, some type of trigger—perhaps a virus or something in the person's environment—brings on the attack against the hair follicles.

Who is most likely to get it?

Alopecia areata affects an estimated four million Americans of both sexes and of all ages and ethnic backgrounds. It often begins in childhood.

If you have a close family member with the disease, your risk of developing it is slightly increased. If your family member lost his or her first patch of hair before age 30, the risk to other family members is greater. Overall, one in five people with the disease have a family member who has it as well.

Is my hair loss a symptom of a serious disease?

Alopecia areata is not a life-threatening disease. It does not cause any physical pain, and people with the condition are generally healthy otherwise. But for most people, a disease that unpredictably affects their appearance the way alopecia areata does is a serious matter.

The effects of alopecia areata are primarily socially and emotionally disturbing. In alopecia universalis, however, loss of eyelashes and eyebrows and hair in the nose and ears can make the person more vulnerable to dust, germs, and foreign particles entering the eyes, nose, and ears.

Alopecia areata often occurs in people whose family members have other autoimmune diseases, such as diabetes, rheumatoid arthritis, thyroid disease, systemic lupus erythematosus, pernicious anemia, or Addison's disease. People who have alopecia areata do not usually have other autoimmune diseases, but they do have a higher occurrence of thyroid disease, atopic eczema, nasal allergies, and asthma.

Will my hair ever grow back?

There is every chance that your hair will regrow, but it may also fall out again. No one can predict when it might regrow or fall out. The course of the disease varies from person to person. Some people lose just a few patches of hair, then the hair regrows, and the condition never recurs. Other people continue to lose and regrow hair for many years. A few lose all the hair on their head; some lose all the hair on their head, face, and body. Even in those who lose all their hair, the possibility for full regrowth remains.

In some, the initial hair regrowth is white, with a gradual return of the original hair color. In most, the regrown hair is ultimately the same color and texture as the original hair.

How is it treated?

While there is neither a cure for alopecia areata nor drugs approved for its treatment, some people find that medications approved for other purposes can help hair grow back, at least temporarily. The following are some treatments for alopecia areata. Keep in mind that while these treatments may promote hair growth, none of them prevent new patches or actually cure the underlying disease. Consult your health care professional about the best option for you.
Note: Brand names included in this chapter are provided as examples only, and their inclusion does not mean that these products are endorsed by the National Institutes of Health or any other Government agency. Also, if a particular brand name is not mentioned, this does not mean or imply that the product is unsatisfactory.

Corticosteroids: Corticosteroids are powerful anti-inflammatory drugs similar to a hormone called cortisol produced in the body. Because these drugs suppress the immune system if given orally, they are often used in the treatment of various autoimmune diseases, including alopecia areata. Corticosteroids may be administered in three ways for alopecia areata:

- *Local injections*: Injections of steroids directly into hairless patches on the scalp and sometimes the brow and beard areas are effective in increasing hair growth in most people. It usually takes about 4 weeks for new hair growth to become visible. Injections deliver small amounts of cortisone to affected areas, avoiding the more serious side effects encountered with long-term oral use. The main side effects of injections are transient pain, mild swelling, and sometimes changes in pigmentation, as well as small indentations in the skin that go away when injections are stopped. Because injections can be painful, they may not be the preferred treatment for children. After 1 or 2 months, new hair growth usually becomes visible, and the injections usually have to be repeated monthly. The cortisone removes the confused immune cells and allows the hair to grow. Large areas cannot be treated, however, because the discomfort and the amount of medicine become too great and can result in side effects similar to those of the oral regimen.
- *Oral corticosteroids:* Corticosteroids taken by mouth are a mainstay of treatment for many autoimmune diseases and may be used in more extensive alopecia areata. But because of the risk

of side effects of oral corticosteroids, such as hypertension and cataracts, they are used only occasionally for alopecia areata and for shorter periods of time.

- *Topical ointments:* Ointments or creams containing steroids rubbed directly onto the affected area are less traumatic than injections and, therefore, are sometimes preferred for children. However, corticosteroid ointments and creams alone are less effective than injections; they work best when combined with other topical treatments, such as minoxidil or anthralin.

Minoxidil (5%) (Rogaine): Topical minoxidil solution promotes hair growth in several conditions in which the hair follicle is small and not growing to its full potential. Minoxidil is FDA-approved for treating male and female pattern hair loss. It may also be useful in promoting hair growth in alopecia areata. The solution, applied twice daily, has been shown to promote hair growth in both adults and children, and may be used on the scalp, brow, and beard areas. With regular and proper use of the solution, new hair growth appears in about 12 weeks.

Anthralin (Psoriatec): Anthralin, a synthetic tar-like substance that alters immune function in the affected skin, is an approved treatment for psoriasis. Anthralin is also commonly used to treat alopecia areata. Anthralin is applied for 20 to 60 minutes ("short contact therapy") to avoid skin irritation, which is not needed for the drug to work. When it works, new hair growth is usually evident in 8 to 12 weeks. Anthralin is often used in combination with other treatments, such as corticosteroid injections or minoxidil, for improved results.

Sulfasalazine: A sulfa drug, sulfasalazine has been used as a treatment for different autoimmune disorders, including psoriasis. It acts on the immune system and has been used to some effect in patients with severe alopecia areata.

Topical Sensitizers: Topical sensitizers are medications that, when applied to the scalp, provoke an allergic reaction that leads to itching, scaling, and eventually hair growth. If the medication works, new hair growth is usually established in 3 to 12 months. Two topical sensitizers are used in alopecia areata: squaric acid dibutyl ester (SADBE) and diphenylcyclopropenone (DPCP). Their safety and consistency of formula are currently under review.

Oral Cyclosporine: Originally developed to keep people's immune systems from rejecting transplanted organs, oral cyclosporine is sometimes used to suppress the immune system response in psoriasis and other immune-mediated skin conditions. But suppressing the immune system can also cause problems, including an increased risk of serious infection and possibly skin cancer. Although oral cyclosporine may regrow hair in alopecia areata, it does not turn the disease off. Most doctors feel the dangers of the drug outweigh its benefits for alopecia areata.

Photochemotherapy: In photochemotherapy, a treatment used most commonly for psoriasis, a person is given a light-sensitive drug called a psoralen either orally or topically and then exposed to an ultraviolet light source. This combined treatment is called PUVA. In clinical trials, approximately 55 percent of people achieve cosmetically acceptable hair growth using photochemotherapy. However, the relapse rate is high, and patients must go to a treatment center where the equipment is available at least two to three times per week. Furthermore, the treatment carries the risk of developing skin cancer.

Alternative Therapies: When drug treatments fail to bring sufficient hair regrowth, some people turn to alternative therapies. Alternatives purported to help alopecia areata include acupuncture, aromatherapy, evening primrose oil, zinc and vitamin supplements, and Chinese herbs.

Because many alternative therapies are not backed by clinical trials, they may or may not be effective for regrowing hair. In fact, some may actually make hair loss worse. Furthermore, just because these therapies are natural does not mean that they are safe. As with any therapy, it is best to discuss these treatments with your doctor before you try them.

In addition to treatments to help hair grow, there are measures that can be taken to minimize the physical dangers or discomforts of lost hair.

- Sunscreens are important for the scalp, face, and all exposed areas.
- Eyeglasses (or sunglasses) protect the eyes from excessive sun, and from dust and debris, when eyebrows or eyelashes are missing.
- Wigs, caps, or scarves protect the scalp from the sun and keep the head warm.

- Antibiotic ointment applied inside the nostrils helps to protect against organisms invading the nose when nostril hair is missing.

Section 62.5

Folliculitis: Infection of the Hair Follicles

Folliculitis is the infection of hair follicles. This can occur anywhere on the skin or scalp. Usually there is some itch and sometimes a little soreness. Folliculitis looks like acne pimples or non-healing, crusty sores. An acute eruption or one present for only a short time is usually due to staphylococcal germs (impetigo of Bockhart). This is treated with oral Keflex, dicloxacillin, or similar oral antibiotic for 10 days.

Topical antibiotic creams or lotions can also be used. Bactroban ointment should be applied into the front of the nose for several days to prevent a carrier state. While this may seem like it makes no sense, the inside front area of the nostrils is often a place where bacteria can survive a course of oral antibiotics. Later, they spread back to the skin to cause a relapse.

Chronic or recurring folliculitis is less likely to clear with just antibiotics. Often this is on the legs of women, but it can occur in any areas of shaving, waxing, hair plucking, or friction. These need to be stopped for at least 3 months to allow the hair to grow in healthy. If shaving is resumed, one should shave with the grain of the hair; it won't **feel** quite as smooth, but it will **look** a whole lot better.

A pill such as tetracycline or minocycline can be given for 4 to 6 weeks. Unless the skin is sensitive, drying antiseptic lotions should be used on the affected areas such as Xerac-AC (aluminum chlorohydrate solution), Cleocin-T solution, or BenzaClin gel. In some cases, the infection with unusual bacteria may be picked up from a dirty hot tub or scrubbing brush.

For those with sensitive skin, friction and rubbing must be avoided. Avoid Lycra workout clothes and tight-fitting rough fabrics like blue jeans in the affected area. Apply a non-greasy moisturizer such as Lac-Hydrin cream (ammonium lactate 12%) plus mild prescription cortisone cream to the area if there is an associated atopic dermatitis (eczema).

Resistant and recurrent cases, especially on the legs, may clear with hair removal laser treatments. This may be expensive and require several treatments, but is helpful when other treatments fail.

Chapter 63

Nail Disorders

Barometers of Health

Nails often serve as barometers of our health; they are diagnostic tools providing the initial signal of the presence or onset of systemic diseases. For example, the pitting of nails and increased nail thickness can be manifestations of psoriasis. Concavity—nails that are rounded inward instead of outward—can foretell iron deficiency anemia. Some nail problems can be conservatively treated with topical or oral medications while others require partial or total removal of the nail. Any discoloration or infection on or about the nail should be evaluated by a podiatric physician.

Nail Ailments

Ingrown Toenails

Ingrown nails, the most common nail impairment, are nails whose corners or sides dig painfully into the soft tissue of nail grooves, often leading to irritation, redness, and swelling. Usually, toenails grow straight out. Sometimes, however, one or both corners or sides curve and grow into the flesh. The big toe is usually the victim of this condition but other toes can also become affected.

Ingrown toenails may be caused by:

"Nail Problems" is reprinted with permission from the American Podiatric Medical Association, www.apma.org.

- Improperly trimmed nails (Trim them straight across, not longer than the tip of the toes.) Do not round off corners. Use toenail clippers.
- Heredity
- Shoe pressure; crowding of toes
- Repeated trauma to the feet from normal activities

If you suspect an infection due to an ingrown toenail, immerse the foot in a warm salt water soak, or a basin of soapy water, then apply an antiseptic and bandage the area.

People with diabetes, peripheral vascular disease, or other circulatory disorders must avoid any form of self-treatment and seek podiatric medical care as soon as possible.

Other "do-it-yourself" treatments, including any attempt to remove any part of an infected nail or the use of over-the-counter medications, should be avoided. Nail problems should be evaluated and treated by your podiatrist, who can diagnose the ailment, and then prescribe medication or another appropriate treatment.

A podiatrist will resect the ingrown portion of the nail and may prescribe a topical or oral medication to treat the infection. If ingrown nails are a chronic problem, your podiatrist can perform a procedure to permanently prevent ingrown nails. The corner of the nail that ingrows, along with the matrix or root of that piece of nail, are removed by use of a chemical, a laser, or by other methods.

Fungal Nails

Fungal infection of the nail, or onychomycosis, is often ignored because the infection can be present for years without causing any pain. The disease is characterized by a progressive change in a nail's quality and color, which is often ugly and embarrassing.

In reality, the condition is an infection underneath the surface of the nail caused by fungi. When the tiny organisms take hold, the nail often becomes darker in color and foul smelling. Debris may collect beneath the nail plate, white marks frequently appear on the nail plate, and the infection is capable of spreading to other toenails, the skin, or even the fingernails. If ignored, the infection can spread and possibly impair one's ability to work or even walk. This happens because the resulting thicker nails are difficult to trim and make walking painful when wearing shoes. Onychomycosis can also be accompanied by a secondary bacterial or yeast infection in or about the nail plate.

Because it is difficult to avoid contact with microscopic organisms like fungi, the toenails are especially vulnerable around damp areas where people are likely to be walking barefoot, such as swimming pools, locker rooms, and showers, for example. Injury to the nail bed may make it more susceptible to all types of infection, including fungal infection. Those who suffer from chronic diseases, such as diabetes, circulatory problems, or immune deficiency conditions, are especially prone to fungal nails. Other contributing factors may be a history of athlete's foot and excessive perspiration.

Prevention

- Proper hygiene and regular inspection of the feet and toes are the first lines of defense against fungal nails.
- Clean and dry feet resist disease.
- Washing the feet with soap and water, remembering to dry thoroughly, is the best way to prevent an infection.
- Shower shoes should be worn when possible in public areas.
- Shoes, socks, or hosiery should be changed more than once daily.
- Toenails should be clipped straight across so that the nail does not extend beyond the tip of the toe.
- Wear shoes that fit well and are made of materials that breathe.
- Avoid wearing excessively tight hosiery, which promote moisture.
- Socks made of synthetic fiber tend to "wick" away moisture faster than cotton or wool socks.
- Disinfect instruments used to cut nails.
- Disinfect home pedicure tools.
- Don't apply polish to nails suspected of infection—those that are red, discolored, or swollen, for example.

Treatment of Fungal Nails

Treatments may vary, depending on the nature and severity of the infection. A daily routine of cleansing over a period of many months may temporarily suppress mild infections. White markings that appear on the surface of the nail can be filed off, followed by the application of an over-the-counter liquid antifungal agent. However, even the best over-the-counter treatments may not prevent a fungal infection from coming back.

A podiatric physician can detect a fungal infection early, culture the nail, determine the cause, and form a suitable treatment plan, which may include prescribing topical or oral medication, and debridement (removal of diseased nail matter and debris) of an infected nail.

Newer oral antifungals, approved by the Food and Drug Administration, may be the most effective treatment. They offer a shorter treatment regimen of approximately three months and improved effectiveness. Podiatrists may also prescribe a topical treatment for onychomycosis, which can be an effective treatment modality for fungal nails.

In some cases, surgical treatment may be required. Temporary removal of the infected nail can be performed to permit direct application of a topical antifungal. Permanent removal of a chronically painful nail that has not responded to any other treatment permits the fungal infection to be cured and prevents the return of a deformed nail.

Trying to solve the infection without the qualified help of a podiatric physician can lead to more problems. With new technical advances in combination with simple preventive measures, the treatment of this lightly regarded health problem can often be successful.

Your podiatric physician/surgeon has been trained specifically and extensively in the diagnosis and treatment of all manner of foot conditions. This training encompasses all of the intricately related systems and structures of the foot and lower leg including neurological, circulatory, skin, and the musculoskeletal system, which includes bones, joints, ligaments, tendons, muscles, and nerves.

Part Nine

Dermatological Medications and Treatments

Chapter 64

Overview of Nonsurgical and Surgical Dermatological Treatments

Chapter Contents

Section 64.1

Getting Ready for Treatment: Seeing a Dermatologist

"Seeing a Dermatologist" is from *National Women's Health Report Online*, Volume 26, Number 3, June 2004. Reproduced with permission of the National Women's Health Resource Center.

If you thought you were finished with dermatologists when you outgrew your teenage acne, think again. Studies find that a physician's ability to identify potentially precancerous lesions is based on the doctor's training in that area, and no one is better trained to spot suspicious spots than a dermatologist.

Different organizations have different recommendations when it comes to skin examinations. The American Academy of Dermatology recommends annual screenings, the American Cancer Society recommends skin exams every three years between ages 20 and 39 and annually after age 40, and the U.S. Preventive Services Task Force says there is insufficient evidence to recommend for or against routine skin examinations. There's no controversy over the fact that the earlier skin cancers are identified, the better the outcome. So talk to your health care professional about when to be screened.

Finding a dermatologist is pretty simple—the American Academy of Dermatology has a search function on its website (http://www.aad.org). As with most medical specialties today, you can also find specialty dermatologists. Some, called Mohs surgeons (named after the creator of a surgical technique for removing skin cancer tumors), specialize in skin cancer surgery.

Dermatopathologists focus on reading dermatological slides to identify cancers and other skin problems, while pediatric dermatologists have additional training in pediatrics. Laser specialists may have received additional training in using lasers, while dermatological immunologists specialize in autoimmune diseases like psoriasis and scleroderma. Then there are cosmetic dermatologists who often limit their practice only to cosmetic procedures.

Your best bet is to start with a general dermatologist, however. "We see all types of patients, and do some surgery, cosmetics, laser procedures, and uncomplicated pathology," says Maryland dermatologist Elizabeth A. Liotta, MD. "If we can't handle a complicated case, we'll happily refer you on."

Section 64.2

Nonsurgical and Surgical Skin Treatments

Excerpted from "Cosmetic Procedures," by the National Women's Health Information Center, August 2004. Available online at http://www.4woman.gov; accessed June 15, 2005.

Trying to fight the effects of aging? Below is a basic guide to the risks involved in both surgical and nonsurgical cosmetic procedures.

Cosmetic Procedures: Surgical

Procedure: Breast Augmentation

Breasts are enlarged by placing an implant behind each breast.

Risks

- implants can rupture, leak, and deflate
- infection
- hardening of scar tissue around implant, causing breast firmness, pain, distorted shape, or implant movement
- bleeding
- pain
- nipples may get more or less sensitive
- numbness near incision
- blood collection around implant/incision
- calcium deposits around implant
- harder-to-find breast lumps

Procedure: Breast Lift

Extra skin is removed from the breast to raise and reshape breast.

Risks

- scarring
- skin loss
- infection
- loss of feeling in nipples or breast
- nipples put in the wrong place
- breasts not symmetrical

Procedure: Breast Reduction

Fat, tissue, and skin is removed from breast.

Risks

- if nipples and areola are detached, may lose sensation and decreased ability to breastfeed
- bleeding
- infection
- scarring
- harder-to-find breast lumps
- poor shape, size, or position of nipples or breasts

Procedure: Eyelid Surgery

Extra fat, skin, and muscle in the upper and/or lower eyelid is removed to correct droopy eyelids.

Risks

- blurred or double vision
- infection
- bleeding under the skin
- swelling
- dry eyes
- whiteheads
- can't close eye completely

- pulling of lower lids
- blindness

Procedure: Facelift

Extra fat is removed, muscles are tightened, and skin is rewrapped around the face and neck to improve sagging facial skin, jowls, and loose neck skin.

Risks
- infection
- bleeding under skin
- scarring
- irregular earlobes
- nerve damage causing numbness or inability to move your face
- hair loss
- skin damage

Procedure: Facial Implant

Implants are used to change the nose, jaws, cheeks, or chin.

Risks
- infection
- feeling of tightness or scarring around implant
- shifting of implant

Procedure: Forehead Lift

Extra skin and muscles that cause wrinkles are removed, eyebrows are lifted, and forehead skin is tightened.

Risks
- infection
- scarring
- bleeding under skin
- eye dryness or irritation
- impaired eyelid function
- loss of feeling in eyelid skin
- injury to facial nerve causing loss of motion or muscle weakness

Procedure: Lip Augmentation

Material is injected or implanted into the lips to create fuller lips and reduce wrinkles around the mouth.

Risks

- infection
- bleeding
- lip asymmetry
- lumping
- scarring

Procedure: Liposuction

Excess fat from a targeted area is removed with a vacuum to shape the body.

Risks

- baggy skin
- skin may change color and fall off
- fluid retention
- shock
- infection
- burning
- fat clots in the lungs
- pain
- damage to organs if punctured
- numbness at the surgery site
- heart problems
- kidney problems
- disability
- death

Procedure: Nose Surgery

Nose is reshaped by resculpting the bone and cartilage in the nose.

Risks

- infection
- bursting blood vessels

- red spots
- bleeding under the skin
- scarring

Procedure: Tummy Tuck

Extra fat and skin in the abdomen is removed, and muscles are tightened to flatten tummy.

Risks

- blood clots
- infection
- bleeding
- scarring
- fluid accumulation under the skin

Cosmetic Procedures: Nonsurgical

Procedure: Botox Injection

Botox is injected into a facial muscle to paralyze it, so lines don't form when a person frowns or squints.

Risks

- face pain
- muscle weakness
- flu-like symptoms
- headaches
- loss of facial expression
- droopy eyelids
- asymmetric smile
- drooling

Procedure: Collagen/Fat Injection

Collagen from a cow or fat from your thigh or abdomen is injected into facial wrinkles, pits, or scars.

Risks

- could trigger an autoimmune disease

- contour problems
- hives
- rash
- swelling
- flu-like symptoms

Procedure: Dermabrasion

A small, spinning wheel or brush with a roughened surface removes the upper layers of facial skin. A new layer of skin appears during healing, giving the face a smoother appearance. Used to treat facial scars, heavy wrinkles, and problems like rosacea.

Risks

- abnormal color
- changes
- whiteheads
- infection
- allergic reaction
- fever blisters
- cold sores
- thickened skin

Procedure: Hyaluronic Acid Injection

This gel is injected into your face to smooth lines, wrinkles, and scars on the skin.

Risks

- swelling
- infection
- redness
- tenderness
- acne
- lumps
- tissue hardening
- risks unknown if used in combination with collagen

Procedure: Laser Hair Removal

Laser light is passed over the skin to remove hair.

Risks

- hair regrowth
- scarring
- change in skin color

Procedure: Laser Skin Resurfacing

Laser light is used to remove wrinkles, lines, age spots, scars, moles, tattoos, and warts from the surface of the skin.

Risks

- burns
- scarring
- change in skin color
- infection
- herpes flare-up (fever, facial pain, and flu-like symptoms)

Procedure: Sclerotherapy

A solution is injected into spider and varicose leg veins (small purple and red blood vessels) to remove the veins.

Risks

- blood clots
- color changes in the skin
- vein removal may not be permanent
- scarring

Procedure: Chemical Peel

A solution is put onto the face (or parts of the face) that causes the skin to blister and peel off. It is replaced with new skin.

Risks

- whiteheads
- infection

- raised scarring
- allergic reaction
- cold sores
- color changes or blotchiness
- heart problems

Section 64.3

Hair Loss Treatments

"Hair Restoration Treatments" is reprinted with permission from the American Society for Dermatologic Surgery, http://asds-net.org.

Hair Loss

Although an abundance of so-called "cures" for thinning hair and baldness are available, the only true way to restore a person's hairline is to seek treatment from a physician. As board-certified specialists trained in hair restoration surgery, dermatologic surgeons are uniquely qualified to diagnose the cause of hair loss and recommend a treatment plan. Since hair restoration procedures greatly rely on the physician's skill and artistry, it's important to see a dermatologic surgeon with training and experience in this area.

Treatment Options

Dermatologic surgeons continue to pioneer the latest advances in the field, such as the use of much smaller and more flexible grafts, innovative tools and high-tech lasers, novel pain-reduction methods and new surgical approaches that make hair restoration treatment a successful solution to hair loss. And, because each case of hair loss or baldness differs in severity and the position of the natural hairline, dermatologic surgeons have further refined the range of hair restoration techniques in order to customize treatment to suit each patient's specific condition. The type of surgery chosen depends on the extent and pattern of hair loss, along with the patient's expectations, situation, and lifestyle. In many cases, a dermatologic surgeon may use a combination of techniques to produce the best results.

Hair Restoration Treatment Techniques

Hair Transplants

Small donor strips of hair-bearing scalp are removed from the back and sides of the head and are divided into grafts for placement in the balding areas. The hair-bearing grafts are carefully inserted into small holes or slits that are made in the balding scalp. These holes or slits are sometimes made with a laser. The grafts can also be inserted between existing hairs to increase the density and thicken the area.

For many years the basic size of the grafts was between 4 and 5 millimeters. Over the last few years smaller and finer grafts, such as micrografts and mini-grafts, have been successfully used.

Initially the donor hair falls out in a few weeks, but regrows about three months later. It continues to grow for as long as the hair would have in the site from which it was removed.

Scalp Reduction

The areas of bald scalp are reduced by surgical excision, then pulling upward and lifting the hair-bearing skin together. Decreasing the size of the bald patch, this option offers a special benefit to patients with extensive balding.

Scalp extenders or tissue expanders are sometimes used to increase the effectiveness of scalp reduction surgery.

Skin Lifts and Grafts

A "flap" of hair-bearing skin is created by making surgical cuts near the balding area. The flap is then rotated onto the balding section.

Minoxidil

This anti-balding drug is applied directly to the scalp. Used in conjunction with surgical treatment, minoxidil can be effective in retaining hair to provide a fuller, more natural look. Minoxidil is not a cure for baldness, but it has been shown to retard recent hair loss and to stimulate new hair growth, particularly in the crown of the scalp in certain, usually younger men.

Finasteride

This drug given orally has been shown under continued usage to help preserve existing hair. It may be combined with minoxidil and other surgical techniques for excellent results.

Chapter 65

Botox: A Look at Looking Good

The promise of a more youthful look was too tempting for 53-year-old Mary Schwallenberg to pass up. So, when the Food and Drug Administration approved a product that temporarily improves the appearance of frown lines between the eyebrows, the Orlando, Florida, resident took a shot at it. And it wasn't long before she became one of many people clamoring for regular treatments that often include refreshments and friendly conversation, as well as injections.

Botulinum Toxin Type A (Botox Cosmetic) is a protein complex produced by the bacterium *Clostridium botulinum*, which contains the same toxin that causes food poisoning. When used in a medical setting as an injectable form of sterile, purified botulinum toxin, small doses block the release of a chemical called acetylcholine by nerve cells that signal muscle contraction. By selectively interfering with the underlying muscles' ability to contract, existing frown lines are smoothed out and, in most cases, are nearly invisible in a week.

Botox injections are the fastest-growing cosmetic procedure in the industry, according to the American Society for Aesthetic Plastic Surgery (ASAPS). In 2001, more than 1.6 million people received injections, an increase of 46 percent over the previous year. More popular than breast enhancement surgery and a potential blockbuster, Botox is regarded by some as the ultimate fountain of youth.

"Botox Cosmetic: A Look at Looking Good," by Carol Lewis, U.S. Food and Drug Administration, *FDA Consumer* magazine, July-August 2002. Available online at http://www.fda.gov; accessed May 13, 2005.

Schwallenberg, a pharmaceutical sales representative who is excited about her next round of injections, says she wants to look her best for her job. "That's corporate America for you," she says. "I have a lot of energy and I just wanted to look good."

Botox was first approved in 1989 to treat two eye muscle disorders—uncontrollable blinking (blepharospasm) and misaligned eyes (strabismus). In 2000, the toxin was approved to treat a neurological movement disorder that causes severe neck and shoulder contractions, known as cervical dystonia. As an unusual side effect of the eye disorder treatment, doctors observed that Botox softened the vertical frown (glabellar) lines between the eyebrows that tend to make people look tired, angry or displeased. But until this improvement was actually demonstrated in clinical studies, Allergan Inc., of Irvine, California, was prohibited from making this claim for the product.

By April 2002, the FDA was satisfied by its review of studies indicating that Botox reduced the severity of frown lines for up to 120 days. The agency then granted approval to use the drug for this condition.

The FDA regulates products, but not how they are used. Approved products are sometimes used by a licensed practitioner for uses other than those stated in the product label. Botox Cosmetic, for example, is currently being used by physicians to treat facial wrinkles other than those specified by the FDA. Consumers should be aware, however, that this off-label use has not been independently reviewed by the agency, and the safety and effectiveness of Botox injections into other regions of the face and neck, alone or in combination with the frown-lines region, have not been clinically evaluated.

Ella L. Toombs, M.D., a dermatologic medical officer in the FDA's Office of Cosmetics and Colors, says, "Careful deliberation, investigation and evaluation is undertaken by the agency before any prescription product is approved." Drugs such as Botox, which are not indicated for serious or life-threatening conditions, "are subject to a greater level of scrutiny because of the benefit-to-risk ratio." Toombs says this means that the FDA may allow someone to incur a greater risk from products that treat medical conditions, rather than from those that are approved for cosmetic purposes.

Botox Parties

The recent rise in the popularity of Botox has much to do with the manner in which it is frequently marketed. Some practitioners buy the toxin in bulk and arrange get-togethers for people receiving their treatments. As in business, volume discounts can be found in medicine.

Plastic surgery events known as Botox parties—also seminars, evenings, and socials—are a key element of Botox marketing in much of the United States. The gatherings are thought to be a convenient means of providing Botox treatments more economically, and may help reduce the anxiety that normally goes along with getting an injection. Doctors are finding that treating people in groups allows them to make the procedure more affordable to their patients.

Here's how a "party" typically works: A group of often nervous, but excited, middle-aged men and women mingle in a common area. Sometimes refreshments are served. One by one, as their name is called, each slips away for about 15 minutes to a private exam room. He or she pays a fee and signs an informed consent agreement. Anesthesia is rarely needed, but sedatives and numbing agents may be available. The practitioner injects about one-tenth of a teaspoon of toxin into specific muscles of the forehead most often targeted for the effect. The person then rejoins the group.

Scott A. Greenberg, M.D., a board-certified plastic surgeon in Winter Park, Florida, has been hosting monthly "Botox Happy Hours" in his medical office since the drug's approval in April. Greenberg feels that these by-invitation-only events to previous patients "are an opportunity to treat a lot of people at one time in a relaxed but professional atmosphere." Greenberg says there is no difference between treating 10 people during individual office visits throughout the day and treating 10 people individually, but in a more socialized setting. "The important thing is that the identical standards of medical care are maintained at these gatherings as in a routine daytime office consultation."

Julianne Clifford, Ph.D., of the FDA's Division of Vaccines and Related Products Applications, explains that "Botox is licensed for marketing and distribution as single-use vials." This means that as packaged, "each vial is intended to be used for a single patient in a single treatment session." Botox does not contain a preservative against potential contamination of the product through repeated use of a single vial. Once opened and diluted, Botox must be used within four hours. Treating multiple people with one vial violates product labeling, which is stated on the package insert, the vial and the carton.

"We lose something when we mass treat," says Franklin L. DiSpaltro, M.D., president of the ASAPS. "One of my concerns is that these parties are a marketing tool—gathering as many patients as possible trivializes a medical treatment, which could deteriorate over time into a nonprofessional environment." DiSpaltro says there's more to medicine "than just dispensing drugs."

Schwallenberg, however, insists that "Dr. Greenberg was very professional. It wasn't a cattle call," she says. "And I don't think I'd go to a doctor I didn't know."

The FDA is concerned that Botox has the potential for being abused. The ASAPS recently reported that unqualified people are dispensing Botox in salons, gyms, hotel rooms, home-based offices, and other retail venues. In such cases, people run the risks of improper technique, inappropriate dosages, and unsanitary conditions. "Botox is a prescription drug that should be administered by a qualified physician in an appropriate medical setting," says Toombs.

Greenberg agrees. "Patient safety has to be of prime concern," he says. "People need to be in the right hands when complications arise." That's why Greenberg does not allow his staff to administer Botox treatments. Even the most skilled health care providers, he says, can have complications as well as dissatisfied customers.

Although there is no chance of contracting botulism from Botox injections, there are some risks associated with the procedure. If too much toxin is injected, for example, or if it is injected into the wrong facial area, a person can end up with droopy eyelid muscles (ptosis) that could last for weeks. This particular complication was observed in clinical trials.

Other common side effects following injection were headache, respiratory infection, flu syndrome, and nausea. Less frequent adverse reactions included pain in the face, redness at the injection site, and muscle weakness. These reactions were generally temporary, but could last several months.

While the effects of Botox Cosmetic don't last, still, people don't seem to mind repeating the procedure every four to six months in order to maintain a wrinkle-free look. Battling the signs of aging in a non-invasive way, after all, is part of the allure of the product—that and the fact that there are no unsightly scars, and that there is very little recovery time with the procedure.

The FDA recommends that Botox Cosmetic be injected no more frequently than once every three months, and that the lowest effective dose should be used.

Considering Botox Cosmetic?

- Be sure that a qualified doctor performs the procedure.

- Make sure that the doctor is trained and qualified in cosmetic skin surgery of the face.
- Ask questions and be informed about the benefits and risks involved in the procedure.
- Avoid alcohol and remain upright for several hours following the procedure.
- Choose a medical setting using sterile techniques. Necessary equipment should be available to respond to any potential problems.

Source: The American Society for Dermatologic Surgery

Chapter 66

Cosmetic Laser Surgery: A High-Tech Weapon in the Fight against Aging Skin

Vaporized.

Normally this is not a good thing where humans are concerned. In science fiction films the characters vaporized by a laser simply disappear. Patients opting for cosmetic laser surgery, however, suffer a less severe fate: Only their wrinkles and other skin imperfections disappear.

In recent years, lasers have shed their science fictional image to become a surgeon's and dermatologist's most promising weapon in the fight against aging skin. According to the American Academy of Cosmetic Surgery in Chicago, nearly 170,000 Americans, men and women, underwent laser resurfacing of the face in 1998, up from 138,891 in 1996—a 64 percent increase. That's nearly twice the number of the more traditional surgical facelifts performed in the same year.

Laser resurfacing is a very controlled burning procedure during which a laser vaporizes superficial layers of facial skin, removing not only wrinkles and lines caused by sun damage and facial expressions, but also acne scars, some folds and creases around the nose and mouth, and even precancerous and benign superficial growths. In a sense, the laser procedure creates a fresh surface over which new skin can grow.

U.S. Food and Drug Administration, *FDA Consumer* magazine, May-June 2000. Revised by David A. Cooke, M.D., on April 27, 2005. Available online at http://www.fda.gov; accessed April 2005.

While the Food and Drug Administration does not regulate how surgeons carry out these procedures, it is responsible for clearing lasers for marketing for the uses requested by the device's manufacturer.

Lasers in Cosmetic Surgery

Since their 1958 discovery, lasers have become a powerful industrial tool, but their applications in medicine have been truly revolutionary. One reason, says Richard Felten, a senior reviewer in FDA's Center for Devices and Radiological Health, is that lasers used as surgical tools can cut through tissue without causing excessive bleeding. In fact, lasers actually can coagulate tissue to stop bleeding. "That's something a knife can't do," Felten says. Also, for many internal procedures, surgeons can get the laser's energy to reach areas within the body more easily than with a scalpel. And finally, the wavelengths of the laser light itself lets surgeons use the device selectively on very specific types of tissues, such as port wine stains or hair follicles, without affecting nearby tissue. (See "Other Laser Treatments.")

But using lasers for facial skin resurfacing was discovered almost by accident, Felten says. In the course of treating acne scars with a laser, surgeons noticed that after resurfacing the skin around the scar to make the scar less visible, small adjacent wrinkles were greatly diminished.

"Resurfacing is very appealing to people," says Stephen W. Perkins, M.D., president of the American Academy of Facial Plastic and Reconstructive Surgery and of the Meridian Plastic Surgery Center of Indianapolis, Ind., "because it is a way of refreshing the skin's surface and getting a new layer of non-sun damaged and more youthful skin."

Collagen is a key fibrous protein in the skin's connective tissue, and it helps give the skin its texture. Natural aging and such factors as sun damage and smoking help break down the collagen layer so that the skin's once smooth surface develops wrinkles. New, more youthful collagen actually forms after laser treatment, says A. Jay Burns, M.D., partner in the Dallas Plastic Surgery Institute and assistant professor of plastic surgery at the University of Texas Southwestern Medical School.

Laser resurfacing can often make patients look 10 to 20 years younger, and the results can last for eight to 10 years, says Tina Alster, M.D., director of the Washington Institute of Dermatologic Laser Surgery in the nation's capital. But she warns that after surgery, patients must avoid sunbathing and destroying their skin again. Patients can have a repeat treatment after one year, but usually the first procedure is so successful a follow-up is not needed.

Lasers cannot rejuvenate skin on other parts of the body nor can laser treatment lift or remove sagging jowls or smooth out "crepey" or sagging neck skin. These conditions only respond to traditional cut-and-stitch surgical methods.

Is Resurfacing for You?

Not everyone makes an ideal candidate for laser resurfacing, Perkins explains. "Certain people with very sensitive skin cannot tolerate the medications and lubricants used on the skin during healing." Perkins also feels that the darker-skinned ethnic groups are not candidates because the laser treatment alters the color of skin too dramatically and unpredictably. Alster, on the other hand, believes that in the hands of a very experienced surgeon, people with darker skin tones, although not ideal candidates, can benefit from surgery.

Alster warns that anyone not mentally prepared for resurfacing or who expects instant results is not a good candidate. "This is not easy in-easy out surgery," she says. "Potential patients have to realize that there will be bruising and swelling and they will be holed up in the house for seven to 10 days," she says. "They will have a crusty, oozy, bruised, scabbed, raw-appearing face." Further, they should not expect unflawed skin. "I can't deliver that," she says. "I am not able to give unlined, unscarred skin." Patients, however, can expect a 50 percent or greater improvement.

They must also plan on at least 10 days of healing before applying any makeup. For satisfactory healing, that means following rigorous after-care treatment, including proper skin cleansing, the application of a skin lubricant, and the frequent changing of dressings.

What Are the Risks?

As with any medical procedure, patients may experience certain complications—most temporary—including a prolonged redness of skin, tenderness, easy flushing, and some pigmentary changes, like hyperpigmentation, when the skin appears darker than normal, says Rox Anderson, M.D., director of the Laser Center at Massachusetts General Hospital in Boston.

Other risks are more serious, and possibly permanent, including hypopigmentation, or lightening of the skin. "Somewhere between one to two years after treatment it becomes clear that there is a permanent lightening of the skin color where the resurfacing was done," he says.

And scarring may occur in about 2 percent of the cases, he adds, from poor postoperative care, during which time an infection may develop. Or a surgeon may go too deep during the procedure, creating an injury the skin cannot repair, says Alster.

Consider the case of Anne Jones (not her real name) in semi-rural Mississippi, a stay-at-home mom and a doctor's wife. Wanting to remove some mild acne scars, she went to a well-respected local plastic surgeon, but after a five-month recovery period, Jones realized that something had gone very wrong. "He had just burned my face," she says. It was red, with scar tissue all over, she adds.

Eventually, Jones went for help to an ophthalmologist who had extensive laser knowledge—many ophthalmologists use lasers for corrective eye surgery. He took one look at her and exclaimed, "Oh, I am so sorry this has happened to you." He told her that the surgeon had been too aggressive and had not used the right settings, so that her skin had retained too much heat and had been severely burned.

Because both qualified and unqualified practitioners are flooding the cosmetic laser surgery field, consumers may face some real hazards. "All of a sudden, there's widespread use of lasers by unqualified people," says Perkins, who notes that some laser manufacturers are so eager to sell their products that they stage one- or two-day meetings, or courses, for training. That means that even dentists, obstetricians, gynecologists, and family doctors are now offering laser surgery, says Alster.

"The person planning to do laser surgery must understand the basic physics of how laser energy is absorbed by tissue and how tissue responds," warns FDA's Felten. "Then that person should go where the surgery is performed and watch a skilled surgeon use the equipment." Besides that, says Anderson, the best people to work with lasers on skin conditions are the professionals who best understand skin and surgery of the skin: dermatologists and plastic surgeons.

"Sometimes people may choose the wrong laser, or a surgeon may believe more is better, which can lead to significant burning," says Alster. And some operators don't know they must keep wiping off the partially desiccated skin or that they must keep moving the hand holding the laser instrument during the procedure.

To date, no national policy exists for credentialing those planning to practice laser surgery. Felten says the FDA is responsible for granting individual manufacturers permission to market their lasers for the specific indications requested. The FDA also often recommends training needed to operate the lasers.

But credentialing is a state function, since states are responsible for the licensing of doctors and nurses, and standards for laser training vary from state to state.

That's bad news for patients like Jones. Two years after her procedure, she has spent nearly $70,000 for both the initial surgery and subsequent consultations and corrective surgeries to remove the scarring. She says she has partially reclaimed her life. But she bitterly regrets undergoing the initial surgery. "I will never look right," says Jones. "I would never do this again."

Finding the Best Surgeon

Selecting a laser surgeon is just like picking a qualified doctor for any medical treatment. "Consumers ask more questions of auto mechanics," says Alster. "This is surgery and with it comes inherent risks and complications. While it is perceived as easy, it is not. When you are talking about skin, it is harder to treat than eyes."

The Internet is a good place to start the search. Consumers can find thousands of websites, including those for specialists, laser and plastic surgery societies, and information pages. But consumers should be wary of assuming the accuracy of any information taken off the Internet because the unscrupulous can put up their own Web pages just as easily as can the qualified.

Alster suggests interviewing several doctors and evaluating their answers and their credentials. After all, she adds, it's the doctor's skill that counts—the laser is just the doctor's tool.

The next step is crucial: asking the right questions. Alster advises asking where the doctor has trained and if he or she owns or rents the equipment—those who own have likely made a commitment to training and to laser surgery. Inquire about how many procedures of this particular type the doctor has performed and how often the doctor performs them. Generally speaking, complication rates are lowest among doctors who have done the procedure many times and who do them frequently. Ask to see before and after pictures of the doctor's cases, and find out how many different types of lasers the doctor owns and how often each piece of equipment is used. "There is not one laser that does everything," she says, cautioning patients to select a surgeon whose practice offers more than one laser system. "One needs to use [the right] laser for the right lesion. So the person examining you must make the correct diagnosis," she says. Alster herself has at least 10 different lasers in her office.

Of course, the final decision may be difficult, since no doctor can guarantee perfection or complete safety, but well-informed patients with reasonable expectations may be one step closer to younger, fresher-looking skin.

Other Laser Treatments

Many skin conditions respond well to laser surgery, including red vascular lesions such as spider veins on the face, hemangiomas, and birthmarks such as port wine stains, says Rox Anderson, M.D., director of the Laser Center at Massachusetts General Hospital in Boston. Lasers also are useful for scars, warts, excessive eye folds, tattoos, and hair removal, along with such conditions as rosacea, brown age spots, and the brown and blue pigmented facial lesions common to Asian skin. "Most Asians are told, 'There's no hope. Live with it,'" Anderson says. But in one or two laser treatments, the facial lesion vanishes. "Lasers really are magic bullets. They can do things deep in the skin without trashing anything else. It's not like surgery where the tools are not microscopically specific." And most significantly, laser resurfacing can remove precancerous lesions caused by sun damage.

—by Alexandra Greeley, a writer in Reston, Va.

Chapter 67

Chemical Peels and Dermabrasion

Chapter Contents

Section 67.1

Chemical Peels

"Facial Rejuvenation by Chemical Peels: Frequently Asked Questions," by the Division of Plastic Surgery, University of Iowa Hospitals and Clinics, published October 2000, revised December 2000. Copyright protected material used with permission of the authors and the University of Iowa's Virtual Hospital, www.vh.org.

When we discuss chemical peels for facial rejuvenation, we are covering a very broad topic. These can vary from very mild peels with very temporary improvements to peels which are quite deep and which may produce long-lasting results. The recovery times from deeper peels can be extensive. [*Note:* The following questions were answered by dermatologists from the University of Iowa Hospitals and Clinics.]

What is a chemical peel?

A chemical peel is the use of some type of chemical, usually an acid, but not always an acid, used to injure the skin to some level with the purpose of producing a reduction in the visibility of wrinkles.

Are there different kinds of peels?

There are many different kinds of peels. Some peels are so mild, that people can buy glycolic types of peels and apply them at home. These peels do not generally produce any lasting results but can improve the general complexion. Stronger peels might include the TCA peel. This stands for trichloroacetic acid. This can vary from a weak concentration, which will only produce mild changes with short duration, or it can be a much more concentrated acid, which will produce a greater degree of redness and swelling, and may improve the fine wrinkles it is intended to treat for a longer period of time. We often use the Obagi blue peel, which is a variation of the TCA peel, for patients who desire a fairly quick recovery time, and only require moderate improvement in fine line wrinkles. For the deep lines that many patients have after many years of sun exposure, smoking and other detrimental acts, will require a much stronger chemical peel. For this we usually use phenolic acid. This chemical in the proper concentration can induce permanent changes in the skin, and can do a great deal to improve the deeper lines that can occur as we get older. There is an old saying, that there is no gain without some pain. The price one must pay for the significant improvements with the phenol peel is the long recovery time. For 10 days to 2 weeks the patient will be quite swollen and extremely red in appearance. And they will basically need to be treated as if they had a second-degree burn. The skin will remain red for a variable period after 2 to 3 weeks. But the patient may begin to apply makeup at that stage.

What is the recovery time after a peel?

Recovery time from a peel depends upon the strength of the treatment. There is almost no recovery time for the mild glycolic acid peel. The TCA peel, depending on its strength, may have a 2 to 7-day recovery, as far as getting back to the normal color of the skin. As previously stated the recovery time from a phenolic peel is quite long.

Can a chemical peel help with age spots?

A chemical peel can help with age spots. The traces here would include the addition of some bleaching agents to the chemical peel. The phenol peel is especially good at eliminating age spots, but as we said, one must endure the long recovery time. I should mention that the laser is also good at removing age spots.

Is anesthesia given during the procedures?

In most circumstances, we do not give a general anesthetic for chemical peels. We do often give some intravenous sedation for the stronger peels such as the phenol peel.

Are some people better candidates for chemical peels?

The chemical peels are most effective and probably least troublesome with patients with very light skin coloration. When one has much darker complexion, either deep Mediterranean or black skin, there is always some concern; there may be some variation in color afterward. It is usually necessary to do a test spot in areas other than the face to evaluate the color changes that might occur from the chemical peel.

What are some of the risks associated with peels?

There are some risks associated with any medical treatment. For the mild chemical peels, the risks are quite low. Patients can have an allergy to an agent and have some type of reaction to the peel, but this is not common in my experience. The major risk associated with the some of the stronger peels is the discoloration after the process. In most cases, a chemical peel will result in a lighter color after the healing process is complete. In some rare instances, a blotchy darker color can occur. This happens most commonly when patients do not take our advice regarding avoiding sun and the use of Sunblock for a period of time after the chemical peel. With the deeper peel, there is a small risk of scarring, if the peel goes too deep. There is also, in the case of a phenol peel, a small risk of cardiac irregularities. For this reason, we always use EKG [electrocardiogram] monitoring during the phenol peel.

What sort of questions should I ask the plastic surgeon? Should he or she be board certified?

I think it is important whether the surgeon has experience in the type of peel that he or she is going to recommend. Plastic surgeons that are board eligible will have been trained in the use of chemical peels. They cannot take their board certification exam unless they have been in practice at least 2 years.

Therefore, I think that board certification or eligibility is one way to check the training of the surgeon.

What's a good peel for acne?

Many people will attempt the phenol peel for acne. Personally, I have had better results using the laser in acne scarring.

Do these peels reduce the risk for possible skin cancers?

A strong chemical peel may kill very early skin cancer cells. I think that if skin cancer is of concern, it is best to have some biopsies of the suspect areas and to treat the skin cancer with more appropriate means. There is certainly some merit to treating some sun damaged skin, which is at high risk for skin cancer, with some of the deeper chemical peels. I cannot say that this method will prevent the development of skin cancer.

Can a laser be used in conjunction with a chemical peel? Say the laser before or after the peel?

I think that it is generally best to discuss the question of laser vs. chemical peel, and then pick the treatment method that will best meet your intended goals for treatment. Certainly one can do repeated Obagi-type peels and then go ahead and do a phenol type peel or the CO_2 laser if that would best achieve your goal.

One must always balance the risk associated with the treatment against the benefits that one hopes to attain.

I have fair skin that has suffered way too much sun damage over my youth. Would a peel help reduce the risk of skin cancer?

As I said earlier, I cannot be certain that a peel would reduce the risk of skin cancer. It may serve to get rid of some cells that are considered precursors to cancer. But over time those problems can reoccur.

So while the discoloration on my face may be "precancerous" (that's what the dermatologist said) I should do biopsy first. He also suggested Renova to help reverse damage. My concerns are not aesthetic, but strictly regard the risk of cancer.

I would agree. Use of a Retin-A product may be useful under the circumstances that you are describing. An experience dermatologist who is quite certain that the changes noted are "precancerous" would certainly feel comfortable with that recommendation and so do I. You should probably be re-examined in at least 6-month intervals to ensure that no changes occur to indicate cancer rather than precancerous conditions.

Is there anything special I need to do to prepare for a chemical peel?

For the deeper chemical peels and for the CO_2 laser, we generally place patients on a Retin-A and hydroxy quinone regimen for at least 4 to 6 weeks. This prepares the skin to achieve maximum benefits from the deep chemical peels. It helps reduce the risk of blotchy dark discoloration after the peel.

We use a similar pretreatment regimen when we are doing CO_2 laser treatment.

Section 67.2

Dermabrasion

"Skin Smoothing Surgery," © 2005 A.D.A.M., Inc.
Reprinted with permission.

Definition

Surgical removal of the top layers of the skin.

Description

Dermabrasion is usually performed on an awake patient using local anesthesia. Extensive procedures, however, may require sedation or general anesthesia. A surgical instrument is used to gently and carefully "sand" the surface of the skin down to normal, healthy skin. The healing tissue is treated with ointments (such as petroleum jelly or antibiotic ointments) to reduce scab formation (crusting) and therefore reduce scar formation.

Dermabrasion is helpful in reducing scars and fine skin creases (wrinkles).

Indications

Dermabrasion may be offered to patients with:

- facial scars from
  - acne
  - accidents
  - previous surgery
- fine facial wrinkles, such as around the mouth
- precancerous growths (keratoses)

For many of these conditions, alternative treatments exist. Always discuss your options with your physician.

Risks

The risks for any anesthesia are:

- reactions to medications
- infrequent but potentially severe heart or breathing problems

The risks for any surgery are:

- bleeding
- infection
- scarring

Additional risks include:

- permanent skin discoloration, either lighter, darker, or pinker

Expectations after Surgery

You will likely be given antibiotic pills to prevent a viral infection (severe cold sores). The skin may be treated with ointment and a wet or waxy dressing. The skin will be quite red and swollen, and eating and talking may be difficult. There may be some aching, tingling, or burning for a while after surgery. Pain can be controlled with medications. The swelling will subside within two to three weeks. The skin will itch as new skin starts to grow. The freckles sometimes disappear in the treated area, but may return.

The dermabraded skin may develop whiteheads (milia) after dermabrasion which usually disappear. Enlarged skin pores may also develop but usually shrink to normal size once the swelling has subsided.

If the treated skin remains red, elevated, and itches after healing has started, this may be a sign that abnormal scars are beginning to form. The surgeon will provide treatment which can be started early.

Convalescence

For men, shaving will be delayed, then an electric razor is used at first. For several weeks, the new skin layer will be a bit swollen, sensitive, and bright pink. Normal activities may be resumed and the patient can be back at work in about two weeks. Avoid any activity that could cause a bump to the treated area for at least 2 weeks; ball sports are to be avoided for 4 to 6 weeks. Stick to indoor pools to avoid sun and wind, and keep the face out of chlorinated water for at least 4 weeks. For 3 to 4 weeks the patient will experience a red flush with alcohol consumption.

It is important to protect the skin from the sun for 6 to 12 months until the pigment has completely returned. The skin pinkness will take about 3 months to fade. Hypoallergenic make-up may be worn to conceal the scar. When full repigmentation occurs, the color should closely match the surrounding skin, making the procedure virtually undetectable.

Chapter 68

Scar Revision Surgery

Alternative Names

Keloid revision; Hypertrophic scar revision; Scar repair

Definition

Surgical procedure to improve or minimize the appearance of scars, restore function, and correct disfigurement resulting from an injury, lesion, or previous surgery.

Description

Scar tissue forms as skin heals after an injury (such as an accident) or surgery. The amount of scarring may be determined by the size, depth, and location of the wound; the age of the person; heredity; and skin characteristics including color (pigmentation).

Surgery to revise scars is done while the patient is awake, sleeping (sedated), or deep asleep and pain-free (local anesthesia or general anesthesia).

Medications (topical corticosteroids, anesthetic ointments, and antihistamine creams) can reduce the symptoms of itching and tenderness. Scars shrink and become less noticeable as they age, therefore, immediate surgical revision is delayed until the scar lightens in color,

---

which is usually several months or even a year after a wound has healed.

A keloid is an abnormal scar that is thicker, different color and texture, extends beyond the edge of the wound, and has a tendency to recur. It often creates a thick, puckered effect simulating a tumor. A keloid is removed at the point where it meets normal tissue.

Massive injuries (such as burns) can cause loss of a large area of skin and may form hypertrophic scars. A hypertrophic scar can cause restricted movement of muscles, joints, and tendons (contracture). Surgical repair includes removing excessive scar tissue and a series of small incisions on both sides of the scar site, which create V-shaped skin flaps (Z-plasty), may be used. The result is a thin, less noticeable scar because the wound closure following a Z-plasty more closely follows the natural skin folds.

Skin grafting involves the taking of a thin (split thickness) layer of skin from another part of the body and placing it over the injured area. Skin flap surgery involves moving an entire thickness (full thickness) of skin, fat, nerves, blood vessels, and muscle from a healthy part of the body to the injured site. These techniques are planned when a considerable amount of skin has been lost in the original injury, when a thin scar will not heal, and when improved function (rather than aesthetic reasons) are the primary concern. Secondary procedures may later be necessary to achieve appropriate aesthetic results.

Indications

No scar can be removed completely. The degree of improvement will depend on variables such as the direction and size of the scar, the age of the person, skin type and color, and hereditary factors that may precondition the extent of the healing process.

Risks

Risks for any anesthesia are:

- reactions to medications;
- problems breathing.

Risks for any surgery are:

- bleeding;
- infection;

- blood clots;
- scar recurrence;
- keloid formation (or recurrence);
- dehiscence (separation) of the wound.

Excessive sun exposure to a scar may cause darkening, which could interfere with future revision.

Expectations after Surgery

A pressure or elastic dressing may be placed over the area following the operation to discourage recurrence of the keloid. For other types of scar revision, a light dressing is applied and sutures are usually removed in 3 to 4 days for the facial area, and 5 to 7 days for incisions on the body elsewhere.

Convalescence

The decision on when to return to normal activities and work depends on the type, degree, and location of the surgery. Most people can resume normal activities soon after surgery. Avoidance of activities that stretch the new immature scar and may widen the scar is usually recommended.

If a long-standing contracture is present, physical therapy may be required in addition to surgery to restore full function.

Exposure to the sun should be avoided for several months following treatment. Sunblockers or a dressing (such as a Band-Aid) will keep the sun from permanently tanning the healing scar.

Part Ten

Skin Hygiene, Care, and Protection

Chapter 69

Caring for Your Skin Year-Round

Chapter Contents

Section 69.1

Dry Skin Care and Treatment

Dry skin, also called xerosis, is a common problem. Your skin needs moisture to stay smooth and supple, and retaining moisture is especially difficult in winter. Central heating of home and other buildings is very drying to the skin.

Simple daily routines, such as bathing and towel drying, may actually remove moisture from the skin. Modifying your bathing routine will help preserve your skin's moisture. Bathing the skin will moisturize temporarily, but it removes the skin's oily lipid layer and in the long run causes more moisture loss than gain.

The wrong moisturizing lotion can have the same effect. Generally, water-based lotions (such as Lubriderm and Keri lotion) are best cosmetically, but oil-based creams are more effective in trapping moisture.

Instructions

1. Each day when you take your bath or shower, try to use lukewarm water. Hot water dries out the skin. Try to limit your time to 15 minutes or less in the bath or shower. Bathing should be done no more than once a day. If you bathe too frequently you will remove the natural oils from the skin, causing dryness.

2. Avoid using harsh soaps that dry the skin. Recommended soaps are Dove, Olay, and Basis. Even better than soap are skin cleansers such as Cetaphil Lotion, Oilatum-AD, and Aquanil.

3. Deodorant soaps are often very harsh and drying. If you need them, limit their use to areas that develop an odor such as the armpits, genital area, and feet.

4. Avoid vigorous use of a washcloth in cleansing. When toweling dry, do not rub the skin. Blot or pat dry so there is still some moisture left on the skin.

5. Next apply a moisturizer to the skin. The best time to do this is immediately after a bath or shower so that the moisturizer holds in the moisture from the shower. Choose either Cetaphil Cream, Moisturel Cream, or Eucerin Cream. If you have severely dry skin, apply an oil to the still moist skin such as Neutrogena Light Sesame Oil, Hermal Body Oil, Alpha-Keri Oil, or RoBathol, then apply a moisturizing cream and also apply the moisturizer at bedtime.

6. All areas that are exposed to the sun, such as the face, ears, hands, and back of the neck should have a moisturizer containing sun block or a sunscreen of SPF 15 or greater applied daily.

7. For laundry, use "All-free," "Tide-free," or "Cheer-free" detergents. Avoid using fabric softeners, especially in the dryer. Keep irritating fabrics away from your skin. Don't wear clothing made of wool or other scratchy fabrics. Use cotton percale sheets on your bed.

8. Use a humidifier in your home during the central heating season. If sweating causes itching, modify your activity and surroundings to minimize sweating. Work and sleep in a fairly constant temperature (68 to 75 degrees Fahrenheit) and humidity (45% to 55% humidity). Remember to keep drinking plenty of water and other liquids to keep your skin moist from the inside, too.

Section 69.2

Winter Skin Care and Frostbite Prevention

Excerpted from "Winter Weather FAQ," Centers for Disease Control and Prevention, December 3, 2004. Available online at http://www.bt.cdc.gov; accessed May 14, 2005.

What is hypothermia?

When exposed to cold temperatures, your body begins to lose heat faster than it can be produced. The result is hypothermia, or abnormally low body temperature. Body temperature that is too low affects the brain, making the victim unable to think clearly or move well. This makes hypothermia particularly dangerous because a person may not know it is happening and won't be able to do anything about it.

Hypothermia occurs most commonly at very cold environmental temperatures, but can occur even at cool temperatures (above 40 degrees Fahrenheit) if a person becomes chilled from rain, sweat, or submersion in cold water.

Who is most at risk for hypothermia?

Victims of hypothermia are most often:

- elderly people with inadequate food, clothing, or heating
- babies sleeping in cold bedrooms
- children left unattended
- adults under the influence of alcohol
- mentally ill individuals
- people who remain outdoors for long periods—the homeless, hikers, hunters, etc.

What are the warning signs for hypothermia?

Adults:

- shivering/exhaustion
- confusion/fumbling hands

- memory loss/slurred speech
- drowsiness

Infants:

- bright red, cold skin
- very low energy

What should I do if I see someone with warning signs of hypothermia?

If you notice signs of hypothermia, take the person's temperature. If it is below 95 degrees Fahrenheit, the situation is an emergency—get medical attention immediately. If medical care is not available, begin warming the person, as follows:

- Get the victim into a warm room or shelter.
- If the victim has on any wet clothing, remove it.
- Warm the center of the body first—chest, neck, head, and groin—using an electric blanket, if available. Or use skin-to-skin contact under loose, dry layers of blankets, clothing, towels, or sheets.
- Warm beverages can help increase the body temperature, but do NOT give alcoholic beverages. Do not try to give beverages to an unconscious person.
- After body temperature has increased, keep the person dry and wrapped in a warm blanket, including the head and neck.
- Get medical attention as soon as possible.

A person with severe hypothermia may be unconscious and may not seem to have a pulse or to be breathing. In this case, handle the victim gently, and get emergency assistance immediately.

Even if the victim appears dead, CPR should be provided. CPR should continue while the victim is being warmed, until the victim responds or medical aid becomes available. In some cases, hypothermia victims who appear to be dead can be successfully resuscitated.

What is frostbite?

Frostbite is an injury to the body that is caused by freezing. Frostbite causes a loss of feeling and color in affected areas. It most often affects the nose, ears, cheeks, chin, fingers, or toes. Frostbite can permanently damage the body, and severe cases can lead to amputation.

What are the warning signs of frostbite?

At the first signs of redness or pain in any skin area, get out of the cold or protect any exposed skin—frostbite may be beginning. Any of the following signs may indicate frostbite:

- a white or grayish-yellow skin area
- skin that feels unusually firm or waxy
- numbness

Note: A victim is often unaware of frostbite until someone else points it out because the frozen tissues are numb.

What should I do if I see someone with warning signs of frostbite?

If you detect symptoms of frostbite, seek medical care. Because frostbite and hypothermia both result from exposure, first determine whether the victim also shows signs of hypothermia, as described previously.

Hypothermia is a more serious medical condition and requires emergency medical assistance.

If there is frostbite but no sign of hypothermia and immediate medical care is not available, proceed as follows:

- Get into a warm room as soon as possible.
- Unless absolutely necessary, do not walk on frostbitten feet or toes—this increases the damage.
- Immerse the affected area in warm—not hot—water (the temperature should be comfortable to the touch for unaffected parts of the body).
- Or, warm the affected area using body heat. For example, the heat of an armpit can be used to warm frostbitten fingers.
- Do not rub the frostbitten area with snow or massage it at all. This can cause more damage.
- Don't use a heating pad, heat lamp, or the heat of a stove, fireplace, or radiator for warming. Affected areas are numb and can be easily burned.

Note: These procedures are not substitutes for proper medical care.

Hypothermia is a medical emergency and frostbite should be evaluated by a health care provider. It is a good idea to take a first aid and emergency resuscitation (CPR) course to prepare for cold-weather health problems. Knowing what to do is an important part of protecting your health and the health of others.

What is the wind chill effect?

As the speed of the wind increases, it can carry heat away from your body much more quickly. When there are high winds, serious weather-related health problems are more likely, even when temperatures are only cool.

Why are infants and older people most at risk for cold-related illness?

Infants lose body heat more easily than adults; additionally, infants can't make enough body heat by shivering. Infants less than one year old should never sleep in a cold room. Provide warm clothing and a blanket for infants and try to maintain a warm indoor temperature. If the temperature cannot be maintained, make temporary arrangements to stay elsewhere. In an emergency, you can keep an infant warm using your own body heat. If you must sleep, take precautions to prevent rolling on the baby. Pillows and other soft bedding can also present a risk of smothering; remove them from the area near the baby.

Older adults often make less body heat because of a slower metabolism and less physical activity. If you are more than 65 years of age, check the temperature in your home often during severely cold weather. Also, check on elderly friends and neighbors frequently to ensure that their homes are adequately heated.

What is the best clothing for cold weather?

Adults and children should wear:

- a hat
- a scarf or knit mask to cover face and mouth
- sleeves that are snug at the wrist
- mittens (they are warmer than gloves)
- water-resistant coat and shoes
- several layers of loose-fitting clothing

Be sure the outer layer of your clothing is tightly woven, preferably wind resistant, to reduce body-heat loss caused by wind. Wool, silk, or polypropylene inner layers of clothing will hold more body heat than cotton. Stay dry—wet clothing chills the body rapidly. Excess perspiration will increase heat loss, so remove extra layers of clothing whenever you feel too warm. Also, avoid getting gasoline or alcohol on your skin while de-icing and fueling your car or using a snow blower. These materials in contact with the skin greatly increase heat loss from the body.

Do not ignore shivering. It's an important first sign that the body is losing heat. Persistent shivering is a signal to return indoors.

Section 69.3

Summer Skin Care

Excerpted from "A Primer on Summer Safety," by Michelle Meadows, U.S. Food and Drug Administration, *FDA Consumer* magazine, May-June 2004. Available online at http://www.fda.gov; accessed May 12, 2005.

When it comes to summer, Olivia Kane, 36, mostly remembers the happy times: eating crabs on the beach, chasing flickering fireflies at night, and playing softball with friends. But there are other memories the Arlington, Virginia, resident wishes she could forget. Like the rash from poison ivy that broke out on her face, neck, and arms two days before she had to walk down the aisle in her sister's wedding. Or the time she went to the beach to get a tan before high school graduation. "What I got was a bright red sunburn," she says. "I had blistered cheeks, a blistered chest, and I was the graduation speaker."

But her worst summer memory was when she took a sip from a can of soda and gulped down a bee that had crawled into the can when she wasn't looking. "I knew I swallowed something," Kane says. "I got so hysterical that I threw up." Out came the bee, and she went straight to the emergency room where she was treated for difficulty breathing.

Experts say there's a lot people can do to minimize the risks of health problems related to summertime activities. "While treatment with FDA-approved products is good, prevention is even better," says Jonathan Wilkin, M.D., director of the Food and Drug Administration's Division of Dermatologic and Dental Drug Products. So before you pack your swimsuit or hit the hiking trail this year, brush up on these summer hazards.

Sunburn

As a child in Pratt, Kansas, Linda Talbott got frequent, blistering sunburns while playing outside all day. Then in her college years, it was cool to be tanned. "Everyone wanted a tan, and I thought tanned skin looked beautiful," Talbott says. "But it's not beautiful when you're 65 and you've had melanoma."

In 1997, Talbott noticed a dark spot under her left eye. "I thought it was mascara, but it grew to the size of a raisin and started to bleed" after about six weeks. Her doctor said it was melanoma, a serious form of skin cancer. Another lesion on her cheek, previously misdiagnosed as an age spot, also turned out to be malignant. She needed immediate surgery on her face to remove the cancerous tissue and save her life.

Everyone is at risk for skin cancer, but especially people with light skin color, light hair or eye color, a family history of skin cancer, chronic sun exposure, a history of sunburns early in life, or freckles, according to the American Cancer Society. Rays from artificial sources of light such as tanning booths also increase the risk of skin cancer.

What you can do: Remember to limit sun exposure, wear protective clothing, and use sunscreen. Sunscreen should be applied 30 minutes before going outdoors and reapplied at least every two hours. Use water-resistant sunscreen with a sun protection factor (SPF) of 15 or higher. The FDA regulates sunscreen as an over-the-counter (OTC) drug and is working on a proposed rule that will specify testing procedures for determining levels of UVA protection in sunscreen products. It will also include labeling for UVA protection to complement existing SPF labeling for UVB. So in the future, consumers will be able to choose a sunscreen based on both UVB and UVA protection levels. Sunscreen is formulated to protect the skin against the sun's ultraviolet light (UV), not to help the skin tan.

Some medications can increase sensitivity to the sun. Examples are tetracycline antibiotics, sulfonamides such as Bactrim, non-steroidal anti-inflammatory drugs such as ibuprofen, and some fluoroquinolones. Cosmetics that contain alpha hydroxy acids (AHAs) may also increase sun sensitivity and the possibility of sunburn. Examples are glycolic acid and lactic acid. It is important to protect your skin from the sun while using AHA-containing products and for a week after discontinuing their use.

According to the American Academy of Dermatology (AAD), along with regularly using sunscreen, it's smart to wear wide-brimmed hats and seek shade under a beach umbrella or a tree. Sunscreens alone may not always protect you. And don't forget sunglasses, which protect the sensitive skin around the eyes and may reduce the long-term risk of developing cataracts. People who wear UV-absorbing contact lenses still should wear UV-absorbing sunglasses since contact lenses don't completely cover the eye.

If you do get a sunburn, don't put ice or butter on it, says Bruce Bonanno, M.D., an emergency physician at Bayshore Community Hospital in Holmdel, New Jersey. "Use a cold compress, and if you don't have that, a pack of frozen vegetables will work." OTC pain relievers may also be helpful. Mild and moderate cases may be helped by topical corticosteroids such as hydrocortisone. Severe cases may require oral steroids such as prednisone.

Be on the lookout for moles that change color or size, bleed, or have an irregular, spreading edge—all potential signs of skin cancer.

Bites from Mosquitoes and Ticks

Rob Baxley, 32, of Savage, Maryland, never saw the tick, but thinks he came into contact with one when he helped his brother build a deck in June 2003. "Soon after that, I noticed a little red spot on my thigh," Baxley says. "But then it grew." He estimates the rash was about the size of a grapefruit when he went to the emergency room in mid-July.

About 80 percent of people who get Lyme disease develop a large rash that looks like a bull's-eye. Baxley experienced other classic Lyme disease symptoms, such as muscle aches and stiff joints. His doctor also found a similar rash on Baxley's calf.

After a blood test confirmed Lyme disease, Baxley took the oral antibiotic doxycycline, followed by intravenous treatment with a second antibiotic called Rocephin (ceftriaxone). In addition to the physical symptoms, he is also experiencing depression for the first time. "The whole thing is frustrating," says Baxley. "It's taken a toll on the whole family."

Ticks are usually harmless. The biggest disease threat from tick bites is Lyme disease, which is caused by the bacterium *Borrelia burgdorferi*. The bacteria are transmitted to humans by the black-legged deer tick, which is about the size of a pinhead and usually lives on deer. According to the Centers for Disease Control and Prevention (CDC), there were 23,763 cases of Lyme disease reported nationwide in 2002.

Another insect-borne illness, West Nile virus, is transmitted by infected mosquitoes and usually produces mild symptoms in healthy people. But the illness can be serious for older people and those with compromised immune systems. In 2002, there were 4,156 cases of West Nile virus in humans reported to the CDC. Less than 1 percent of people infected with West Nile virus develop severe illness. The symptoms are flu-like and can include fever, headache, body aches, and skin rash.

What you can do: There are no vaccines on the market for West Nile virus or Lyme disease. If you're spending time in tall grass or woody areas, use insect repellent with DEET to ward off mosquitoes and ticks. But insect repellent should not be used on babies, and repellent used on children should contain no more than 10 percent DEET.

Check yourself and your children for ticks before bedtime. If you find a tick, remove it with tweezers, drop it in a plastic bag and throw it away. You don't have to save the tick to show it to doctors. People who want to get a tick tested for diseases or other information could check with their local health departments, but not all of them offer tick testing. The CDC recommends cleansing the area of the tick bite with antiseptic. Early removal is important because a tick generally has to be on the skin for 36 hours or more to transmit Lyme disease.

OTC antihistamines, such as Benadryl or Claritin, can bring itch relief. Topical anti-itch cream on the affected area also may help, especially for children, says Edward Lamay, M.D., a physician in the emergency department at Durham Regional Hospital in Durham, N.C. You may also want to keep their nails short. "Some kids scratch bites, break the skin, and then get a bacterial infection," Lamay says.

Bee Stings

In the summer of 2003, the Nebraska Poison Center in Omaha received a call about a 4-year-old girl who was stung on the tongue by a bee while sipping from a soda can. She was treated in the emergency room for swelling not only to the tongue, but to her lips and up to her eyes.

"It's a concern any time there is swelling in the face or an area other than where the sting occurred," says Charles Pattavina, M.D., an emergency physician at The Miriam Hospital in Providence, Rhode Island. Other symptoms of an allergic reaction are hives, itching, rash, difficulty breathing, and shock. Most reactions to bees are mild, but severe allergic reactions lead to between 40 and 50 deaths each year. An allergic reaction can occur even if a person has been stung before with no complications.

What you can do: To keep bees away, wear light-colored clothing and avoid scented soaps and perfumes. Don't leave food, drinks, and garbage out uncovered. Treat a bee sting by scraping the stinger away in a side-to-side motion with a credit card or fingernail, and then washing the area with soap and water. Pulling the stinger or using tweezers may push more venom into the skin. For any bug bite or sting, ice or a cold compress and OTC pain-relieving creams or oral medications can help.

Because bees puncture the skin with their stingers, there is a risk of tetanus infection. After getting the regular series of childhood tetanus shots, adults should have a tetanus booster shot every 10 years.

Watch for signs of allergic reaction to stings, which typically happen within the first few hours. If you or your child has ever had an allergic reaction to a sting, experts recommend carrying epinephrine, a prescription hormone given by injection to support blood pressure, increase heart rate, and relax airways.

Burns from Fireworks and Grills

Sia Karpinski, 10, of Akron, Ohio, hasn't been interested in playing with sparklers since July 4, 2002, when she stepped on a discarded sparkler while in bare feet. She was treated for serious burns at the Burn Center at Akron Children's Hospital as an outpatient for about six weeks.

The U.S. Consumer Product Safety Commission estimates that about 8,800 people were treated in emergency rooms in 2002 for injuries associated with fireworks. Most injuries involved the hands, head, and eyes. Lee Duffner, M.D., an ophthalmologist in Hollywood, Florida, says, "Unfortunately, I've treated burns of the cornea and eyelids and hemorrhages inside the eye caused by hand-held sparklers and other fireworks."

Mary Mondozzi, a nurse at the Akron Children's Hospital Burn Center, says she also sees burns from grills and campfires. "Children get hurt playing around grills or they get burned when they throw objects into campfires," she says.

What you can do: Stick with public firework displays handled by professionals. Children should always be closely supervised when food is being cooked indoors or outdoors. Be aware that gas leaks, blocked tubes, and overfilled propane tanks cause most gas grill fires and explosions. "Teach children to cover their faces, stop, drop, and roll if their clothes catch fire," Mondozzi says.

Generally, minor burns smaller than a person's palm can be treated at home. But burns bigger than that, and burns on the hands, feet, face, genitals, and major joints usually require emergency treatment. "For a minor injury, run cool water over it and cover it with a clean, dry cloth," says Mondozzi. Don't apply ice, which can worsen a burn. Don't apply petroleum jelly or butter, which can hold heat in the tissue. Consult your family doctor if a minor burn does not heal in a couple of days or if there are signs of infection, such as redness and swelling.

Poison Ivy, Poison Oak, and Poison Sumac

Betsy Dunphy, 44, enjoys living in a woody area in Herndon, Virginia. But she could do without the poison ivy. She once missed a week of work when a rash from the vine spread all over her face and chest. In the summer of 2002, she developed a poison ivy rash on her wrist after moving azalea plants, and was careful to keep it from spreading.

Rashes from poison ivy, oak, or sumac are all caused by urushiol, a substance in the sap of the plants. Poison plant rashes can't be spread from person to person, but it's possible to pick up a rash from urushiol that sticks to clothing, tools, balls, and pets.

What you can do: Dunphy says she's been able to avoid an outbreak in the last two years mainly by learning what poison ivy looks like and avoiding it. According to the American Academy of Dermatology, while "leaves of three, beware of me," is the old saying, "leaflets of three, beware of me" is even better because each leaf has three smaller leaflets.

"I also wash my garden tools regularly, especially if there is the slightest chance that they've come into contact with poison ivy," Dunphy says. If you know you will be working around poison ivy, wear long pants, long sleeves, boots, and gloves.

Hikers, emergency workers, and others who have a difficult time avoiding poison ivy may benefit from a product called Ivy Block, made by EnviroDerm Pharmaceuticals Inc., of Louisville, Kentucky. It's the only FDA-approved product for preventing or reducing the severity of rashes from poison ivy, oak, or sumac. The OTC lotion contains bentoquatam, a substance that forms a clay-like coating on the skin.

If you come into contact with poison ivy, oak, or sumac, wash the skin in cool water as soon as possible to prevent the spread of urushiol. If you get a rash, oatmeal baths and calamine lotion can dry up blisters and bring relief from itching. Treatment may include OTC or prescription corticosteroids and antihistamines.

Chapter 70

Caring for Your Skin If You Have Diabetes

What are diabetes problems?

Too much glucose (sugar) in the blood for a long time can cause diabetes problems. This high blood glucose (also called blood sugar) can damage many parts of the body, such as the heart, blood vessels, eyes, and kidneys. Heart and blood vessel disease can lead to heart attacks and strokes. You can do a lot to prevent or slow down diabetes problems.

This chapter is about feet and skin problems caused by diabetes. You will learn the things you can do each day and during each year to stay healthy and prevent diabetes problems.

How can diabetes hurt my feet?

High blood glucose from diabetes causes two problems that can hurt your feet.

Nerve damage. One problem is damage to nerves in your legs and feet. With damaged nerves, you might not feel pain, heat, or cold in your legs and feet. A sore or cut on your foot may get worse because you do not know it is there. This lack of feeling is caused by nerve

---

Excerpted from "Prevent Diabetes Problems: Keep Your Feet and Skin Healthy," National Institute of Diabetes and Digestive and Kidney Diseases (NIDDK), September 2003. Available online at http://www.niddk.nih.gov; accessed May 17, 2005.

damage, also called diabetic neuropathy. It can lead to a large sore or infection.

Poor blood flow. The second problem happens when not enough blood flows to your legs and feet. Poor blood flow makes it hard for a sore or infection to heal. This problem is called peripheral vascular disease. Smoking when you have diabetes makes blood flow problems much worse.

These two problems can work together to cause a foot problem. For example, you get a blister from shoes that do not fit. You do not feel the pain from the blister because you have nerve damage in your foot. Next, the blister gets infected. If blood glucose is high, the extra glucose feeds the germs. Germs grow and the infection gets worse. Poor blood flow to your legs and feet can slow down healing. Once in a while a bad infection never heals. The infection might cause gangrene. If a person has gangrene, the skin and tissue around the sore die. The area becomes black and smelly.

To keep gangrene from spreading, a doctor may have to do surgery to cut off a toe, foot, or part of a leg. Cutting off a body part is called an amputation.

What can I do to take care of my feet?

- Wash your feet in warm water every day. Make sure the water is not too hot by testing the temperature with your elbow. Do not soak your feet. Dry your feet well, especially between your toes.
- Look at your feet every day to check for cuts, sores, blisters, redness, calluses, or other problems. Checking every day is even more important if you have nerve damage or poor blood flow. If you cannot bend over or pull your feet up to check them, use a mirror. If you cannot see well, ask someone else to check your feet.
- If your skin is dry, rub lotion on your feet after you wash and dry them. Do not put lotion between your toes.
- File corns and calluses gently with an emery board or pumice stone. Do this after your bath or shower.
- Cut your toenails once a week or when needed. Cut toenails when they are soft from washing. Cut them to the shape of the toe and not too short. File the edges with an emery board.

- Always wear shoes or slippers to protect your feet from injuries.
- Always wear socks or stockings to avoid blisters. Do not wear socks or knee-high stockings that are too tight below your knee.
- Wear shoes that fit well. Shop for shoes at the end of the day when your feet are bigger. Break in shoes slowly. Wear them 1 to 2 hours each day for the first 1 to 2 weeks.
- Before putting your shoes on, feel the insides to make sure they have no sharp edges or objects that might injure your feet.
- Take off your shoes and socks so your doctor will check your feet.

What are common diabetes foot problems?

Anyone can have corns, blisters, and athlete's foot. If you have diabetes and your blood glucose stays high, these foot problems can lead to infections.

- Corns and calluses are thick layers of skin caused by too much rubbing or pressure on the same spot. Corns and calluses can become infected.
- Blisters can form if shoes always rub the same spot. Wearing shoes that do not fit or wearing shoes without socks can cause blisters. Blisters can become infected.
- Ingrown toenails happen when an edge of the nail grows into the skin. The skin can get red and infected. Ingrown toenails can happen if you cut into the corners of your toenails when you trim them. If toenail edges are sharp, smooth them with an emery board. You can also get an ingrown toenail if your shoes are too tight.
- A bunion forms when your big toe slants toward the small toes and the place between the bones near the base of your big toe grows big. This spot can get red, sore, and infected. Bunions can form on one or both feet. Pointy shoes may cause bunions. Bunions often run in the family. Surgery can remove bunions.
- Plantar warts are caused by a virus. The warts usually form on the bottoms of the feet.
- Hammertoes form when a foot muscle gets weak. The weakness may be from diabetic nerve damage. The weakened muscle

makes the tendons in the foot shorter and makes the toes curl under the feet. You may get sores on the bottoms of your feet and on the tops of your toes. The feet can change their shape. Hammertoes can cause problems with walking and finding shoes that fit well. Hammertoes can run in the family. Wearing shoes that are too short can also cause hammertoes.

- Dry and cracked skin can happen because the nerves in your legs and feet do not get the message to keep your skin soft and moist. Dry skin can become cracked and allow germs to enter. If your blood glucose is high, it feeds the germs and makes the infection worse.
- Athlete's foot is a fungus that causes redness and cracking of the skin. It is itchy. The cracks between the toes allow germs to get under the skin. If your blood glucose is high, it feeds the germs and makes the infection worse. The infection can spread to the toenails and make them thick, yellow, and hard to cut.

All of these foot problems can be taken care of. Tell your doctor about any foot problem as soon as you see it.

How can diabetes hurt my skin?

Diabetes can hurt your skin in two ways:

- If your blood glucose is high, your body loses fluid. With less fluid in your body, your skin can get dry. Dry skin can be itchy, causing you to scratch and make it sore. Also, dry skin can crack. Cracks allow germs to enter and cause infection. If your blood glucose is high, it feeds germs and makes infections worse. Skin can get dry on your legs, feet, elbows, and other places on your body.
- Nerve damage can decrease the amount you sweat. Sweating helps keep your skin soft and moist. Decreased sweating in your feet and legs can cause dry skin.

What can I do to take care of my skin?

- After you wash with a mild soap, make sure you rinse and dry yourself well. Check places where water can hide, such as under the arms, under the breasts, between the legs, and between the toes.

- Keep your skin moist by using a lotion or cream after you wash. Ask your doctor to suggest one.
- Drink lots of fluids, such as water, to keep your skin moist and healthy.
- Wear all-cotton underwear. Cotton allows air to move around your body better.
- Check your skin after you wash. Make sure you have no dry, red, or sore spots that might lead to an infection.
- Tell your doctor about any skin problems.

Chapter 71

Caring for Your Skin If You Have Lupus

Skin problems are very common in people with lupus. Some skin rashes and sores (also called lesions or ulcers) are very specific to lupus, while others can occur in other diseases as well. A sensitivity to and too much exposure to the ultraviolet (UV) rays of sun and some types of artificial light are responsible for aggravating some rashes and lesions. Many types of skin conditions are common in lupus.

Butterfly rash: This rash over the nose and cheeks can range from a faint blush to a rash that is very severe, with scaling. It is very sensitive to light and appears to gets worse when skin is exposed to sun or certain types of artificial light. The rash may be permanent or may come and go.

Discoid lesions: These scarring, coin-shaped lesions are seen on areas of the skin that have been exposed to UV light. They may also occur on the scalp and produce a scarring, localized baldness that is permanent.

Subacute cutaneous lesions: These nonscarring, red, coin-shaped lesions are very sensitive to UV light. They can appear scaly and can mimic the lesions seen in psoriasis. They may occur only on the face or cover large areas of the body.

Excerpted from "Lupus: A Patient Care Guide for Nurses and Other Health Professionals," Patient Information Patient Information Sheet #7, May 2001. Available online at http://www.niams.nih.gov; accessed June 4, 2005.

Mucous membrane lesions: Mouth ulcers are sometimes seen in lupus patients. Nose and vaginal ulcers may also occur. These lesions are usually painless.

Hair loss: In addition to losing hair because of discoid lesions, some lupus patients may develop a temporary, generalized hair loss followed by the growth of new hair. Hair loss may also be caused by infection or by use of corticosteroids or other lupus medications. A severe lupus flare could result in defective hair growth, causing the hair to be fragile and break easily.

Vasculitis: This is a condition in which the blood vessels become inflamed. Very small blood vessels can break and cause bleeding into the tissues, resulting in tiny, reddish-purple spots on the skin known as petechiae. Larger spots are called purpura and may look like a bruise. Vasculitis can also cause blood clots to form, skin ulcers to develop, and small black areas to appear around fingers and toenails. These black areas are a sign of serious tissue damage. If they begin to develop, see your doctor immediately.

Raynaud phenomenon: This is a condition in which the blood vessels of the fingers and toes react in an extreme way to cold or stress. They suddenly get very narrow (vasoconstrict). This decreases the blood supply going through the vessel. As a result, the fingers and toes become cold and can become pale or bluish. Pain or tingling can occur when the hands and feet warm up and circulation returns to normal.

Drug-induced skin changes: Some drugs used to treat lupus, such as corticosteroids, immunosuppressives, and antineoplastics, can affect the skin. Your doctor or nurse will review these side effects with you if one of these drugs has been prescribed.

Caring for Yourself

- Reduce your exposure to the sun and to some sources of artificial light (especially fluorescent and halogen bulbs). The skin of people with lupus is very sensitive to the UV light that comes from these sources.
- Limit outdoor activity between the hours of 10 a.m. and 4 p.m. This may mean a big change in your lifestyle if you work or play outdoors a lot.

- Wear a sunscreen on exposed areas of skin. It should have a sun protection factor (SPF) of 15 or higher. Be sure that the sunscreen protects against both UVB and UVA rays.
- Wear sunscreen all year round and on cloudy days as well as on sunny days. Also wear it indoors if you spend a lot of time in a room with many windows (glass does not filter out UV rays).
- Wear protective clothing, such as hats with wide brims and clothing made of tightly woven material. Thin, loosely woven material allows UV light to penetrate to the skin.
- Be aware of fluorescent light and halogen lamps. They can be found in many places and include floor lamps, overhead lights, photocopiers, and slide projectors. Sunscreen and protective clothing can help.
- Tell your doctor immediately if any rash or sore appears or gets worse.
- If your doctor prescribes a medication for your skin condition, be sure to take it as directed.
- Try rinsing your mouth with salt water and eating soft foods if you have mouth ulcers. A number of other treatments and preparations are available to treat mouth ulcers as well as those in the nose and vagina.
- Avoid preparations or medications you know will make your skin condition worse. These might include hair dyes, skin creams, certain drugs that can make you more sensitive to the sun (for example, tetracyclines or diuretics), and things you are allergic to.
- It's okay to wear makeup, but try hypoallergenic brands. A brand that also includes UV protection would be good to use.
- If you have Raynaud's phenomenon, dress warmly in cold weather. Pay particular attention to keeping your hands and feet warm. Keeping your home warm will also help prevent an attack.
- Avoid smoking, caffeine, and stress—all of these can contribute to Raynaud phenomenon.
- If you have trouble maintaining a positive attitude about your appearance or your lupus, call your doctor or nurse to discuss your feelings and concerns.

Chapter 72

Don't Be in the Dark about Tanning

Some think turning light skin darker gives off an aura of good health. But a suntan actually signals skin damage. When exposed to the sun's ultraviolet radiation, the skin produces a pigment called melanin to protect itself from burning. And while indoor or "sunless" tanning may seem like convenient alternatives, especially during the winter months, these practices may not be risk free. Before stepping into a tanning booth or buying over-the-counter (OTC) tanning products, consider these facts.

Indoor tanning can be as harmful as outdoor tanning. More than 1 million people visit tanning salons on an average day, according to the American Academy of Dermatology (AAD). But many don't know that indoor tanning devices, such as tanning beds and sunlamps, emit ultraviolet (UV) radiation that's similar to and sometimes more powerful than the sun. The Food and Drug Administration discourages the use of tanning beds and sunlamps.

Be wary of claims about "safe rays" because there is no such thing. Both types of ultraviolet light, UVB and UVA, can cause wrinkling and other signs of premature skin aging, skin cancer, and damage to the eyes and the immune system.

The FDA enforces regulations related to the labeling and use of these products, while the Federal Trade Commission focuses on false, misleading, and deceptive advertising claims.

"Don't Be in the Dark About Tanning," by Michelle Meadows, U.S. Food and Drug Administration, *FDA Consumer* magazine, November-December 2003. Available online at http://www.fda.gov; accessed May 29, 2005.

Also remember that some medical conditions such as lupus and diabetes can make skin more sensitive to light, as can some drugs such as birth control pills and medications such as the antibiotic tetracycline.

Some suntanning products don't contain sunscreen. It only takes a few bad sunburns to raise the risk of skin cancer, and skin damage builds up over years even when no burning occurs. This is why sunscreen, which blocks UVA and UVB, is recommended. The FDA has expressed concern about suntanning products without sunscreen, and encourages consumers to check the labels. Tanning products without sunscreen must display a warning that the product does not protect against sunburn.

Sunscreen is regulated by the FDA as an OTC drug. Cosmetics that make sun-protection claims are regulated as both drugs and cosmetics. Look for products with a sun protection factor (SPF) of 15 or more. The higher the number, the better the protection. Sunscreen should be liberally applied to skin 30 minutes before going out in the sun, and then every two hours after that.

DHA-containing sunless spray is approved only for external use. During the last few years, some companies have offered a sunless option that involves spraying customers in a tanning booth with the color additive dihydroxyacetone (DHA). DHA interacts with the dead surface cells in the outermost layer of the skin to darken skin color.

DHA has been approved by the FDA for use as a tanner since 1977, and has typically been used in OTC lotions and creams. Its use is restricted to external application, which means that it shouldn't be sprayed in or on the mouth, eyes, or nose, says Linda Katz, M.D., director of the FDA's Office of Cosmetics and Colors in the Center for Food Safety and Applied Nutrition. "DHA should not be inhaled, ingested, or used in such a way that the eyes and eye area are exposed to it because the risks, if any, are unknown," Katz says. For consumers who choose to get DHA spray in tanning booths, the FDA recommends protective measures for the eyes, nose, and mucous membranes.

There are no tanning pills approved by the FDA. Some companies have marketed tanning pills that contain the color additive canthaxanthin. When large amounts of canthaxanthin are ingested, the substance can turn the skin a range of colors, from orange to brown. The additive is not listed for use in tanning pills in the United States, but rather is approved for use as a food color additive, and only in small amounts. Imported tanning pills that contain canthaxanthin may be refused entry into the United States because they contain non-permitted color additives.

Tanning pills have been associated with health problems, including an eye disorder called canthaxanthin retinopathy, which is the formation of yellow deposits on the eye's retina. Canthaxanthin has also been reported to cause liver injury and a severe itching condition called urticaria, according to the AAD.

Chapter 73

Discuss with Teens the Dangers of Tanning

Parents of teenagers are strongly encouraged by public health experts and medical professionals to discuss with their kids the dangers of indoor tanning equipment, and even to discourage its use. In fact, legislators in some states are proposing to make it illegal for a teen to tan in a commercial salon without parental consent.

According to the American Cancer Society (ACS), exposure to the sun's ultraviolet (UV) rays appears to be the most important environmental factor in developing skin cancer. Consequently, the dangers from exposure to UV rays from artificial sources of light, such as tanning beds and sunlamps, are similar to the dangers of exposure to sunlight. Moreover, some experts strongly believe that the sharp rise in the rates of the most serious type of skin cancer—malignant melanoma—may be due to increased exposure to UV radiation, whether from natural sunlight or artificial sources of light.

When exposed to UV radiation, the skin begins to produce a pigment called melanin to protect itself from burning. It is the production of melanin that causes the skin to darken and produce the tan. The production of new melanin takes three to five days.

Joshua L. Fox, M.D., a dermatologist in Fresh Meadows, N.Y., says, "Continued use of a tanning bed or sunlamp can be quite dangerous, particularly during the teenage years." Teens are at greater risk, he

---

"Teen Tanning Hazards," by Carol Rados, U.S. Food and Drug Administration, *FDA Consumer* magazine, March-April 2005. Available online at http://www.fda.gov; accessed May 28, 2005.

says, because they are still experiencing tremendous growth at the cellular level, and, like other cells in the body, the skin cells are dividing more rapidly than they do during adulthood.

W. Howard Cyr, Ph.D., and Sharon A. Miller, both laboratory leaders in the Food and Drug Administration's Center for Devices and Radiological Health, say that the agency has regulated the manufacture of sunlamp products—sunlamps, tanning beds, tanning booths, and other related equipment—since 1979. Initially, there was a widespread acute risk from sunlamp products, as indicated by a large number of skin and eye injuries treated annually in hospital emergency rooms. Federal performance standards for sunlamp products were established to protect people from acute burns and exposure to hazardous shortwave UV radiation that was unnecessary for tanning.

In 1985, the agency decided to amend the standards to make the requirements more compatible with then-current products. When sunlamp technology changed and sunlamps emitting primarily UVA radiation—longer-wave, less efficient at producing a sunburn—became prevalent, longer exposure times were allowed, Miller says.

In 1986, the FDA published a policy letter that described how the maximum timer limit should be determined and provided guidance on recommended exposure schedules. The manufacturers of sunlamp products are required to include a recommended exposure schedule in their labeling. This schedule should be clearly visible to users before they begin their exposure session.

"FDA does not recommend the use of indoor tanning equipment," Miller says. Fox agrees. "There is no such thing as a safe tan," he says. "Just one sunburn increases your risk for skin cancer."

However, Miller says that if people insist on using tanning devices, there are things they can do to reduce the potential dangers.

"Start slowly, with short exposure times, and build up to a tan. If you get the maximum exposure the first time, you will probably get burned," Miller says. And, she adds, often people don't even know they are burned until it's too late. "Remember that a sunburn doesn't usually show up until several hours after the exposure," she says. In addition, the recommended exposure schedules do not allow for tanning more frequently than every other day. After a tan is developed, tanning frequency should be reduced to no more than twice a week.

Cyr and Miller warn that, in practice, tanning salon operators control the exposure time and that they may allow the customer to exceed exposure times written on the label. This is especially true for the beginning of the tanning course when users are advised to start off with very short exposures, usually five minutes or less. Fox says that people who use these products should always ask to see the information contained in the label. Be wary, he adds, if tanning salon operators can't produce it.

Miller says that the use of FDA-compliant eyewear that blocks UV rays is absolutely essential for tanning bed users to protect their eyes from corneal burns and cataracts from long-term exposure.

A study done by researchers at Wake Forest University, published in the July 2004 issue of the *Journal of the American Academy of Dermatology*, found that participants thought UV exposure was not only desirable for improving appearances, but also was somewhat addictive. The study concluded that "The relaxing and reinforcing effects of UV exposure contribute to tanning behavior in frequent tanners and should be explored in greater detail."

Fox advises parents to explore safer, alternative means for their children to acquire a tan. "Teens should know about the options," he says, which include self-tanners in the form of creams and gels. "Get the look you like without the damage that can occur with tanning equipment."

Chapter 74

Cosmetics and Your Health

What are cosmetics? How are they different from over-the-counter (OTC) drugs?

Cosmetics are put on the body for these purposes:

- cleanse it
- make it beautiful
- make it attractive
- change its appearance or the way it looks

Cosmetic products include the following:

- skin creams
- lotions
- perfumes
- lipsticks
- fingernail polishes
- eye and face makeup products
- permanent waves
- hair dyes

Excerpted from "Frequently Asked Questions about Cosmetics and Your Health," National Women's Health Information Center, November 2004. Available online at http://www.4woman.gov; accessed June 2, 2005.

- toothpastes
- deodorants

Unlike drugs, which are used to treat or prevent disease in the body, cosmetics do not change or affect the body's structure or functions.

What's in cosmetics?

Fragrances and preservatives are the main ingredients in cosmetics. Fragrances are the most common cause of skin problems. More than 5,000 different kinds are used in products. Products marked "fragrance-free" or "without perfume" mean that no fragrances have been added to make the product smell good.

Preservatives in cosmetics are the second most common cause of skin problems. They prevent bacteria and fungus from growing in the product and protect products from damage caused by air or light. But preservatives can also cause the skin to become irritated and infected. The following are some examples of preservatives:

- paraben
- imidazolidinyl urea
- Quaternium-15
- DMDM [dimethylol dimethyl] hydantoin
- phenoxyethanol
- formaldehyde

The ingredients below cannot be used, or their use is limited, in cosmetics. They may cause cancer or other serious health problems.

- bithionol
- mercury compounds
- vinyl chloride
- halogenated salicylanilides
- zirconium complexes in aerosol sprays
- chloroform
- methylene chloride
- chlorofluorocarbon propellants
- hexachlorophene

Are cosmetics safe?

Yes, for the most part. Serious problems from cosmetics are rare. But sometimes problems can happen.

The most common injury from cosmetics is from scratching the eye with a mascara wand. Eye infections can result if the scratches go untreated. These infections can lead to ulcers on the cornea (clear covering of the eye), loss of lashes, or even blindness. To play it safe, never try to apply mascara while riding in a car, bus, train, or plane.

Sharing makeup can also lead to serious problems. Cosmetic brushes and sponges pick up bacteria from the skin. And if you moisten brushes with saliva, the problem can be worse. Washing your hands before using makeup will help prevent this problem.

Sleeping while wearing eye makeup can cause problems, too. If mascara flakes into your eyes while you sleep, you might wake up with itching, bloodshot eyes, infections, or eye scratches. So be sure to remove all makeup before going to bed.

Cosmetic products that come in aerosol containers also can be a hazard. For example, it is dangerous to use aerosol hairspray near heat, fire, or while smoking. Until hairspray is fully dry, it can catch on fire and cause serious burns. Fires related to hairsprays have caused injuries and death. Aerosol sprays or powders also can cause lung damage if they are deeply inhaled into the lungs.

How can I protect myself against the dangers of cosmetics?

- Never drive and put on makeup. Not only does this make driving a danger, hitting a bump in the road and scratching your eyeball can cause serious eye injury.
- Never share makeup. Always use a new sponge when trying products at a store. Insist that salespersons clean container openings with alcohol before applying to your skin.
- Keep makeup containers closed tight when not in use.
- Keep makeup out of the sun and heat. Light and heat can kill the preservatives that help to fight bacteria. Don't keep cosmetics in a hot car for a long time.
- Don't use cosmetics if you have an eye infection, such as pinkeye. Throw away any makeup you were using when you first found the problem.
- Never add liquid to a product unless the label tells you to do so.

- Throw away any makeup if the color changes or it starts to smell.
- Never use aerosol sprays near heat or while smoking, because they can catch on fire.
- Don't deeply inhale hairsprays or powders. This can cause lung damage.
- Avoid color additives that are not approved for use in the eye area, such as "permanent" eyelash tints and kohl (color additive that contains lead salts and is still used in eye cosmetics in other countries). Be sure to keep kohl away from children. It may cause lead poisoning.

What are "cosmeceuticals?"

Some products can be both cosmetics and drugs. This may happen when a product has two uses. For example, a shampoo is a cosmetic because it's used to clean the hair. But, an antidandruff treatment is a drug because it's used to treat dandruff. So an antidandruff shampoo is both a cosmetic and a drug. Here are some other examples:

- toothpastes that contain fluoride
- deodorants that are also antiperspirants
- moisturizers and makeup that provide sun protection

These products must meet the standards for both cosmetics (color additives) and drugs.

Some cosmetic makers use the term "cosmeceutical" to refer to products that have drug-like benefits. FDA does not recognize this term. A product can be a drug, a cosmetic, or a combination of both. But the term "cosmeceutical" has no meaning under the law.

While drugs are reviewed and approved by FDA, FDA does not approve cosmetics. If a product acts like a drug, FDA must approve it as a drug.

How long do cosmetics last?

You may not be able to use eye makeup, such as mascara, eyeliner, and eye shadow, for as long as other products. This is because of the risk of eye infection. Some experts recommend replacing mascara three months after purchase. If mascara becomes dry, throw it away.

Don't add water or, even worse, saliva to moisten it. That will bring bacteria into the product.

You may also need to watch certain "all natural" products that contain substances taken from plants. These products may be more at risk for bacteria. Since these products contain no preservatives or have non-traditional ones, your risk of infection may be greater.

If you don't store these products as directed, they may expire before the expiration date. For example, cosmetics stored in high heat may go bad faster than the expiration date. On the other hand, products stored the way they should be can be safely used until they expire.

What are hypoallergenic cosmetics?

Hypoallergenic cosmetics are products that makers claim cause fewer allergic reactions than other products. Women with sensitive skin, and even those with "normal" skin, may think these products will be gentler. But there are no federal standards for using the term hypoallergenic. The term can mean whatever a company wants it to mean. Cosmetic makers do not have to prove their claims to the FDA.

Some products that have "natural" ingredients can cause allergic reactions. If you have an allergy to certain plants or animals, you could have an allergic reaction to cosmetics with those things in them. For example, lanolin from sheep wool is found in many lotions. But it's a common cause of allergies too.

Can cosmetics cause acne?

Some skin and hair care products can cause acne. To help prevent and control acne flare-ups, take good care of your skin. For example, use a mild soap or cleanser to gently wash your face twice a day. Choose "non-comedogenic" makeup and hair care products. This means that they don't close up the pores.

Are cosmetic products with alpha hydroxy acids safe?

Alpha hydroxy acids (AHAs) come from fruit and milk sugars. They are found in many creams and lotions. Many people buy products with AHAs, because they claim to reduce wrinkles, spots, sun-damaged skin, and other signs of aging. Some studies suggest they may work.

But are these products safe? FDA has received reports of reactions in people using AHA products. Their complaints include the following:

- severe redness

- swelling (especially in the area of the eyes)
- burning
- blistering
- bleeding
- rash
- itching
- skin discoloration

AHAs may also increase your skin's risk of sunburn.

To find out if a product contains an AHA, look on the list of ingredients. By law, all cosmetics have ingredients on their outer label. AHAs may be called other names, like glycolic acid and lactic acid.

What precautions should I follow when using AHA products?

If you want to use AHA products, follow these safety tips:

- Always protect your skin before going out during the day. Use a sunscreen with an SPF (sun protection factor) of at least 15. Wear a hat with a brim. Cover up with lightweight, loose-fitting long-sleeved shirts and pants.
- Buy products with good label information: a list of ingredients to see which AHA or other chemical acids are in the product; the name and address of the maker; and a statement about the product's AHA and pH levels

The first two have to be on the label. The third is one is by choice. You can call or write the maker to find about a product's AHA and pH levels.

- Buy only products with an AHA level of 10 percent or less and a pH of 3.5 or more.
- Test a small area of skin to see if it is sensitive to any AHA product before using a lot of it.
- Stop using the product right away if you have a reaction, such as stinging, redness, or bleeding.
- Talk with your doctor or dermatologist (a doctor that treats skin problems) if you have a problem.

Chapter 75

Tattoos and Your Health

Chapter Contents

Section 75.1

The Health Risks of Tattoos and Permanent Makeup

"Tattoos and Permanent Makeup," U.S. Food and Drug Administration, Center for Food Safety and Applied Nutrition, July 1, 2004. Available online at http://vm.cfsan.fda.gov; accessed June 1, 2005.

The inks used in tattoos and permanent makeup (also known as micropigmentation) and the pigments in these inks are subject to FDA [U.S. Food and Drug Administration] regulation as cosmetics and color additives. However, FDA has not attempted to regulate the use of tattoo inks and the pigments used in them and does not control the actual practice of tattooing. Rather, such matters have been handled through local laws and by local jurisdictions.

But with the growth in popularity of tattooing and permanent makeup, FDA has begun taking a closer look at related safety questions. Among the issues under consideration are tattoo removal, adverse reactions to tattoo colors, and infections that result from tattooing.

Another concern is the increasing variety of pigments and diluents being used in tattooing—more than fifty different pigments and shades, and the list continues to grow. Although a number of color additives are approved for use in cosmetics, none is approved for injection into the skin. Using an unapproved color additive in a tattoo ink makes the ink adulterated. Many pigments used in tattoo inks are not approved for skin contact at all. Some are industrial grade colors that are suitable for printers' ink or automobile paint.

Nevertheless, many individuals choose to undergo tattooing in its various forms. For some, it is an aesthetic choice or an initiation rite. Some choose permanent makeup as a time saver or because they have physical difficulty applying regular, temporary makeup. For others, tattooing is an adjunct to reconstructive surgery, particularly of the face or breast, to simulate natural pigmentation. People who have lost their eyebrows due to alopecia (a form of hair loss) may choose to have "eyebrows" tattooed on, whereas people with vitiligo (a lack of pigmentation in areas of the skin) may try tattooing to help camouflage the condition.

Whatever their reason, consumers should be aware of the risks involved in order to make an informed decision.

What Risks Are Involved in Tattooing?

The following are the primary complications that can result from tattooing:

Infection

Unsterile tattooing equipment and needles can transmit infectious diseases, such as hepatitis. The risk of infection is the reason the American Association of Blood Banks requires a one-year wait between getting a tattoo and donating blood.

It is extremely important to make sure that all tattooing equipment is clean and sterilized before use. Even if the needles are sterilized or never have been used, it is important to understand that in some cases the equipment that holds the needles cannot be sterilized reliably due to its design. In addition, the person who receives a tattoo must be sure to care for the tattooed area properly during the first week or so after the pigments are injected.

Removal Problems

Despite advances in laser technology, removing a tattoo is a painstaking process, usually involving several treatments and considerable expense. Complete removal without scarring may be impossible.

Allergic Reactions

Although allergic reactions to tattoo pigments are rare, when they happen they may be particularly troublesome because the pigments can be hard to remove. Occasionally, people may develop an allergic reaction to tattoos they have had for years.

Granulomas

These are nodules that may form around material that the body perceives as foreign, such as particles of tattoo pigment.

Keloid Formation

If you are prone to developing keloids—scars that grow beyond normal boundaries—you are at risk of keloid formation from a tattoo.

Keloids may form any time you injure or traumatize your skin, and according to Office of Cosmetics and Colors (OCAC) dermatologist Ella Toombs, M.D., tattooing or micropigmentation is a form of trauma. *Micropigmentation: State of the Art*, a book written by Charles Zwerling, M.D., Annette Walker, R.N., and Norman Goldstein, M.D., states that keloids occur more frequently as a consequence of tattoo removal.

MRI Complications

There have been reports of people with tattoos or permanent makeup who experienced swelling or burning in the affected areas when they underwent magnetic resonance imaging (MRI). This seems to occur only rarely and apparently without lasting effects.

There also have been reports of tattoo pigments interfering with the quality of the image. This seems to occur mainly when a person with permanent eyeliner undergoes MRI of the eyes. Mascara may produce a similar effect. The difference is that mascara is easily removable.

The cause of these complications is uncertain. Some have theorized that they result from an interaction with the metallic components of some pigments.

However, the risks of avoiding an MRI when your doctor has recommended one are likely to be much greater than the risks of complications from an interaction between the MRI and tattoo or permanent makeup. Instead of avoiding an MRI, individuals who have tattoos or permanent makeup should inform the radiologist or technician of this fact in order to take appropriate precautions, avoid complications, and assure the best results.

The Most Common Problem: Dissatisfaction

According to Dr. Toombs, the most common problem that develops with tattoos is the desire to remove them. Removing tattoos and permanent makeup can be very difficult.

Skill levels vary widely among people who perform tattooing. According to an article by J.K. Chiang, S. Barsky, and D.M. Bronson in the June 1999 issue of the *Journal of the American Academy of Dermatology*, the main complication with eyelid tattooing is improperly placed pigment. You may want to ask the person performing the procedure for references and ask yourself how willing you are to risk permanently wearing someone else's mistake.

Although tattoos may be satisfactory at first, they sometimes fade. Also, if the tattooist injects the pigments too deeply into the skin, the pigments may migrate beyond the original sites, resulting in a blurred appearance.

Another cause of dissatisfaction is that the human body changes over time, and styles change with the season. The permanent makeup that may have looked flattering when first injected may later clash with changing skin tones and facial or body contours. People who plan to have facial cosmetic surgery are advised that the appearance of their permanent makeup may become distorted. The tattoo that seemed stylish at first may become dated and embarrassing. And changing tattoos or permanent makeup is not as easy as changing your mind.

Removal Techniques

Methods for removing tattoos include laser treatments, abrasion, scarification, and surgery. Some people attempt to camouflage an objectionable tattoo with a new one. Each approach has drawbacks.

Laser treatments can lighten many tattoos, some more easily and effectively than others. Generally, several visits are necessary over a span or weeks or months, and the treatments can be expensive. Some individuals experience hypopigmentation—a lightening of the natural skin coloring—in the affected area. Laser treatments also can cause some tattoo pigments to change to a less desirable shade.

Unfortunately, knowing what pigments are in your tattoo or permanent makeup has always been difficult and has become more so as the variety of tattoo inks has multiplied. Inks are often sold by brand name only, not by chemical composition. Because the pigments are sold to tattoo parlors and salons, not on a retail basis to consumers, manufacturers are not required by law to list the ingredients on the labels. Furthermore, because manufacturers may consider the identity and grade of their pigments "proprietary," neither the tattooist nor the customer may be able to obtain this information.

There also have been reports of individuals suffering allergic reactions after laser treatments to remove tattoos, apparently because the laser caused allergenic substances in the tattoo ink to be released into the body.

Dermabrasion involves abrading layers of skin with a wire brush or diamond fraise (a type of sanding disc). This process itself may leave a scar.

Salabrasion, in which a salt solution is used to remove the pigment, is sometimes used in conjunction with dermabrasion, but has become less common.

Scarification involves removing the tattoo with an acid solution and creating a scar in its place.

Surgical removal sometimes involves the use of tissue expanders (balloons inserted under the skin, so that when the tattoo is cut away, there is less scarring). Larger tattoos may require repeated surgery for complete removal.

Camouflaging a tattoo entails the injection of new pigments either to form a new pattern or cover a tattoo with skin-toned pigments. Dr. Toombs notes, however, that injected pigments tend not to look natural because they lack the skin's natural translucence.

What about Temporary Tattoos?

Temporary tattoos, such as those applied to the skin with a moistened wad of cotton, fade several days after application. Most contain color additives approved for cosmetic use on the skin. However, the agency has issued an import alert for several foreign-made temporary tattoos.

According to OCAC [Office of Cosmetics and Colors] Consumer Safety Officer Allen Halper, the temporary tattoos subject to the import alert are not allowed into the United States because they don't carry the FDA-mandated ingredient labels or they contain colors not permitted by FDA for use in cosmetics applied to the skin. FDA has received reports of allergic reactions to temporary tattoos.

In a similar action, FDA has issued an import alert for henna intended for use on the skin. Henna is approved only for use as a hair dye, not for direct application to the skin. Also, henna typically produces a reddish brown tint, raising questions about what ingredients are added to produce the varieties of colors labeled as "henna," such as "black henna" and "blue henna."

Reporting Adverse Reactions

FDA urges consumers and healthcare providers to report adverse reactions to tattoos and permanent makeup, problems with removal, or adverse reactions to temporary tattoos. Consumers and healthcare providers can register complaints by contacting their FDA district office (see the blue pages of your local phone directory) or by contacting FDA's Center for Food Safety and Applied Nutrition (CFSAN) Adverse Events Reporting System (CAERS) by phone at (301) 436-2405 or by e-mail at CAERS@cfsan.fda.gov.

Section 75.2

Tattoo Removal

Tattoos

A tattoo used to be a permanent and irreversible adornment to one's skin. However, in recent years dermatologic surgeons have developed safe and effective techniques to successfully remove unwanted tattoos.

Patients request removal of a tattoo for a variety of reasons—social, cultural, or physical. Some patients develop an allergic reaction to a tattoo several years after the initial application. Because each tattoo is unique, removal techniques must be tailored to suit each individual case. For instance, professionally applied tattoos tend to penetrate the deeper layers of the skin at uniform levels. This uniformity allows dermatologic surgeons to use techniques that remove broader areas of inked skin at the same depth.

Homemade tattoos are often applied with an uneven hand and their removal may be more difficult. Deeper blue and black ink colors are particularly difficult to remove. Professional tattoos made with some of the newer inks and pastel colors may also be difficult to remove entirely.

Removing Tattoos

Tattoos can be removed by a dermatologic surgeon on an outpatient basis with local anesthesia. The most common techniques used are:

Laser Surgery

The surgeon removes the tattoo by selectively treating the pigment colors with a high-intensity laser beam. Lasers have become the standard treatment because they offer a "bloodless," low risk, highly effective approach with minimal side effects. The type of laser used generally depends upon the pigment colors. In many cases, multiple treatments may be required.

Dermabrasion

The surgeon "sands" the skin, removing the surface and middle layers of the tattoo. The combination of surgical and dressing techniques helps to raise and absorb the tattoo inks.

Surgical Excision

The surgeon removes the tattoo with a scalpel and closes the wound with stitches. This technique proves highly effective in removing some tattoos and allows the surgeon to excise inked areas with great control.

Are There Side Effects or Complications?

Side effects are generally minor, but may include skin discoloration at the treatment site, infection of the tattoo site, lack of complete pigment removal, or some scarring. A raised or thickened scar may appear three to six months after the tattoo is removed.

Chapter 76

Body Piercings

Over the past few years, body art has become popular, and it's hard to walk down the street, go to the mall, or watch TV without seeing someone with a piercing or a tattoo. Whether it's ears, lips, nostrils, eyebrows, belly buttons, tongues, or even cheeks, you've probably seen piercings—maybe multiple piercings—on lots of people. You might think body piercings look cool and you've thought about getting one. But are they safe? Are they a good idea? And what should you be aware of if you do decide to get one?

What Is a Body Piercing and What Can You Expect?

A body piercing is exactly that—a piercing or puncture made in your body by a needle. After that, a piece of jewelry is inserted into the puncture. The most popular pierced body parts seem to be the ears, the nostrils, and the belly button.

If the person performing the piercing provides a safe, clean, and professional environment, this is what you can expect from getting a body part pierced:

This information was provided by KidsHealth, one of the largest resources online for medically reviewed health information written for parents, kids, and teens. For more articles like this one, visit www.KidsHealth.org, or www.TeensHealth.org. Reviewed by Renee K. Kottenhahn, M.D., April 2004.

- The area you've chosen to be pierced (except for the tongue) is cleaned with a germicidal soap (a soap that kills disease-causing bacteria and microorganisms).
- Your skin is then punctured with a very sharp, clean needle.
- The piece of jewelry, which has already been sterilized, is attached to the area.
- The person performing the piercing disposes of the needle in a special container so that there is no risk of the needle or blood touching someone else.
- The pierced area is cleaned.
- The person performing the piercing checks and adjusts the jewelry.
- The person performing the piercing gives you instructions on how to make sure your new piercing heals correctly and what to do if there is a problem.

Before You Pierce That Part

If you're thinking about getting pierced, do your research first. If you're under 18, some places won't allow you to get a piercing without a parent's consent. It's a good idea to find out what risks are involved and how best to protect yourself from infections and other complications.

Certain sites on the body can cause more problems than others—infection is a common complication of mouth and nose piercings because of the millions of bacteria that live in those areas. Tongue piercings can damage teeth over time. And tongue, cheek, and lip piercings can cause gum problems.

Studies have shown that people with certain types of heart disease might have a higher risk of developing a heart infection after body piercing. If you have a medical problem such as allergies, diabetes, skin disorders, a condition that affects your immune system, or infections—or if you are pregnant—ask your doctor if there are any special concerns you should have or precautions you should take beforehand. Also, it's not a good idea to get a body piercing if you're prone to getting keloids (an overgrowth of scar tissue).

If you decide to get a body piercing:

- Make sure you're up to date with your immunizations (especially hepatitis and tetanus).

- Plan where you will get medical care if your piercing becomes infected (signs of infection include excessive redness/tenderness around the piercing site; prolonged bleeding; pus; or change in your skin color around the piercing area).

Also, if you plan to get a tongue or mouth piercing, make sure your teeth and gums are healthy.

Making Sure the Piercing Shop Is Safe and Sanitary

Body piercing is regulated in some states but not others. Although most piercing shops try to provide a clean and healthy environment, some shops might not take proper precautions against infections or other health hazards.

If you decide to get a body piercing, do a little investigative work about a shop's procedures and find out whether they provide a clean and safe environment for their customers. Every shop should have an autoclave (a sterilizing machine) and should keep instruments in sealed packets. Ask questions and make sure:

- the shop is clean
- the person doing the piercing washes his or her hands with a germicidal soap
- the person doing the piercing wears fresh disposable gloves (like those worn at a doctor's office)
- the person doing the piercing uses disposable or sterilized instruments
- the person doing the piercing does not use a piercing gun (they're not sterile)
- the needle being used is new and is being used for the first time
- the needle is disposed of in a special sealed container after the piercing
- there are procedures for the proper handling and disposal of waste (like needles or gauze with blood on it)

It's also a good idea to ask about the types of jewelry the shop offers because some people have allergic reactions to some types of metals. Before you get a piercing, make sure you know if you're allergic to certain metals or not. Only non-toxic metals such as the following should be used for body piercings:

- surgical steel
- solid 14-karat or 18-karat gold
- niobium
- titanium
- platinum

If you think the shop isn't clean enough, if all your questions aren't answered, or if you feel in any way uncomfortable, go somewhere else to get your piercing.

Some Health Risks

If all goes well, you should be fine after a body piercing except for some temporary symptoms, including some pain, swelling at the pierced area, and in the case of a tongue piercing, increased saliva. But be aware that several things, including the following, can go wrong in some cases:

- chronic infection
- uncontrollable or prolonged bleeding
- scarring
- hepatitis B and C
- tetanus
- skin allergies to the jewelry that's used
- abscesses or boils (collections of pus that can form under your skin at the site of the piercing)
- inflammation or nerve damage

Depending on the body part, healing times can take anywhere from a few weeks to more than a year. If you do get a piercing, make sure you take good care of it afterward—don't pick or tug at it, keep the area clean with soap (not alcohol), and don't touch it without washing your hands first. Never use hydrogen peroxide because it can break down newly formed tissue. If you have a mouth piercing, use an antibacterial mouthwash after eating.

If you're thinking of donating blood, keep in mind some organizations won't accept blood donations from anyone who has had a body piercing or tattoo within the last year because both procedures can transmit blood-borne diseases.

If your piercing doesn't heal correctly or you feel something might be wrong, it's important to have someone help you get medical attention. Most importantly—don't pierce yourself or have a friend do it—make sure it's done by a professional in a safe and clean environment.

Chapter 77

Heading off Hair-Care Disasters: Use Caution with Relaxers and Dyes

According to the Food and Drug Administration's Office of Cosmetics and Colors, hair straighteners and hair dyes are among its top consumer complaint areas. Complaints range from hair breakage to symptoms warranting an emergency room visit. Reporting such complaints is voluntary, and the reported problem is often due to incorrect use of a product rather than the product itself. FDA encourages consumers to understand the risks that come with using hair chemicals, and to take a proactive approach in ensuring their proper use. The agency doesn't have authority under the Federal Food, Drug, and Cosmetic Act to require premarket approval for cosmetics, but it can take action when safety issues surface.

Safer Straightening

FDA has received complaints about scalp irritation and hair breakage related to both lye and "no lye" relaxers. Some consumers falsely assume that compared to lye relaxers, no-lye relaxers take all the worry out of straightening.

"People may think because it says 'no lye' that it's not caustic," says FDA biologist Lark Lambert. But both types of relaxers contain ingredients that work by breaking chemical bonds of the hair, and both can burn the scalp if used incorrectly. Lye relaxers contain sodium

---

Excerpted from the article by Michelle Meadows, U.S. Food and Drug Administration, *FDA Consumer*, January-February 2001. Available online at http://www.fda.gov; accessed April 2005.

hydroxide as the active ingredient. With no-lye relaxers, calcium hydroxide and guanidine carbonate are mixed to produce guanidine hydroxide.

Research has shown that this combination in no-lye relaxers results in less scalp irritation than lye relaxers, but the same safety rules apply for both. They should be used properly, left on no longer than the prescribed time, carefully washed out with neutralizing shampoo, and followed up with regular conditioning. For those who opt to straighten their own hair, it's wise to enlist help simply because not being able to see and reach the top and back of the head makes proper application of the chemical and thorough rinsing more of a challenge.

Some stylists recommend applying a layer of petroleum jelly on the scalp before applying a relaxer because it creates a protective barrier between the chemical and the skin. Scratching, brushing, and combing can make the scalp more susceptible to chemical damage and should be avoided right before using a relaxer. Parents should be especially cautious when applying chemicals to children's hair and should keep relaxers out of children's reach. There have been reports of small children ingesting straightening chemicals and suffering injuries that include burns to the face, tongue, and esophagus.

Hair Dye Reactions

As with hair relaxers, some consumers have reported hair loss, burning, redness, and irritation from hair dyes. Allergic reactions to dyes include itching, swelling of the face, and even difficulty breathing.

Coal tar hair dye ingredients are known to cause allergic reactions in some people, FDA's Lambert says. Synthetic organic chemicals, including hair dyes and other color additives, were originally manufactured from coal tar, but today manufacturers primarily use materials derived from petroleum. The use of the term "coal tar" continues because historically that language has been incorporated into the law and regulations.

The law does not require that coal tar hair dyes be approved by FDA, as is required for other uses of color additives. In addition, the law does not allow FDA to take action against coal tar hair dyes that are shown to be harmful, if the product is labeled with the prescribed caution statement indicating that the product may cause irritation in certain individuals, that a patch test for skin sensitivity should be done, and that the product must not be used for dyeing the eyelashes or eyebrows. The patch test involves putting a dab of hair dye behind the ear or inside the elbow, leaving it there for two days, and looking for itching, burning, redness, or other reactions.

"The problem is that people can become sensitized—that is, develop an allergy—to these ingredients," Lambert says. "They may do the patch test once, and then use the product for 10 years" before having an allergic reaction. "But you're supposed to do the patch test every time," he says, even in salons.

When using all hair chemicals, it's critical to keep them away from children to prevent ingestion and other accidents, and to follow product directions carefully. It sounds basic, but some people don't do it, says FDA's Halper. "If it says leave on hair for five minutes, seven minutes doesn't make it better," he says. "In fact, it could do damage."

Look out for Your Eyes

Whether applying hair chemicals at home or in a hair salon, consumers and beauticians should be careful to keep them away from the eyes. FDA has received reports of injuries from hair relaxers and hair dye accidentally getting into eyes. And while it may be tempting to match a new hair color to eyebrows and eyelashes, consumers should resist the urge. The use of permanent eyelash and eyebrow tinting and dyeing has been known to cause serious eye injuries and even blindness. There are no color additives approved by FDA for dyeing or tinting eyelashes and eyebrows.

The law does not require that coal tar hair dyes be approved by FDA, as is required for other uses of color additives. In addition, the law does not allow FDA to take action against coal tar hair dyes that are shown to be harmful, if the product is labeled with the following caution statement: "Caution—This product contains ingredients which may cause skin irritation on certain individuals and a preliminary test according to accompanying directions should first be made. This product must not be used for dyeing the eyelashes or eyebrows; to do so may cause blindness."

—by Michelle Meadows, a staff writer for FDA Consumer

Chapter 78

Safe Hair Removal

You've got it, you know you don't want it, and it can appear anywhere.

Unwanted hair is common on the upper lip, the chin, cheeks, on the back, legs, fingers, feet, or toes. It can be caused by a variety of factors, including genetics, certain medications such as hormones or steroids, or even medical abnormalities, such as higher androgen (male hormone) levels or conditions of the endocrine system, such as polycystic ovarian syndrome. Have you already tried plucking? Most people can get used to this painful method, but it won't work on large areas covered with unwanted hair. There are several hair removal strategies to treat unwanted hair, but be warned: None is 100% permanent.

Hair Removal Strategies

There are several ways to remove your unwanted hair, including over-the-counter methods and those administered under a doctor's care. With most of these methods, the hair eventually grows back.

"Hair Removal," © 2003 The Cleveland Clinic Foundation, 9500 Euclid Avenue, Cleveland, OH 44195, www.clevelandclinic.org. Additional information is available from the Cleveland Clinic Health Information Center, 216-444-3771, toll-free 800-223-2273 extension 43771, or at http://www.clevelandclinic.org/health.

Shaving

Your hair growth rate will determine how often you have to shave the affected region. This is best for legs, arms, or facial hair. This hair removal method can cause ingrown hairs in the pubic region, however.

Plucking

Plucking is the most painful method, but may be the most worthwhile for those few hairs you want to remove to reshape your eyebrows or to pull out those few stray hairs that may appear on your face, especially for a woman. You should not use this hair removal method for large areas because it can cause ingrown hairs or scarring.

Depilation

Be cautious when selecting hair removal creams over the counter: all creams are not the same. For instance, a hair removal cream designated for pubic hair should not be used to remove facial hair. The chemicals in these products dissolve the hair shaft. But here are the drawbacks: the chemicals can also cause superficial burns. If you have a history of allergic reactions, you may want to seek the advice of your doctor before trying any hair removal creams.

Hot Waxing

You can do this at home or you can also have it performed by a professional in a salon. Hot waxing can be messy, and may leave some hairs behind because they can break off. Infection is one side effect to watch for. Still, many women use this hair removal method in the bikini area and for hair on the upper lip.

Laser Hair Removal

This is one of the longest-lasting methods, and generally requires 3 to 4 or more treatment sessions. The laser beam or a light pulse works to destroy the hair bulb. This hair removal treatment can be expensive and sometimes painful. Be sure to select a doctor or technician who is highly trained and knowledgeable. Laser treatment is not for everyone: your hair must be dark in color. Laser treatment also requires multiple sessions, but can be used on many parts of the body where unwanted hair may appear.

Electrolysis

There are two primary hair removal methods of electrolysis: galvanic and thermolytic.

- **Galvanic:** chemically destroys hair follicle; oldest method used, but requires several treatments.
- **Thermolytic:** uses heat to destroy the hair follicle.

In either case, be sure to find a professional who is highly trained and knowledgeable with this hair removal method. Electrolysis can be used on all parts of the body to remove unwanted hair.

Oral Medications

If none of these hair removal methods seem to address your particular problems, ask your doctor about oral medications to inhibit hair growth.

There is a topical cream called Vaniqa, recently approved by the Food and Drug Administration, for the slowing of facial hair growth in women. This cream slows growth, but will not remove the hair.

Chapter 79

Caring for Your Nails

Healthy nails are an important part of overall health. When nails are in good physical shape, they are not only aesthetically pleasing, but make it easier to perform everyday tasks. Regular visits to nail salons cost consumers in America more than six billion dollars each year. In addition, consumers also spend millions on retail nail cosmetics at drugstores and cosmetic counters. While the number of problems associated with nail cosmetics and services is small, there are some health risks associated with all that soaking, buffing, massaging, and polishing.

Dermatologist Phoebe Rich, M.D., Clinical Associate Professor of Dermatology, Oregon Health Sciences University, Portland, OR, discussed the best ways for consumers to keep their nails healthy both in the salon and at home.

"Nail cosmetics and salon services are generally quite safe, but there are four potential problem areas associated with the use of nail cosmetics and salon services: allergic reactions, irritant reaction, mechanical damage to the nail, and infection," said Dr. Rich. "While these are fairly rare occurrences, they can be serious. Consumers are urged to take some simple measures to guard against these potential health concerns."

"Healthy Nails at Your Fingertips—and on Your Toes: Simple Tips to Keep Your Nails Attractive and Infection-Free at Home and in the Salon," October 22, 2003, is reprinted with permission from the American Academy of Dermatology.

Allergic Reactions

Allergic reactions occur when a nail cosmetic ingredient sensitizes the skin so that every time the ingredient is used, itching, redness, blisters, and pain may result. The most common ingredient that can create an allergic reaction is methylmethacrylate, or MMA, which is used in the application of acrylic nails.

"Although MMA has been banned by many states and the FDA has issued warnings about its hazards, the substance is still being used in some discount salons because it costs so much less than the safer acrylate alternatives such as ethyl methacrylate," stated Dr. Rich. "If consumers notice a strong odor associated with acrylic nail application, MMA is probably being used and that salon should be avoided. Consumers should also report that salon to the state medical board."

Tosylamide formaldehyde resin is an ingredient found in some nail polishes that can create an allergic reaction. If consumers experience itching or burning of the skin following a nail salon service or the application of nail cosmetics at home, Dr. Rich recommends removing the product as soon as possible and visiting a dermatologist to determine which ingredient is responsible for the allergy. A dermatologist can provide treatment options to ensure resolution of the allergy and continued nail health.

Irritant Reactions

When the nails are dehydrated due to excessive exposure to irritating substances including chemicals and soapy water, the nails may split, peel, and become brittle. A few of the most dehydrating substances the nails are exposed to include nail polish remover and formaldehyde, which is a common ingredient in nail hardeners.

"Consumers should not use nail polish remover more than once a week and should moisturize their hands often, especially after using any dehydrating products and after washing the hands," recommended Dr. Rich. "One of the best ways to protect your nails from irritants is to wear gloves when doing wet work, such as cleaning with harsh products, or when gardening."

Mechanical Damage to the Nail and Infections

The nail plate is designed to bend or break when stressed, but if consumers wear nail enhancements that are too long and put too much pressure on the nail, such as opening soda cans with the nails, the force of the stress will be transferred to the nail bed. This results in separation of the nail from the nail bed, creating a moist, warm space under the nail where bacteria or yeast can grow.

"Fungal infections make up approximately 50 percent of all nail disorders and since the infection occurs under the nail plate or in the nail bed, it can be difficult to treat," said Dr. Rich. "One way to reduce the risk of contracting toenail fungus is to wear shower slippers in public showers, lockers rooms, and around swimming pools. Overall, it's important when caring for the nails at home or having a service in a salon, to make sure that the nails are being treated gently and safely."

The cuticle is another important part of a healthy nail because it forms a seal between the nail and the skin at the top of the finger so that irritants cannot gain access. When the cuticle is clipped or removed with small nippers or metal scrapers during a manicure or pedicure, it can result in an infection.

"It's important that consumers do not let their cuticles be cut, scraped or pushed to the point of breaking the seal between the nail and the skin," stated Dr. Rich. "The best time to push back the dead cuticle is after soaking or showering when the cuticle is soft and use a soft towel or an appropriate nail-care implement, such as an orange stick."

Avoiding ingrown nails is also an important part of maintaining healthy nails. Consumers should always clip or cut their nails straight across. Certain shoes can also irritate ingrown toenails, especially if the shoes are tight or if the front of the shoe comes to a point and forces the toes close together or on top of each other.

Contracting an infection is the most serious health risk related to nail cosmetics particularly from manicure and pedicure tools and implements that have not been properly sterilized. Viral infections such as HIV, hepatitis B and C, and warts can be transmitted to unsuspecting consumers from improperly sterilized implements. "Most nail salons take sanitation very seriously and follow strict sanitation and disinfection guidelines, but consumers should not be afraid to ask how implements are cleaned," said Dr. Rich. "Look at the salon with cleanliness in mind and ask yourself these questions: Are the stations clean? Does the nail technician wash her hands between clients? Are there dirty implements lying around? If the salon does not appear clean, then move on." Dr. Rich also recommends that in order to protect against infection consumers bring their own tools and implements to be used at the salon.

Keeping the nails healthy and neat looking can enhance a person's appearance and self-esteem and has become an important grooming ritual for both men and women. "As more and more consumers frequent nail salons and use nail cosmetics at home, the potential for infection and irritation grows as well," stated Dr. Rich. "Savvy consumers who follow these simple guidelines can protect their nails and overall health and continue to enjoy the appearance of well-kept finger and toenails."

Part Eleven

Additional Help and Information

Chapter 80

Glossary of Terms Related to the Skin, Hair, and Nails

Acne: An inflammatory follicular, papular, and pustular eruption involving the pilosebaceous apparatus.

Acne vulgaris: An eruption, predominantly of the face, upper back, and chest, composed of comedones, cysts, papules, and pustules on an inflammatory base; the condition occurs in a majority of people during puberty and adolescence. Follicular suppuration may lead to scarring. Topical treatments include tretinoin, benzoyl peroxide, and antibiotics. Sunlight, systemic antibiotics, and oral 13-cis-retinoic acid (except in pregnancy) are also effective.

Actinic keratosis: A premalignant warty lesion occurring on the sun-exposed skin of the face or hands in aged light-skinned persons; hyperkeratosis may form a cutaneous horn, and squamous cell carcinoma of low-grade malignancy may develop in a small proportion of untreated patients.

Alopecia: Absence or loss of hair.

Candidiasis: Infection with, or disease caused by, *Candida*, especially *C. albicans*. This disease usually results from debilitation (as in immunosuppression and especially AIDS), physiologic change, prolonged administration of antibiotics, and iatrogenic and barrier breakage.

Definitions in this chapter were taken from *Stedman's Medical Dictionary*, 27th Edition.

Carbuncle: Deep-seated pyogenic infection of the skin and subcutaneous tissues, usually arising in several contiguous hair follicles, with formation of connecting sinuses.

Carcinoma: Any of various types of malignant neoplasm derived from epithelial cells, chiefly glandular (adenocarcinoma) or squamous (squamous cell carcinoma); the most commonly occurring kind of cancer.

Chemical peel: A chemosurgical technique designed to remove acne scars or treat chronic skin changes caused by exposure to sunlight.

Collagen: The major protein (comprising over half of that in mammals) of the white fibers of connective tissue, cartilage, and bone, that is insoluble in water but can be altered to easily digestible, soluble gelatins by boiling in water, dilute acids, or alkalis.

Dermabrasion: Operative procedure to efface acne scars or pits performed with sandpaper, rotating wire brushes, or other abrasive materials.

Dermatitis: Inflammation of the skin.

Dermatologist: A physician who specializes in the diagnosis and treatment of cutaneous diseases and related systemic diseases.

Dermatology: The branch of medicine concerned with the study of the skin, diseases of the skin, and the relationship of cutaneous lesions to systemic disease.

Dermis: A layer of skin composed of a superficial thin layer that interdigitates with the epidermis, the stratum papillare, and the stratum reticulare; it contains blood and lymphatic vessels, nerves and nerve endings, glands, and, except for glabrous skin, hair follicles.

Eczema: Generic term for inflammatory conditions of the skin, particularly with vesiculation in the acute stage, typically erythematous, edematous, papular, and crusting; followed often by lichenification and scaling and occasionally by duskiness of the erythema and, infrequently, hyperpigmentation; often accompanied by sensations of itching and burning; often hereditary and associated with allergic rhinitis and asthma.

Edema: An accumulation of an excessive amount of watery fluid in cells or intercellular tissues.

Epidermis: The superficial epithelial portion of the skin (cutis). The thick epidermis of the palms and soles contains the following strata from the surface: stratum corneum (keratin layer), stratum lucidum (clear layer), stratum granulosum (granular layer), stratum spinosum (prickle cell layer), and stratum basale (basal cell layer); in other parts of the body, the stratum lucidum may be absent.

Epidermolysis bullosa: A group of inherited chronic noninflammatory skin diseases in which large bullae and erosions result from slight mechanical trauma.

Furuncle (boil): A localized pyogenic infection, most frequently by *Staphylococcus aureus*, originating deep in a hair follicle.

Hair follicle: A tubelike invagination of the epidermis from which the hair shaft develops and into which the sebaceous glands open; the follicle is lined by a cellular inner and outer root sheath of epidermal origin and is invested with a fibrous sheath derived from the dermis.

Hemangioma: A congenital anomaly, in which proliferation of blood vessels leads to a mass that resembles a neoplasm; it can occur anywhere in the body but is most frequently noticed in the skin and subcutaneous tissues.

Hirsutism: Presence of excessive bodily and facial hair, usually in a male pattern, especially in women; may be present in normal adults as an expression of an ethnic characteristic or may develop in children or adults as the result of androgen excess due to tumors or drugs, or nonandrogenetic drugs.

Hypertrophic scar: An elevated scar resembling a keloid but which does not spread into surrounding tissues, is rarely painful, and regresses spontaneously; collagen bundles run parallel to the skin surface.

Keloid: A nodular, firm, movable, nonencapsulated, often linear mass of hyperplastic scar tissue, tender and frequently painful, consisting of wide irregularly distributed bands of collagen; occurs in the dermis and adjacent subcutaneous tissue, usually after trauma, surgery, a burn, or severe cutaneous disease such as cystic acne, and is more common in blacks.

Keratin: Collective name for a group of proteins that form the intermediate filaments in epithelial cells.

Lesion: A wound or injury or a pathologic change in the tissues.

Melanoma: A malignant neoplasm, derived from cells that are capable of forming melanin, arising most commonly in the skin of any part of the body, or in the eye, and, rarely, in the mucous membranes of the genitalia, anus, oral cavity, or other sites; occurs mostly in adults and may originate de novo or from a pigmented nevus or lentigo maligna. Melanomas frequently metastasize widely; regional lymph nodes, skin, liver, lungs, and brain are likely to be involved. Intense, intermittent sun exposure, especially of fair-skinned children, increases the risk of melanoma later in life.

Nevus (mole): A benign localized overgrowth of melanin-forming cells of the skin present at birth or appearing early in life.

Onychomycosis: Very common fungus infections of the nails, causing thickening, roughness, and splitting, often caused by *Trichophyton rubrum or T. mentagrophytes*, *Candida*, and occasionally molds.

Pediculosis: The state of being infested with lice.

Pemphigus: A nonspecific term for blistering skin diseases.

Porphyria: A group of disorders involving heme biosynthesis, characterized by excessive excretion of porphyrins or their precursors; may be inherited or may be acquired, as from the effects of certain chemical agents.

Port-wine stain: A large congenital vascular malformation nevus having a purplish color; it is usually found on the head and neck and persists throughout life.

Pressure sore (bedsore): A chronic ulcer that appears in pressure areas of skin overlying a bony prominence in debilitated patients confined to bed or otherwise immobilized, due to a circulatory defect.

Psoriasis: A common multifactorial inherited condition characterized by the eruption of circumscribed, discrete and confluent, reddish, silvery-scaled maculopapules; the lesions occur predominantly on the elbows, knees, scalp, and trunk, and microscopically show characteristic parakeratosis and elongation of rete ridges with shortening of epidermal keratinocyte transit time due to decreased cyclic guanosine monophosphate.

Pustule: A circumscribed, superficial elevation of the skin, up to 1.0 cm in diameter, containing purulent material.

Rosacea: Chronic vascular and follicular dilation involving the nose and contiguous portions of the cheeks; may vary from mild but persistent erythema to extensive hyperplasia of the sebaceous glands, seen especially in men as rhinophyma and by deep-seated papules and pustules; accompanied by telangiectasia at the affected erythematous sites.

Scabies: An eruption due to the mite *Sarcoptes scabiei* var. hominis; the female of the species burrows into the skin, producing a vesicular eruption with intense pruritus between the fingers, on the male or female genitalia, buttocks, and elsewhere on the trunk and extremities.

Scleroderma: Thickening and induration of the skin caused by new collagen formation, with atrophy of pilosebaceous follicles; either a manifestation of progressive systemic sclerosis or localized (morphea).

Sebaceous glands: Numerous holocrine glands in the dermis that usually open into the hair follicles and secrete an oily semifluid, sebum.

Sebum: The secretion of the sebaceous glands.

Shingles: An infection caused by a herpesvirus (varicella-zoster virus), characterized by an eruption of groups of vesicles on one side of the body following the course of a nerve due to inflammation of ganglia and dorsal nerve roots resulting from activation of the virus, which in many instances has remained latent for years following a primary chickenpox infection; the condition is self-limited but may be accompanied by or followed by severe postherpetic pain.

Tinea: A fungus infection (dermatophytosis) of the keratin component of hair, skin, or nails.

Ultraviolet A (UVA): Ultraviolet radiation that causes skin tanning but is very weakly sunburn-producing and carcinogenic.

Ultraviolet B (UVB): Ultraviolet radiation that most effectively causes sunburning and tanning; excessive UVB exposure is a cause of cancer of fair skin.

Urticaria: An eruption of itching wheals, usually of systemic origin; it may be due to a state of hypersensitivity to foods or drugs, foci of infection, physical agents (heat, cold, light, friction), or psychic stimuli.

Varicella (chickenpox): An acute contagious disease, usually occurring in children, caused by the varicella-zoster virus genus, Varicellovirus, a member of the family *Herpesviridae*, and marked by a sparse eruption of papules, which become vesicles and then pustules, like that of smallpox although less severe and varying in stages, usually with mild constitutional symptoms; incubation period is about 14–17 days.

Varicose veins: Permanent dilation and tortuosity of veins, most commonly seen in the legs, probably as a result of congenitally incomplete valves; there is a predisposition to varicose veins among persons in occupations requiring long periods of standing, and in pregnant women.

Vitiligo: The appearance on otherwise normal skin of nonpigmented white patches of varied sizes, often symmetrically distributed and usually bordered by hyperpigmented areas; hair in the affected areas is usually white. Epidermal melanocytes are completely lost in depigmented areas by an autoimmune process.

Wart: A flesh-colored growth characterized by circumscribed hypertrophy of the papillae of the dermis.

Chapter 81

Directory of Dermatology Organizations and Resources

Government Agencies and Organizations

Agency for Healthcare Research and Quality
540 Gaither Road
Rockville, MD 20850
Phone: (301) 427-1364
Website: http://www.ahrq.gov
E-mail: info@ahrq.gov

Centers for Disease Control and Prevention
1600 Clifton Road
Atlanta, GA 30333
Toll-Free: (800) 311-3435
Phone: (404) 639-3311
Website: http://www.cdc.gov
E-mail: ccdinfo@cdc.gov

Federal Trade Commission
600 Pennsylvania Avenue, NW
Washington, DC 20580
Toll-Free: (877) 382-4357
Phone: (202) 326-2222
Website: http://www.ftc.gov

Healthfinder.gov
U.S. Department of Health and Human Services
P.O. Box 1133
Washington, DC 20013-1133
Website: http://www.healthfinder.gov
E-mail: healthfinder@nhic.org

Resources in this chapter were compiled from several sources deemed reliable; all contact information was verified and updated in May 2005.

National Cancer Institute
6116 Executive Boulevard,
MSC8322
Suite 3036A
Bethesda, MD 20892-8322
Toll-Free: (800) 422-6237
TTY Toll-Free: (800) 332-8615
Website: http://www.cancer.gov
E-mail:
cancergovstaff@mail.nih.gov

National Center for Alternative and Complementary Medicine
P.O. Box 7923
Gaithersburg, MD 20898
Toll-Free: (888) 644-6226
Phone: (301) 519-3153
TTY: (866) 464-3615
Fax: (866) 464-3616
Website: http://nccam.nih.gov
E-mail: info@nccam.nih.gov

National Center for Infectious Diseases
Centers for Disease Control
and Prevention
Mailstop C-14
1600 Clifton Road
Atlanta, GA 30333
Website: http://www.cdc.gov/
ncidod
E-mail: ncid@cdc.gov

National Institute of Allergy and Infectious Diseases
6610 Rockledge Drive
MSC 6612
Bethesda, MD 20892-6612
Phone: (301) 402-1663
Website: http://
www.niaid.nih.gov

National Institute of Arthritis and Musculoskeletal and Skin Diseases
1 AMS Circle
Bethesda, MD 20892-3675
Toll-Free: (877) 22-NIAMS (226-4267)
Phone: (301) 495-4484
TTY: (301) 565-2966
Fax: (301) 718-6366
Website: http://
www.niams.nih.gov
E-mail: niamsinfo@mail.nih.gov

National Institute of Neurological Disorders and Stroke (NINDS)
P.O. Box 5801
Bethesda, MD 20824
Toll-Free: (800) 352-9424
Phone: (301) 496-5751
TTY: (301) 468-5981
Website: http://
www.ninds.nih.gov

National Institutes of Health Clinical Trials
National Library of Medicine
8600 Rockville Pike
Bethesda, MD 20894
Toll-Free: (888) 346-3656
Phone: (301) 594-5983
Fax: (301) 496-2809
Website: http://
www.clinicaltrials.gov

National Women's Health Information Center
8550 Arlington Boulevard
Suite 300
Fairfax, VA 22031
Toll-Free: (800) 994-WOMAN (994-9662)
TTY: (888) 220-5446
Website: http://www.4woman.gov

Office of Dietary Supplements
National Institutes of Health
6100 Executive Blvd., Room 3B01, MSC 7517
Bethesda, MD 20892
Phone: (301)435-2920
Fax: (301) 480-1845
Website: http://ods.od.nih.gov
E-mail: ods@nih.gov

U.S. Food and Drug Administration
5600 Fishers Lane
Rockville, MD 20857-0001
Toll-Free: (888) 463-6332
Website: http://www.fda.gov

U.S. National Library of Medicine
8600 Rockville Pike
Bethesda, MD 20894
Toll-Free: (888)346-3656
Phone: (301) 594-5983
Fax: (301) 402-1384
Website: http://www.nlm.nih.gov

Private and Nonprofit Organizations

American Academy of Dermatology
P.O. Box 4014
Schaumburg, IL 60168-4014
Toll-Free: (888) 462-DERM (426-3376)
Phone: (847) 330-0230
Fax: (847) 330-0050
Website: http://www.aad.org

American Academy of Family Physicians
11400 Tomahawk Creek Parkway
Leawood, KS 66211-2672
Toll-Free: (800) 274-2237
Phone: (913) 906-6000
Website: http://www.aafp.org
E-mail: fp@aafp.org

American Cancer Society
P.O. Box 102454
Atlanta, GA 30368-2454
Toll-Free: (800) ACS-2345 (227-2345)
TTY: (866)228-4327
Website: http://www.cancer.org

American Celiac Society
59 Crystal Avenue
West Orange, NJ 07052
Phone: (504) 737-3293
Fax: (973) 669-8808
E-mail: AmerCeliacSoc@netscape.net

American College of Allergy, Asthma, and Immunology
555 East Wells Street
Suite 1100
Milwaukee, WI 53202-3823
Toll-Free: (800) 822-2762
Phone: (414) 272-6071
Website: http://www.aaaai.org
E-mail: info@aaaai.org

American Hair Loss Council
125 Seventh Street
Suite 625
Pittsburgh, PA 15222
Website: http://www.ahlc.org
E-mail: ahlc@e-zign.com

American Medical Association/Medem
649 Mission Street
2nd Floor
San Francisco, CA 94105
Toll-Free: (877) 926-3336
Phone: (415) 644-3800
Fax: (415) 644-3950
Website: http://
www.medem.com
E-mail: info@medem.com

American Melanoma Foundation
2160 Fletcher Parkway
Suite O
El Cajon, CA 92020
Phone: (619) 448-0991
Fax: (619) 448-2902
Website: http://
www.melanomafoundation.org
E-mail: sunsmartz
@melanomafoundation.org

American Osteopathic College of Dermatology
1501 East Illinois Street
P.O. Box 7525
Kirksville, MO 63501
Toll-Free: (800) 449-2623
Phone: (660) 665-2184
Fax: (660) 627-2623
Website: http://www.aocd.org
E-mail: info@aocd.org

American Podiatric Medical Association
9312 Old Georgetown Road
Bethesda, MD 20814-1621
Toll-Free: (800) FOOTCARE
(366-8273)
Phone: (301) 571-9200
Fax: (301) 530-2752
Website: http://www.apma.org

American Porphyria Foundation
P.O. Box 22712
Houston, TX 77227
Phone: (713) 266-9617
Fax: (713) 840-9552
Website: http://
www.porphyriafoundation.com
E-mail: porphyrus@juno.com

American Skin Association, Inc.
346 Park Avenue South, 4th
Floor
New York, NY 10010
Toll-Free: (800) 499-SKIN (7546)
Phone: (212) 889-4858
Fax: (212) 889-4959
Website: http://
www.americanskin.org
E-mail: info@americanskin.org

American Vitiligo Research Foundation
P.O. Box 7540
Clearwater, FL 33758
Phone: (727) 461-3899
Fax: (727) 461-4796
Website: http://www.avrf.org
E-mail: vitiligo@avrf.org

Celiac Disease Foundation
13251 Ventura Boulevard
Suite 1
Studio City, CA 91604-1838
Phone: (818) 990-2354
Fax: (818) 990-2379
Website: http://www.celiac.org
E-mail: cdf@celiac.org

Celiac Sprue Association/ USA
P.O. Box 31700
Omaha, NE 68131
Toll-Free: (877) CSA-4CSA
Phone: (402) 558-0600
Fax: (402) 558-1347
Website: http://www.csaceliacs.org
E-mail: celiacs@csaceliacs.org

Children's Tumor Foundation
95 Pine Street
16th Floor
New York, NY 10005
Toll-Free: (800) 323-7938
Phone: (212) 344-6633
Fax: (212) 747-0004
Website: http://www.ctf.org
E-mail: info@ctf.org

Cleveland Clinic
9500 Euclid Avenue
Cleveland, OH 44195
Toll-Free: (800) 223-2273, ext. 48950
Phone: (216) 444-2200
TTY: (216) 444-0261
Website: http://www.clevelandclinic.org

DebRA of America, Inc. (Dystrophic Epidermolysis Bullosa Research Association of America)
5 West 36th Street
Suite 404
New York, NY 10018
Phone: (212) 868-1573
Website: http://www.debra.org
E-mail: staff@debra.org

Foundation for Ichthyosis and Related Skin Types
1601 Valley Forge Road
Lansdale, PA 19446
Toll-Free: (800) 545-3286
Phone: (215) 631-1411
Fax: (215) 631-1413
Website: http://www.scalyskin.org
E-mail: info@scalyskin.org

Gluten Intolerance Group
15110 10th Avenue SW, Suite A
Seattle, WA 98166
Phone: (206) 246-6652
Fax: (206) 246-6531
Website: http://www.gluten.net
E-mail: info@gluten.net

Inflammatory Skin Disease Institute
P.O. Box 1074
Newport News, VA 23601
Phone: (757) 223-0795
Fax: (757) 595-1842
Website: http://www.isdionline.org
E-mail: ExDirISDI@aol.com

International Pemphigus Foundation
828 San Pablo Ave., Suite 210
Albany, CA 94706
Phone: (510) 527-4970
Fax: (510) 527-8497
Website: http://www.pemphigus.org
E-mail: pemphigus@pemphigus.org

Leukemia & Lymphoma Society
1311 Mamaroneck Avenue
White Plains, NY 10605
Toll-Free: (800) 955-4572
Phone: (914) 949-5213
Fax: (914) 949-6691
Website: http://www.leukemia-lymphoma.org

Lupus Foundation of America, Inc.
2000 L Street NW, Suite 710
Washington, DC 20036
Toll-Free: (800) 558-0121
Phone: (202) 349-1155
Fax: (202) 349-1156
Website: http://www.lupus.org
E-mail: info@lupus.org

Mayo Foundation for Medical Education and Research
200 First Street SW
Rochester, MN 55905
Website: http://www.mayoclinic.com
E-mail: comments@mayoclinic.com

Melanoma Education Foundation
P.O. Box 2023
Peabody, MA 01960
Phone: (978) 535-3080
Fax: (978) 535-5602
Website: http://www.skincheck.org
E-mail: mef@skincheck.org

Myositis Association
1233 20th St. NW
Suite 402
Washington, DC 20036
Phone: (202) 887-0088
Fax: (202) 466-8940
Website: http://www.myositis.org
E-mail: tma@myositis.org

National Alopecia Areata Foundation
P.O. Box 150760
San Rafael, CA 94915-0760
Phone: (415) 472-3780
Fax: (415) 472-5343
Website: http://www.naaf.org
E-mail: info@naaf.org

National Ataxia Foundation
2600 Fernbrook Lane
Suite 119
Minneapolis, MN 55447-4752
Phone: (763) 553-0020
Fax: (763) 553-0167
Website: http://www.ataxia.org
E-mail: mnaf@ataxia.org

National Eczema Association
4460 Redwood Highway
Suite 16D
San Rafael, CA 94903-1953
Toll-Free: (800) 818-7546
Phone: (415) 499-3474
Fax: (415) 472-5345
Website: http://www.nationaleczema.org
E-mail: info@nationaleczema.org

National Foundation for Cancer Research
4600 East West Highway
Suite 525
Bethesda, Maryland 20814
Toll-Free: (800) 321-CURE (2873)
Phone: (301) 654-1250
Fax: (301) 654-5824
Website: http://www.nfcr.org
E-mail: cure@nfcr.org

National Jewish Medical and Research Center
1400 Jackson Street
Denver, CO 80206
Toll-Free: (800) 222-LUNG (5864)
Phone: (303) 388-4461 (7700)
Website: http://www.njc.org
E-mail: lungline@njc.org

National Organization for Albinism & Hypopigmentation
P.O. Box 959
East Hampstead, NH 03826-0959
Toll-Free: (800) 473-2310
Phone: (603) 887-2310
Fax: (800) 648-2310
Website: http://www.albinism.org
E-mail: info@albinism.org

National Organization for Rare Disorders
55 Kenosia Avenue
P.O. Box 1968
Danbury, CT 06813-1968
Toll-Free: (800) 999-6673
Phone: (203) 744-0100
TTY: (203) 797-9590
Fax: (203) 798-2291
Website: http://www.rarediseases.org
E-mail: orphan@rarediseases.org

National Psoriasis Foundation
6600 SW 92nd
Suite 300
Portland, OR 97223
Toll-Free: (800) 723-9166
Phone: (503) 244-7404
Fax: (503) 245-0626
Website: http://www.psoriasis.org
E-mail: getinfo@psoriasis.org

National Rosacea Society
800 South Northwest Highway, Suite 200
Barrington, IL 60010
Toll-Free: (888) NO BLUSH (662-5874)
Phone: (847) 382-8971
Fax: (847) 382-5567
Website: http://www.rosacea.org
E-mail: rosaceas@aol.com

National Vitiligo Foundation
700 Olympic Plaza Circle
Suite 404
Tyler, TX 75701
Phone: (903) 595-3713
Fax: (903) 593-1545
Website: http://www.vitiligofoundation.org
E-mail: vitiligo@trimofran.org

Nemours Foundation Center for Children's Health Media
1600 Rockland Road
Wilmington, DE 19803
Phone: (302) 651-4000
Fax: (302) 651-4055
Website: http://www.kidshealth.org
E-mail: info@kidshealth.org

Nevus Outreach, Inc.
1601 Madison Boulevard
Bartlesville, OK 74006
Toll-Free: (877) 426-3887
Phone: (918) 331-0595
Fax: (918) 331-0595
Website: http://www.nevus.org
E-mail: info@nevus.org

Nevus Network
P.O. Box 305
West Salem, OH 44287
Phone: (419) 853-4525
Website: http://www.nevusnetwork.org
E-mail: info@nevusnetwork.org

Scleroderma Foundation
12 Kent Way
Suite 101
Byfiled, MA 01922
Toll-Free: (800) 722-4673
Phone: (978) 463-5843
Fax: (978) 463-5809
Website: http://www.scleroderma.org
E-mail: sfinfo@scleroderma.org

Scleroderma Research Foundation
220 Montgomery Street
Suite 1411
San Francisco, CA 94104
Phone: (415) 834-9444
Fax: (415) 834-9177
Website: http://www.srfcure.org

Sjögren's Syndrome Foundation
8120 Woodmont Avenue
Suite 530
Bethesda, MD 20814
Toll-Free: (800) 475-6473
Phone: (301) 718-0300
Fax: (301) 718-0322
Website: http://www.sjogrens.org
E-mail: ssf@sjogrens.org

Skin Cancer Foundation
245 Fifth Avenue, Suite 1403
New York, NY 10016
Toll-Free: (800) SKIN-490 (754-6490)
Phone: (212) 725-5176
Fax: (212) 725-5751
Website: http://www.skincancer.org
E-mail: info@skincancer.org

Sturge-Weber Foundation
P.O. Box 418
Mt. Freedom, NJ 07970
Toll-Free: (800) 627-5482
Phone: (973) 895-4445
Fax: (973) 895-4846
Website: http://www.sturge-weber.com
E-mail: swf@sturge-weber.com

Society for Pediatric Dermatology
5422 North Bernard
Chicago, IL 60625
Phone: (773) 583-9780
Fax: (773) 583-9765
Website: http://www.pedsderm.net
E-mail: Patrici107@aol.com

Tuberous Sclerosis Alliance
801 Roeder Road, Suite 750
Silver Spring, MD 20910
Toll-Free: (800) 225-6872
Phone: (301) 562-9890
Fax: (301) 562-9870
Website: http://www.tsalliance.org
E-mail: info@tsalliance.org

Xeroderma Pigmentosum Society
437 Snydertown Road
Craryville, NY 12521
Toll-Free: (877) 977-2873
Phone: (518) 851-2612
Fax: (518) 851-2612
Website: http://www.xps.org
E-mail: xps@xps.org

Vascular Birthmark Foundation
P.O. Box 106
Latham, NY 12110
Phone: (877) VBF-LOOK
Website: http://www.birthmark.org

Dermatological Surgery Organizations

American Academy of Facial and Reconstructive Plastic Surgery
310 S. Henry Street
Alexandria, VA 22314
Phone: (703) 299-9291
Fax: (703) 299-8898
Website: http://www.facemd.org
E-mail: info@aafprs.org

American Society for Dermatologic Surgery (ASDS)
5550 Meadowbrook Drive
Suite 120
Rolling Meadows, IL 60008
Phone: (847) 956-0900
Fax: (847) 956-0999
Website: http://www.aboutskinsurgery.com
E-mail: info@asds.net

American Society for Laser Medicine and Surgery
2404 Stewart Avenue
Wausau, WI 54401
Phone: (715) 845-9283
Fax: (715) 848-2493
Website: http://www.aslms.org
E-mail: information@aslms.org

American Society of Aesthetic Plastic Surgery
Phone: (212) 921-0500
Fax: (212) 921-0011
Toll-Free: (888) 272-7711
Website: http://www.surgery.org
E-mail: findasurgeon@surgery.org

American Society of Plastic Surgeons
444 E. Algonquin Road
Arlington Heights, IL 60005
Toll-Free: (888) 4-PLASTIC (475-2784)
Phone: (847) 228-9900
Website: http://www.plasticsurgery.org
E-mail: hr@plasticsurgery.org

Index

Index

Page numbers followed by 'n' indicate a footnote. Page numbers in *italics* indicate a table or illustration.

A

B

C

D

E

F

G

H

I

M

T

U

V

W

X

Y

Z

Health Reference Series

COMPLETE CATALOG

List price $87 per volume. **School and library price $78 per volume.**

Adolescent Health Sourcebook

Basic Consumer Health Information about Common Medical, Mental, and Emotional Concerns in Adolescents, Including Facts about Acne, Body Piercing, Mononucleosis, Nutrition, Eating Disorders, Stress, Depression, Behavior Problems, Peer Pressure, Violence, Gangs, Drug Use, Puberty, Sexuality, Pregnancy, Learning Disabilities, and More

Along with a Glossary of Terms and Other Resources for Further Help and Information

Edited by Chad T. Kimball. 658 pages. 2002. 0-7808-0248-9.

"It is written in clear, nontechnical language aimed at general readers. . . . Recommended for public libraries, community colleges, and other agencies serving health care consumers."
—*American Reference Books Annual, 2003*

"Recommended for school and public libraries. Parents and professionals dealing with teens will appreciate the easy-to-follow format and the clearly written text. This could become a 'must have' for every high school teacher." —*E-Streams, Jan '03*

"A good starting point for information related to common medical, mental, and emotional concerns of adolescents." —*School Library Journal, Nov '02*

"This book provides accurate information in an easy to access format. It addresses topics that parents and caregivers might not be aware of and provides practical, useable information." —*Doody's Health Sciences Book Review Journal, Sep-Oct '02*

"Recommended reference source."
—*Booklist, American Library Association, Sep '02*

AIDS Sourcebook, 3rd Edition

Basic Consumer Health Information about Acquired Immune Deficiency Syndrome (AIDS) and Human Immunodeficiency Virus (HIV) Infection, Including Facts about Transmission, Prevention, Diagnosis, Treatment, Opportunistic Infections, and Other Complications, with a Section for Women and Children, Including Details about Associated Gynecological Concerns, Pregnancy, and Pediatric Care

Along with Updated Statistical Information, Reports on Current Research Initiatives, a Glossary, and Directories of Internet, Hotline, and Other Resources

Edited by Dawn D. Matthews. 664 pages. 2003. 0-7808-0631-X.

ALSO AVAILABLE: *AIDS Sourcebook, 1st Edition.* Edited by Karen Bellenir and Peter D. Dresser. 831 pages. 1995. 0-7808-0031-1.

AIDS Sourcebook, 2nd Edition. Edited by Karen Bellenir. 751 pages. 1999. 0-7808-0225-X.

"The 3rd edition of the *AIDS Sourcebook*, part of Omnigraphics' *Health Reference Series*, is a welcome update. . . . This resource is highly recommended for academic and public libraries."
—*American Reference Books Annual, 2004*

"Excellent sourcebook. This continues to be a highly recommended book. There is no other book that provides as much information as this book provides."
—*AIDS Book Review Journal, Dec-Jan 2000*

"Recommended reference source."
—*Booklist, American Library Association, Dec '99*

"A solid text for college-level health libraries."
—*The Bookwatch, Aug '99*

Cited in *Reference Sources for Small and Medium-Sized Libraries, American Library Association, 1999*

Alcoholism Sourcebook

Basic Consumer Health Information about the Physical and Mental Consequences of Alcohol Abuse, Including Liver Disease, Pancreatitis, Wernicke-Korsakoff Syndrome (Alcoholic Dementia), Fetal Alcohol Syndrome, Heart Disease, Kidney Disorders, Gastrointestinal Problems, and Immune System Compromise and Featuring Facts about Addiction, Detoxification, Alcohol Withdrawal, Recovery, and the Maintenance of Sobriety

Along with a Glossary and Directories of Resources for Further Help and Information

Edited by Karen Bellenir. 613 pages. 2000. 0-7808-0325-6.

"This title is one of the few reference works on alcoholism for general readers. For some readers this will be a welcome complement to the many self-help books on the market. Recommended for collections serving general readers and consumer health collections."
—*E-Streams, Mar '01*

"This book is an excellent choice for public and academic libraries."
—*American Reference Books Annual, 2001*

"Recommended reference source."
—*Booklist, American Library Association, Dec '00*

"Presents a wealth of information on alcohol use and abuse and its effects on the body and mind, treatment, and prevention." —*SciTech Book News, Dec '00*

"Important new health guide which packs in the latest consumer information about the problems of alcoholism." —*Reviewer's Bookwatch, Nov '00*

SEE ALSO *Drug Abuse Sourcebook, Substance Abuse Sourcebook*

Allergies Sourcebook, 2nd Edition

Basic Consumer Health Information about Allergic Disorders, Triggers, Reactions, and Related Symptoms, Including Anaphylaxis, Rhinitis, Sinusitis, Asthma, Dermatitis, Conjunctivitis, and Multiple Chemical Sensitivity

Along with Tips on Diagnosis, Prevention, and Treatment, Statistical Data, a Glossary, and a Directory of Sources for Further Help and Information

Edited by Annemarie S. Muth. 598 pages. 2002. 0-7808-0376-0.

ALSO AVAILABLE: *Allergies Sourcebook, 1st Edition.* Edited by Allan R. Cook. 611 pages. 1997. 0-7808-0036-2.

"This book brings a great deal of useful material together. . . . This is an excellent addition to public and consumer health library collections."

—*American Reference Books Annual, 2003*

"This second edition would be useful to laypersons with little or advanced knowledge of the subject matter. This book would also serve as a resource for nursing and other health care professions students. It would be useful in public, academic, and hospital libraries with consumer health collections." —*E-Streams, Jul '02*

Alternative Medicine Sourcebook, 2nd Edition

Basic Consumer Health Information about Alternative and Complementary Medical Practices, Including Acupuncture, Chiropractic, Herbal Medicine, Homeopathy, Naturopathic Medicine, Mind-Body Interventions, Ayurveda, and Other Non-Western Medical Traditions

Along with Facts about such Specific Therapies as Massage Therapy, Aromatherapy, Qigong, Hypnosis, Prayer, Dance, and Art Therapies, a Glossary, and Resources for Further Information

Edited by Dawn D. Matthews. 618 pages. 2002. 0-7808-0605-0.

ALSO AVAILABLE: *Alternative Medicine Sourcebook, 1st Edition.* Edited by Allan R. Cook. 737 pages. 1999. 0-7808-0200-4.

"Recommended for public, high school, and academic libraries that have consumer health collections. Hospital libraries that also serve the public will find this to be a useful resource." —*E-Streams, Feb '03*

"Recommended reference source."

—*Booklist, American Library Association, Jan '03*

"An important alternate health reference."

—*MBR Bookwatch, Oct '02*

"A great addition to the reference collection of every type of library." —*American Reference Books Annual, 2000*

Alzheimer's Disease Sourcebook, 3rd Edition

Basic Consumer Health Information about Alzheimer's Disease, Other Dementias, and Related Disorders, Including Multi-Infarct Dementia, AIDS Dementia Complex, Dementia with Lewy Bodies, Huntington's Disease, Wernicke-Korsakoff Syndrome (Alcohol-Reated Dementia), Delirium, and Confusional States

Along with Information for People Newly Diagnosed with Alzheimer's Disease and Caregivers, Reports Detailing Current Research Efforts in Prevention, Diagnosis, and Treatment, Facts about Long-Term Care Issues, and Listings of Sources for Additional Information

Edited by Karen Bellenir. 645 pages. 2003. 0-7808-0666-2.

ALSO AVAILABLE: *Alzheimer's, Stroke & 29 Other Neurological Disorders Sourcebook, 1st Edition.* Edited by Frank E. Bair. 579 pages. 1993. 1-55888-748-2.

ALSO AVAILABLE: *Alzheimer's Disease Sourcebook, 2nd Edition.* Edited by Karen Bellenir. 524 pages. 1999. 0-7808-0223-3.

"This very informative and valuable tool will be a great addition to any library serving consumers, students and health care workers."

—*American Reference Books Annual, 2004*

"This is a valuable resource for people affected by dementias such as Alzheimer's. It is easy to navigate and includes important information and resources."

—*Doody's Review Service, Feb. 2004*

"Recommended reference source."

—*Booklist, American Library Association, Oct '99*

SEE ALSO *Brain Disorders Sourcebook*

Arthritis Sourcebook, 2nd Edition

Basic Consumer Health Information about Osteoarthritis, Rheumatoid Arthritis, Other Rheumatic Disorders, Infectious Forms of Arthritis, and Diseases with Symptoms Linked to Arthritis, Featuring Facts about Diagnosis, Pain Management, and Surgical Therapies

Along with Coping Strategies, Research Updates, a Glossary, and Resources for Additional Help and Information

Edited by Amy L. Sutton. 593 pages. 2004. 0-7808-0667-0.

ALSO AVAILABLE: *Arthritis Sourcebook, 1st Edition.* Edited by Allan R. Cook. 550 pages. 1998. 0-7808-0201-2.

". . . accessible to the layperson."

—*Reference and Research Book News, Feb '99*

Asthma Sourcebook

Basic Consumer Health Information about Asthma, Including Symptoms, Traditional and Nontraditional Remedies, Treatment Advances, Quality-of-Life Aids,

Medical Research Updates, and the Role of Allergies, Exercise, Age, the Environment, and Genetics in the Development of Asthma

Along with Statistical Data, a Glossary, and Directories of Support Groups, and Other Resources for Further Information

Edited by Annemarie S. Muth. 628 pages. 2000. 0-7808-0381-7.

"A worthwhile reference acquisition for public libraries and academic medical libraries whose readers desire a quick introduction to the wide range of asthma information." —*Choice, Association of College & Research Libraries, Jun '01*

"Recommended reference source."
—*Booklist, American Library Association, Feb '01*

"Highly recommended." —*The Bookwatch, Jan '01*

"There is much good information for patients and their families who deal with asthma daily."
—*American Medical Writers Association Journal, Winter '01*

"This informative text is recommended for consumer health collections in public, secondary school, and community college libraries and the libraries of universities with a large undergraduate population."
—*American Reference Books Annual, 2001*

■

Attention Deficit Disorder Sourcebook

Basic Consumer Health Information about Attention Deficit/Hyperactivity Disorder in Children and Adults, Including Facts about Causes, Symptoms, Diagnostic Criteria, and Treatment Options Such as Medications, Behavior Therapy, Coaching, and Homeopathy

Along with Reports on Current Research Initiatives, Legal Issues, and Government Regulations, and Featuring a Glossary of Related Terms, Internet Resources, and a List of Additional Reading Material

Edited by Dawn D. Matthews. 470 pages. 2002. 0-7808-0624-7.

"Recommended reference source."
—*Booklist, American Library Association, Jan '03*

"This book is recommended for all school libraries and the reference or consumer health sections of public libraries." —*American Reference Books Annual, 2003*

■

Back & Neck Sourcebook, 2nd Edition

Basic Consumer Health Information about Spinal Pain, Spinal Cord Injuries, and Related Disorders, Such as Degenerative Disk Disease, Osteoarthritis, Scoliosis, Sciatica, Spina Bifida, and Spinal Stenosis, and Featuring Facts about Maintaining Spinal Health, Self-Care, Pain Management, Rehabilitative Care, Chiropractic Care, Spinal Surgeries, and Complementary Therapies

Along with Suggestions for Preventing Back and Neck Pain, a Glossary of Related Terms, and a Directory of Resources

Edited by Amy L. Sutton. 633 pages. 2004. 0-7808-0738-3

ALSO AVAILABLE: *Back & Neck Disorders Sourcebook, 1st Edition.* Edited by Karen Bellenir. 548 pages. 1997. 0-7808-0202-0.

"The strength of this work is its basic, easy-to-read format. Recommended."
—*Reference and User Services Quarterly, American Library Association, Winter '97*

■

Blood & Circulatory Disorders Sourcebook, 2nd Edition

Basic Consumer Health Information about the Blood and Circulatory System and Related Disorders, Such as Anemia and Other Hemoglobin Diseases, Cancer of the Blood and Associated Bone Marrow Disorders, Clotting and Bleeding Problems, and Conditions That Affect the Veins, Blood Vessels, and Arteries, Including Facts about the Donation and Transplantation of Bone Marrow, Stem Cells, and Blood and Tips for Keeping the Blood and Circulatory System Healthy

Along with a Glossary of Related Terms and Resources for Additional Help and Information

Edited by Amy L. Sutton. 659 pages. 2005. 0-7808-0746-4.

ALSO AVAILABLE: *Blood and Circulatory Disorders Sourcebook, 1st Edition.* Edited by Karen Bellenir and Linda M. Shin. 554 pages. 1998. 0-7808-0203-9.

"Recommended reference source."
—*Booklist, American Library Association, Feb '99*

"An important reference sourcebook written in simple language for everyday, non-technical users."
—*Reviewer's Bookwatch, Jan '99*

■

Brain Disorders Sourcebook, 2nd Edition

Basic Consumer Health Information about Acquired and Traumatic Brain Injuries, Infections of the Brain, Epilepsy and Seizure Disorders, Cerebral Palsy, and Degenerative Neurological Disorders, Including Amyotrophic Lateral Sclerosis (ALS), Dementias, Multiple Sclerosis, and More

Along with Information on the Brain's Structure and Function, Treatment and Rehabilitation Options, Reports on Current Research Initiatives, a Glossary of Terms Related to Brain Disorders and Injuries, and a Directory of Sources for Further Help and Information

Edited by Sandra J. Judd. 625 pages. 2005. 0-7808-0744-8.

ALSO AVAILABLE: *Brain Disorders Sourcebook, 1st Edition.* Edited by Karen Bellenir. 481 pages. 1999. 0-7808-0229-2.

"Belongs on the shelves of any library with a consumer health collection." —*E-Streams, Mar '00*

"Recommended reference source."
—*Booklist, American Library Association, Oct '99*

***SEE ALSO** Alzheimer's Disease Sourcebook*

Breast Cancer Sourcebook, 2nd Edition

Basic Consumer Health Information about Breast Cancer, Including Facts about Risk Factors, Prevention, Screening and Diagnostic Methods, Treatment Options, Complementary and Alternative Therapies, Post-Treatment Concerns, Clinical Trials, Special Risk Populations, and New Developments in Breast Cancer Research

Along with Breast Cancer Statistics, a Glossary of Related Terms, and a Directory of Resources for Additional Help and Information

Edited by Sandra J. Judd. 595 pages. 2004. 0-7808-0668-9.

***ALSO AVAILABLE:** Breast Cancer Sourcebook, 1st Edition.* Edited by Edward J. Prucha and Karen Bellenir. 580 pages. 2001. 0-7808-0244-6.

"It would be a useful reference book in a library or on loan to women in a support group."
—*Cancer Forum, Mar '03*

"Recommended reference source."
—*Booklist, American Library Association, Jan '02*

"This reference source is highly recommended. It is quite informative, comprehensive and detailed in nature, and yet it offers practical advice in easy-to-read language. It could be thought of as the 'bible' of breast cancer for the consumer." —*E-Streams, Jan '02*

"The broad range of topics covered in lay language make the *Breast Cancer Sourcebook* an excellent addition to public and consumer health library collections."
—*American Reference Books Annual 2002*

"From the pros and cons of different screening methods and results to treatment options, *Breast Cancer Sourcebook* provides the latest information on the subject."
—*Library Bookwatch, Dec '01*

"This thoroughgoing, very readable reference covers all aspects of breast health and cancer. . . . Readers will find much to consider here. Recommended for all public and patient health collections."
—*Library Journal, Sep '01*

***SEE ALSO** Cancer Sourcebook for Women, Women's Health Concerns Sourcebook*

Breastfeeding Sourcebook

Basic Consumer Health Information about the Benefits of Breastmilk, Preparing to Breastfeed, Breastfeeding as a Baby Grows, Nutrition, and More, Including Information on Special Situations and Concerns Such as Mastitis, Illness, Medications, Allergies, Multiple Births, Prematurity, Special Needs, and Adoption

Along with a Glossary and Resources for Additional Help and Information

Edited by Jenni Lynn Colson. 388 pages. 2002. 0-7808-0332-9.

***SEE ALSO** Pregnancy & Birth Sourcebook*

"Particularly useful is the information about professional lactation services and chapters on breastfeeding when returning to work. . . . *Breastfeeding Sourcebook* will be useful for public libraries, consumer health libraries, and technical schools offering nurse assistant training, especially in areas where Internet access is problematic."
—*American Reference Books Annual, 2003*

Burns Sourcebook

Basic Consumer Health Information about Various Types of Burns and Scalds, Including Flame, Heat, Cold, Electrical, Chemical, and Sun Burns

Along with Information on Short-Term and Long-Term Treatments, Tissue Reconstruction, Plastic Surgery, Prevention Suggestions, and First Aid

Edited by Allan R. Cook. 604 pages. 1999. 0-7808-0204-7.

"This is an exceptional addition to the series and is highly recommended for all consumer health collections, hospital libraries, and academic medical centers."
—*E-Streams, Mar '00*

"This key reference guide is an invaluable addition to all health care and public libraries in confronting this ongoing health issue."
—*American Reference Books Annual, 2000*

"Recommended reference source."
—*Booklist, American Library Association, Dec '99*

***SEE ALSO** Skin Disorders Sourcebook*

Cancer Sourcebook, 4th Edition

Basic Consumer Health Information about Major Forms and Stages of Cancer, Featuring Facts about Head and Neck Cancers, Lung Cancers, Gastrointestinal Cancers, Genitourinary Cancers, Lymphomas, Blood Cell Cancers, Endocrine Cancers, Skin Cancers, Bone Cancers, Sarcomas, and Others, and Including Information about Cancer Treatments and Therapies, Identifying and Reducing Cancer Risks, and Strategies for Coping with Cancer and the Side Effects of Treatment

Along with a Cancer Glossary, Statistical and Demographic Data, and a Directory of Sources for Additional Help and Information

Edited by Karen Bellenir. 1,119 pages. 2003. 0-7808-0633-6.

***ALSO AVAILABLE:** Cancer Sourcebook, 1st Edition.* Edited by Frank E. Bair. 932 pages. 1990. 1-55888-888-8.

New Cancer Sourcebook, 2nd Edition. Edited by Allan R. Cook. 1,313 pages. 1996. 0-7808-0041-9.

Cancer Sourcebook, 3rd Edition. Edited by Edward J. Prucha. 1,069 pages. 2000. 0-7808-0227-6.

"With cancer being the second leading cause of death for Americans, a prodigious work such as this one, which locates centrally so much cancer-related information, is clearly an asset to this nation's citizens and others." —*Journal of the National Medical Association, 2004*

"This title is recommended for health sciences and public libraries with consumer health collections." —*E-Streams, Feb '01*

"... can be effectively used by cancer patients and their families who are looking for answers in a language they can understand. Public and hospital libraries should have it on their shelves." —*American Reference Books Annual, 2001*

"Recommended reference source." —*Booklist, American Library Association, Dec '00*

Cited in *Reference Sources for Small and Medium-Sized Libraries, American Library Association, 1999*

"The amount of factual and useful information is extensive. The writing is very clear, geared to general readers. Recommended for all levels." —*Choice, Association of College & Research Libraries, Jan '97*

SEE ALSO *Breast Cancer Sourcebook, Cancer Sourcebook for Women, Pediatric Cancer Sourcebook, Prostate Cancer Sourcebook*

■

Cancer Sourcebook for Women, 2nd Edition

Basic Consumer Health Information about Gynecologic Cancers and Related Concerns, Including Cervical Cancer, Endometrial Cancer, Gestational Trophoblastic Tumor, Ovarian Cancer, Uterine Cancer, Vaginal Cancer, Vulvar Cancer, Breast Cancer, and Common Non-Cancerous Uterine Conditions, with Facts about Cancer Risk Factors, Screening and Prevention, Treatment Options, and Reports on Current Research Initiatives

Along with a Glossary of Cancer Terms and a Directory of Resources for Additional Help and Information

Edited by Karen Bellenir. 604 pages. 2002. 0-7808-0226-8.

ALSO AVAILABLE: *Cancer Sourcebook for Women, 1st Edition.* Edited by Allan R. Cook and Peter D. Dresser. 524 pages. 1996. 0-7808-0076-1.

"An excellent addition to collections in public, consumer health, and women's health libraries." —*American Reference Books Annual, 2003*

"Overall, the information is excellent, and complex topics are clearly explained. As a reference book for the consumer it is a valuable resource to assist them to make informed decisions about cancer and its treatments." —*Cancer Forum, Nov '02*

"Highly recommended for academic and medical reference collections." —*Library Bookwatch, Sep '02*

"This is a highly recommended book for any public or consumer library, being reader friendly and containing accurate and helpful information." —*E-Streams, Aug '02*

"Recommended reference source." —*Booklist, American Library Association, Jul '02*

SEE ALSO *Breast Cancer Sourcebook, Women's Health Concerns Sourcebook*

■

Cardiovascular Diseases & Disorders Sourcebook, 3rd Edition

Basic Consumer Health Information about Heart and Vascular Diseases and Disorders, Such as Angina, Heart Attacks, Arrhythmias, Cardiomyopathy, Valve Disease, Atherosclerosis, and Aneurysms, with Information about Managing Cardiovascular Risk Factors and Maintaining Heart Health, Medications and Procedures Used to Treat Cardiovascular Disorders, and Concerns of Special Significance to Women

long with Reports on Current Research Initiatives, a Glossary of Related Medical Terms, and a Directory of Sources for Further Help and Information

Edited by Sandra J. Judd. 713 pages. 2005. 0-7808-0739-1.

ALSO AVAILABLE: *Heart Diseases & Disorders Sourcebook, 2nd Edition.* Edited by Karen Bellenir. 612 pages. 2000. 0-7808-0238-1.

Cardiovascular Diseases & Disorders Sourcebook, 1st Edition. Edited by Karen Bellenir and Peter D. Dresser. 683 pages. 1995. 0-7808-0032-X.

"This work stands out as an imminently accessible resource for the general public. It is recommended for the reference and circulating shelves of school, public, and academic libraries." —*American Reference Books Annual, 2001*

"Recommended reference source." —*Booklist, American Library Association, Dec '00*

"Provides comprehensive coverage of matters related to the heart. This title is recommended for health sciences and public libraries with consumer health collections." —*E-Streams, Oct '00*

SEE ALSO *Healthy Heart Sourcebook for Women*

■

Caregiving Sourcebook

Basic Consumer Health Information for Caregivers, Including a Profile of Caregivers, Caregiving Responsibilities and Concerns, Tips for Specific Conditions, Care Environments, and the Effects of Caregiving

Along with Facts about Legal Issues, Financial Information, and Future Planning, a Glossary, and a Listing of Additional Resources

Edited by Joyce Brennfleck Shannon. 600 pages. 2001. 0-7808-0331-0.

"Essential for most collections." —*Library Journal, Apr 1, 2002*

"An ideal addition to the reference collection of any public library. Health sciences information professionals may also want to acquire the *Caregiving Source-*

book **for their hospital or academic library for use as a ready reference tool by health care workers interested in aging and caregiving."** —*E-Streams, Jan '02*

"Recommended reference source."
—*Booklist, American Library Association, Oct '01*

■

Child Abuse Sourcebook

Basic Consumer Health Information about the Physical, Sexual, and Emotional Abuse of Children, with Additional Facts about Neglect, Munchausen Syndrome by Proxy (MSBP), Shaken Baby Syndrome, and Controversial Issues Related to Child Abuse, Such as Withholding Medical Care, Corporal Punishment, and Child Maltreatment in Youth Sports, and Featuring Facts about Child Protective Services, Foster Care, Adoption, Parenting Challenges, and Other Abuse Prevention Efforts

Along with a Glossary of Related Terms and Resources for Additional Help and Information

Edited by Dawn D. Matthews. 620 pages. 2004. 0-7808-0705-7.

■

Childhood Diseases & Disorders Sourcebook

Basic Consumer Health Information about Medical Problems Often Encountered in Pre-Adolescent Children, Including Respiratory Tract Ailments, Ear Infections, Sore Throats, Disorders of the Skin and Scalp, Digestive and Genitourinary Diseases, Infectious Diseases, Inflammatory Disorders, Chronic Physical and Developmental Disorders, Allergies, and More

Along with Information about Diagnostic Tests, Common Childhood Surgeries, and Frequently Used Medications, with a Glossary of Important Terms and Resource Directory

Edited by Chad T. Kimball. 662 pages. 2003. 0-7808-0458-9.

"This is an excellent book for new parents and should be included in all health care and public libraries."
—*American Reference Books Annual, 2004*

■

Colds, Flu & Other Common Ailments Sourcebook

Basic Consumer Health Information about Common Ailments and Injuries, Including Colds, Coughs, the Flu, Sinus Problems, Headaches, Fever, Nausea and Vomiting, Menstrual Cramps, Diarrhea, Constipation, Hemorrhoids, Back Pain, Dandruff, Dry and Itchy Skin, Cuts, Scrapes, Sprains, Bruises, and More

Along with Information about Prevention, Self-Care, Choosing a Doctor, Over-the-Counter Medications, Folk Remedies, and Alternative Therapies, and Including a Glossary of Important Terms and a Directory of Resources for Further Help and Information

Edited by Chad T. Kimball. 638 pages. 2001. 0-7808-0435-X.

"A good starting point for research on common illnesses. It will be a useful addition to public and consumer health library collections."
—*American Reference Books Annual 2002*

"Will prove valuable to any library seeking to maintain a current, comprehensive reference collection of health resources. . . . Excellent reference."
—*The Bookwatch, Aug '01*

"Recommended reference source."
—*Booklist, American Library Association, July '01*

■

Communication Disorders Sourcebook

Basic Information about Deafness and Hearing Loss, Speech and Language Disorders, Voice Disorders, Balance and Vestibular Disorders, and Disorders of Smell, Taste, and Touch

Edited by Linda M. Ross. 533 pages. 1996. 0-7808-0077-X.

"This is skillfully edited and is a welcome resource for the layperson. It should be found in every public and medical library." —*Booklist Health Sciences Supplement, American Library Association, Oct '97*

■

Congenital Disorders Sourcebook

Basic Information about Disorders Acquired during Gestation, Including Spina Bifida, Hydrocephalus, Cerebral Palsy, Heart Defects, Craniofacial Abnormalities, Fetal Alcohol Syndrome, and More

Along with Current Treatment Options and Statistical Data

Edited by Karen Bellenir. 607 pages. 1997. 0-7808-0205-5.

"Recommended reference source."
—*Booklist, American Library Association, Oct '97*

SEE ALSO *Pregnancy & Birth Sourcebook*

■

Consumer Issues in Health Care Sourcebook

Basic Information about Health Care Fundamentals and Related Consumer Issues, Including Exams and Screening Tests, Physician Specialties, Choosing a Doctor, Using Prescription and Over-the-Counter Medications Safely, Avoiding Health Scams, Managing Common Health Risks in the Home, Care Options for Chronically or Terminally Ill Patients, and a List of Resources for Obtaining Help and Further Information

Edited by Karen Bellenir. 618 pages. 1998. 0-7808-0221-7.

"Both public and academic libraries will want to have a copy in their collection for readers who are interested in self-education on health issues."
—*American Reference Books Annual, 2000*

"The editor has researched the literature from government agencies and others, saving readers the time and effort of having to do the research themselves. Recommended for public libraries."

—*Reference and User Services Quarterly, American Library Association, Spring '99*

"Recommended reference source."

—*Booklist, American Library Association, Dec '98*

Contagious Diseases Sourcebook

Basic Consumer Health Information about Infectious Diseases Spread by Person-to-Person Contact through Direct Touch, Airborne Transmission, Sexual Contact, or Contact with Blood or Other Body Fluids, Including Hepatitis, Herpes, Influenza, Lice, Measles, Mumps, Pinworm, Ringworm, Severe Acute Respiratory Syndrome (SARS), Streptococcal Infections, Tuberculosis, and Others

Along with Facts about Disease Transmission, Antimicrobial Resistance, and Vaccines, with a Glossary and Directories of Resources for More Information

Edited by Karen Bellenir. 643 pages. 2004. 0-7808-0736-7.

Contagious & Non-Contagious Infectious Diseases Sourcebook

Basic Information about Contagious Diseases like Measles, Polio, Hepatitis B, and Infectious Mononucleosis, and Non-Contagious Infectious Diseases like Tetanus and Toxic Shock Syndrome, and Diseases Occurring as Secondary Infections Such as Shingles and Reye Syndrome

Along with Vaccination, Prevention, and Treatment Information, and a Section Describing Emerging Infectious Disease Threats

Edited by Karen Bellenir and Peter D. Dresser. 566 pages. 1996. 0-7808-0075-3.

Death & Dying Sourcebook

Basic Consumer Health Information for the Layperson about End-of-Life Care and Related Ethical and Legal Issues, Including Chief Causes of Death, Autopsies, Pain Management for the Terminally Ill, Life Support Systems, Insurance, Euthanasia, Assisted Suicide, Hospice Programs, Living Wills, Funeral Planning, Counseling, Mourning, Organ Donation, and Physician Training

Along with Statistical Data, a Glossary, and Listings of Sources for Further Help and Information

Edited by Annemarie S. Muth. 641 pages. 1999. 0-7808-0230-6.

"Public libraries, medical libraries, and academic libraries will all find this sourcebook a useful addition to their collections."

—*American Reference Books Annual, 2001*

"An extremely useful resource for those concerned with death and dying in the United States."

—*Respiratory Care, Nov '00*

"Recommended reference source."

—*Booklist, American Library Association, Aug '00*

"This book is a definite must for all those involved in end-of-life care." —*Doody's Review Service, 2000*

Dental Care & Oral Health Sourcebook, 2nd Edition

Basic Consumer Health Information about Dental Care, Including Oral Hygiene, Dental Visits, Pain Management, Cavities, Crowns, Bridges, Dental Implants, and Fillings, and Other Oral Health Concerns, Such as Gum Disease, Bad Breath, Dry Mouth, Genetic and Developmental Abnormalities, Oral Cancers, Orthodontics, and Temporomandibular Disorders

Along with Updates on Current Research in Oral Health, a Glossary, a Directory of Dental and Oral Health Organizations, and Resources for People with Dental and Oral Health Disorders

Edited by Amy L. Sutton. 609 pages. 2003. 0-7808-0634-4.

ALSO AVAILABLE: *Oral Health Sourcebook, 1st Edition.* Edited by Allan R. Cook. 558 pages. 1997. 0-7808-0082-6.

"This book could serve as a turning point in the battle to educate consumers in issues concerning oral health."

—*American Reference Books Annual, 2004*

"Unique source which will fill a gap in dental sources for patients and the lay public. A valuable reference tool even in a library with thousands of books on dentistry. Comprehensive, clear, inexpensive, and easy to read and use. It fills an enormous gap in the health care literature." —*Reference and User Services Quarterly, American Library Association, Summer '98*

"Recommended reference source."

—*Booklist, American Library Association, Dec '97*

Depression Sourcebook

Basic Consumer Health Information about Unipolar Depression, Bipolar Disorder, Postpartum Depression, Seasonal Affective Disorder, and Other Types of Depression in Children, Adolescents, Women, Men, the Elderly, and Other Selected Populations

Along with Facts about Causes, Risk Factors, Diagnostic Criteria, Treatment Options, Coping Strategies, Suicide Prevention, a Glossary, and a Directory of Sources for Additional Help and Information

Edited by Karen Belleni. 602 pages. 2002. 0-7808-0611-5.

"*Depression Sourcebook* is of a very high standard. Its purpose, which is to serve as a reference source to the lay reader, is very well served."

—*Journal of the National Medical Association, 2004*

"Invaluable reference for public and school library collections alike." —*Library Bookwatch, Apr '03*

"Recommended for purchase."

—*American Reference Books Annual, 2003*

Dermatological Disorders Sourcebook, 2nd Edition

Basic Consumer Health Information about Conditions and Disorders Affecting the Skin, Hair, and Nails, Such as Acne, Rosacea, Rashes, Dermatitis, Pigmentation Disorders, Birthmarks, Skin Cancer, Skin Injuries, Psoriasis, Scleroderma, and Hair Loss, Including Facts about Medications and Treatments for Dermatological Disorders and Tips for Maintaining Healthy Skin, Hair, and Nails

Along with Information about How Aging Affects the Skin, a Glossary of Related Terms, and a Directory of Resources for Additional Help and Information

Edited by Amy L. Sutton. 645 pages. 2005. 0-7808-0795-2.

ALSO AVAILABLE: *Skin Disorders Sourcebook, 1st Edition.* Edited by Allan R. Cook. 647 pages. 1997. 0-7808-0080-X.

"... comprehensive, easily read reference book."
—Doody's Health Sciences Book Reviews, Oct '97

■

Diabetes Sourcebook, 3rd Edition

Basic Consumer Health Information about Type 1 Diabetes (Insulin-Dependent or Juvenile-Onset Diabetes), Type 2 Diabetes (Noninsulin-Dependent or Adult-Onset Diabetes), Gestational Diabetes, Impaired Glucose Tolerance (IGT), and Related Complications, Such as Amputation, Eye Disease, Gum Disease, Nerve Damage, and End-Stage Renal Disease, Including Facts about Insulin, Oral Diabetes Medications, Blood Sugar Testing, and the Role of Exercise and Nutrition in the Control of Diabetes

Along with a Glossary and Resources for Further Help and Information

Edited by Dawn D. Matthews. 622 pages. 2003. 0-7808-0629-8.

ALSO AVAILABLE: *Diabetes Sourcebook, 1st Edition.* Edited by Karen Bellenir and Peter D. Dresser. 827 pages. 1994. 1-55888-751-2.

Diabetes Sourcebook, 2nd Edition. Edited by Karen Bellenir. 688 pages. 1998. 0-7808-0224-1.

"This edition is even more helpful than earlier versions. . . . It is a truly valuable tool for anyone seeking readable and authoritative information on diabetes."
—American Reference Books Annual, 2004

"An invaluable reference." *—Library Journal, May '00*

Selected as one of the 250 "Best Health Sciences Books of 1999." *—Doody's Rating Service, Mar-Apr 2000*

"Provides useful information for the general public."
—Healthlines, University of Michigan Health Management Research Center, Sep/Oct '99

"... provides reliable mainstream medical information ... belongs on the shelves of any library with a consumer health collection." *—E-Streams, Sep '99*

"Recommended reference source."
—Booklist, American Library Association, Feb '99

Diet & Nutrition Sourcebook, 2nd Edition

Basic Consumer Health Information about Dietary Guidelines, Recommended Daily Intake Values, Vitamins, Minerals, Fiber, Fat, Weight Control, Dietary Supplements, and Food Additives

Along with Special Sections on Nutrition Needs throughout Life and Nutrition for People with Such Specific Medical Concerns as Allergies, High Blood Cholesterol, Hypertension, Diabetes, Celiac Disease, Seizure Disorders, Phenylketonuria (PKU), Cancer, and Eating Disorders, and Including Reports on Current Nutrition Research and Source Listings for Additional Help and Information

Edited by Karen Bellenir. 650 pages. 1999. 0-7808-0228-4.

ALSO AVAILABLE: *Diet & Nutrition Sourcebook, 1st Edition.* Edited by Dan R. Harris. 662 pages. 1996. 0-7808-0084-2.

"This book is an excellent source of basic diet and nutrition information." *—Booklist Health Sciences Supplement, American Library Association, Dec '00*

"This reference document should be in any public library, but it would be a very good guide for beginning students in the health sciences. If the other books in this publisher's series are as good as this, they should all be in the health sciences collections."
—American Reference Books Annual, 2000

"This book is an excellent general nutrition reference for consumers who desire to take an active role in their health care for prevention. Consumers of all ages who select this book can feel confident they are receiving current and accurate information." *—Journal of Nutrition for the Elderly, Vol. 19, No. 4, '00*

"Recommended reference source."
—Booklist, American Library Association, Dec '99

SEE ALSO *Digestive Diseases & Disorders Sourcebook, Eating Disorders Sourcebook, Gastrointestinal Diseases & Disorders Sourcebook, Vegetarian Sourcebook*

■

Digestive Diseases & Disorders Sourcebook

Basic Consumer Health Information about Diseases and Disorders that Impact the Upper and Lower Digestive System, Including Celiac Disease, Constipation, Crohn's Disease, Cyclic Vomiting Syndrome, Diarrhea, Diverticulosis and Diverticulitis, Gallstones, Heartburn, Hemorrhoids, Hernias, Indigestion (Dyspepsia), Irritable Bowel Syndrome, Lactose Intolerance, Ulcers, and More

Along with Information about Medications and Other Treatments, Tips for Maintaining a Healthy Digestive Tract, a Glossary, and Directory of Digestive Diseases Organizations

Edited by Karen Bellenir. 335 pages. 2000. 0-7808-0327-2.

"This title would be an excellent addition to all public or patient-research libraries."
—American Reference Books Annual, 2001

"This title is recommended for public, hospital, and health sciences libraries with consumer health collections." —*E-Streams, Jul-Aug '00*

"Recommended reference source."
—*Booklist, American Library Association, May '00*

SEE ALSO *Diet & Nutrition Sourcebook, Eating Disorders Sourcebook, Gastrointestinal Diseases & Disorders Sourcebook*

Disabilities Sourcebook

Basic Consumer Health Information about Physical and Psychiatric Disabilities, Including Descriptions of Major Causes of Disability, Assistive and Adaptive Aids, Workplace Issues, and Accessibility Concerns

Along with Information about the Americans with Disabilities Act, a Glossary, and Resources for Additional Help and Information

Edited by Dawn D. Matthews. 616 pages. 2000. 0-7808-0389-2.

"It is a must for libraries with a consumer health section." —*American Reference Books Annual 2002*

"A much needed addition to the Omnigraphics ***Health Reference Series.*** A current reference work to provide people with disabilities, their families, caregivers or those who work with them, a broad range of information in one volume, has not been available until now. . . . It is recommended for all public and academic library reference collections." —*E-Streams, May '01*

"An excellent source book in easy-to-read format covering many current topics; highly recommended for all libraries." —*Choice, Association of College and Research Libraries, Jan '01*

"Recommended reference source."
—*Booklist, American Library Association, Jul '00*

Domestic Violence Sourcebook, 2nd Edition

Basic Consumer Health Information about the Causes and Consequences of Abusive Relationships, Including Physical Violence, Sexual Assault, Battery, Stalking, and Emotional Abuse, and Facts about the Effects of Violence on Women, Men, Young Adults, and the Elderly, with Reports about Domestic Violence in Selected Populations, and Featuring Facts about Medical Care, Victim Assistance and Protection, Prevention Strategies, Mental Health Services, and Legal Issues

Along with a Glossary of Related Terms and Resources for Additional Help and Information

Edited by Dawn D. Matthews. 628 pages. 2004. 0-7808-0669-7.

ALSO AVAILABLE: *Domestic Violence & Child Abuse Sourcebook, 1st Edition.* Edited by Helene Henderson. 1,064 pages. 2001. 0-7808-0235-7.

"Interested lay persons should find the book extremely beneficial. . . . A copy of ***Domestic Violence and Child Abuse Sourcebook*** should be in every public library in the United States."
—*Social Science & Medicine, No. 56, 2003*

"This is important information. The Web has many resources but this sourcebook fills an important societal need. I am not aware of any other resources of this type." —*Doody's Review Service, Sep '01*

"Recommended for all libraries, scholars, and practitioners." —*Choice, Association of College & Research Libraries, Jul '01*

"Recommended reference source."
—*Booklist, American Library Association, Apr '01*

"Important pick for college-level health reference libraries." —*The Bookwatch, Mar '01*

"Because this problem is so widespread and because this book includes a lot of issues within one volume, this work is recommended for all public libraries."
—*American Reference Books Annual, 2001*

Drug Abuse Sourcebook, 2nd Edition

Basic Consumer Health Information about Illicit Substances of Abuse and the Misuse of Prescription and Over-the-Counter Medications, Including Depressants, Hallucinogens, Inhalants, Marijuana, Stimulants, and Anabolic Steroids

Along with Facts about Related Health Risks, Treatment Programs, Prevention Programs, a Glossary of Abuse and Addiction Terms, a Glossary of Drug-Related Street Terms, and a Directory of Resources for More Information

Edited by Catherine Ginther. 607 pages. 2004. 0-7808-0740-5.

ALSO AVAILABLE: Drug Abuse Sourcebook, 1st Edition. Edited by Karen Bellenir. 629 pages. 2000. 0-7808-0242-X.

"Containing a wealth of information . . . . This resource belongs in libraries that serve a lower-division undergraduate or community college clientele as well as the general public." —*Choice, Association of College and Research Libraries, Jun '01*

"Recommended reference source."
—*Booklist, American Library Association, Feb '01*

"Highly recommended." —*The Bookwatch, Jan '01*

"Even though there is a plethora of books on drug abuse, this volume is recommended for school, public, and college libraries."
—*American Reference Books Annual, 2001*

SEE ALSO *Alcoholism Sourcebook, Substance Abuse Sourcebook*

Ear, Nose & Throat Disorders Sourcebook

Basic Information about Disorders of the Ears, Nose, Sinus Cavities, Pharynx, and Larynx, Including Ear Infections, Tinnitus, Vestibular Disorders, Allergic and Non-Allergic Rhinitis, Sore Throats, Tonsillitis, and Cancers That Affect the Ears, Nose, Sinuses, and Throat

Along with Reports on Current Research Initiatives, a Glossary of Related Medical Terms, and a Directory of Sources for Further Help and Information

Edited by Karen Bellenir and Linda M. Shin. 576 pages. 1998. 0-7808-0206-3.

"Overall, this sourcebook is helpful for the consumer seeking information on ENT issues. It is recommended for public libraries."

—*American Reference Books Annual, 1999*

"Recommended reference source."

—*Booklist, American Library Association, Dec '98*

■

Eating Disorders Sourcebook

Basic Consumer Health Information about Eating Disorders, Including Information about Anorexia Nervosa, Bulimia Nervosa, Binge Eating, Body Dysmorphic Disorder, Pica, Laxative Abuse, and Night Eating Syndrome

Along with Information about Causes, Adverse Effects, and Treatment and Prevention Issues, and Featuring a Section on Concerns Specific to Children and Adolescents, a Glossary, and Resources for Further Help and Information

Edited by Dawn D. Matthews. 322 pages. 2001. 0-7808-0335-3.

"Recommended for health science libraries that are open to the public, as well as hospital libraries. This book is a good resource for the consumer who is concerned about eating disorders." —*E-Streams, Mar '02*

"This volume is another convenient collection of excerpted articles. Recommended for school and public library patrons; lower-division undergraduates; and two-year technical program students." —*Choice, Association of College & Research Libraries, Jan '02*

"Recommended reference source." —*Booklist, American Library Association, Oct '01*

SEE ALSO *Diet & Nutrition Sourcebook, Digestive Diseases & Disorders Sourcebook, Gastrointestinal Diseases & Disorders Sourcebook*

■

Emergency Medical Services Sourcebook

Basic Consumer Health Information about Preventing, Preparing for, and Managing Emergency Situations, When and Who to Call for Help, What to Expect in the Emergency Room, the Emergency Medical Team, Patient Issues, and Current Topics in Emergency Medicine

Along with Statistical Data, a Glossary, and Sources of Additional Help and Information

Edited by Jenni Lynn Colson. 494 pages. 2002. 0-7808-0420-1.

"Handy and convenient for home, public, school, and college libraries. Recommended."

—*Choice, Association of College and Research Libraries, Apr '03*

"This reference can provide the consumer with answers to most questions about emergency care in the United States, or it will direct them to a resource where the answer can be found."

—*American Reference Books Annual, 2003*

"Recommended reference source."

—*Booklist, American Library Association, Feb '03*

■

Endocrine & Metabolic Disorders Sourcebook

Basic Information for the Layperson about Pancreatic and Insulin-Related Disorders Such as Pancreatitis, Diabetes, and Hypoglycemia; Adrenal Gland Disorders Such as Cushing's Syndrome, Addison's Disease, and Congenital Adrenal Hyperplasia; Pituitary Gland Disorders Such as Growth Hormone Deficiency, Acromegaly, and Pituitary Tumors; Thyroid Disorders Such as Hypothyroidism, Graves' Disease, Hashimoto's Disease, and Goiter; Hyperparathyroidism; and Other Diseases and Syndromes of Hormone Imbalance or Metabolic Dysfunction

Along with Reports on Current Research Initiatives

Edited by Linda M. Shin. 574 pages. 1998. 0-7808-0207-1.

"Omnigraphics has produced another needed resource for health information consumers."

—*American Reference Books Annual, 2000*

"Recommended reference source."

—*Booklist, American Library Association, Dec '98*

■

Environmental Health Sourcebook, 2nd Edition

Basic Consumer Health Information about the Environment and Its Effect on Human Health, Including the Effects of Air Pollution, Water Pollution, Hazardous Chemicals, Food Hazards, Radiation Hazards, Biological Agents, Household Hazards, Such as Radon, Asbestos, Carbon Monoxide, and Mold, and Information about Associated Diseases and Disorders, Including Cancer, Allergies, Respiratory Problems, and Skin Disorders

Along with Information about Environmental Concerns for Specific Populations, a Glossary of Related Terms, and Resources for Further Help and Information

Edited by Dawn D. Matthews. 673 pages. 2003. 0-7808-0632-8.

ALSO AVAILABLE: *Environmentally Induced Disorders Sourcebook, 1st Edition.* Edited by Allan R. Cook. 620 pages. 1997. 0-7808-0083-4.

"This recently updated edition continues the level of quality and the reputation of the numerous other volumes in Omnigraphics' ***Health Reference Series.***"
—*American Reference Books Annual, 2004*

"Recommended reference source."
—*Booklist, American Library Association, Sep '98*

"This book will be a useful addition to anyone's library." —*Choice Health Sciences Supplement, Association of College and Research Libraries, May '98*

". . . a good survey of numerous environmentally induced physical disorders . . . a useful addition to anyone's library."
—*Doody's Health Sciences Book Reviews, Jan '98*

". . . provide[s] introductory information from the best authorities around. Since this volume covers topics that potentially affect everyone, it will surely be one of the most frequently consulted volumes in the ***Health Reference Series.***" —*Rettig on Reference, Nov '97*

Environmentally Induced Disorders Sourcebook, 1st Edition

SEE *Environmental Health Sourcebook, 2nd Edition*

Ethnic Diseases Sourcebook

Basic Consumer Health Information for Ethnic and Racial Minority Groups in the United States, Including General Health Indicators and Behaviors, Ethnic Diseases, Genetic Testing, the Impact of Chronic Diseases, Women's Health, Mental Health Issues, and Preventive Health Care Services

Along with a Glossary and a Listing of Additional Resources

Edited by Joyce Brennfleck Shannon. 664 pages. 2001. 0-7808-0336-1.

"Recommended for health sciences libraries where public health programs are a priority."
—*E-Streams, Jan '02*

"Not many books have been written on this topic to date, and the ***Ethnic Diseases Sourcebook*** is a strong addition to the list. It will be an important introductory resource for health consumers, students, health care personnel, and social scientists. It is recommended for public, academic, and large hospital libraries."
—*American Reference Books Annual 2002*

"Recommended reference source."
—*Booklist, American Library Association, Oct '01*

"Will prove valuable to any library seeking to maintain a current, comprehensive reference collection of health resources. . . . An excellent source of health information about genetic disorders which affect particular ethnic and racial minorities in the U.S."
—*The Bookwatch, Aug '01*

Eye Care Sourcebook, 2nd Edition

Basic Consumer Health Information about Eye Care and Eye Disorders, Including Facts about the Diagnosis, Prevention, and Treatment of Common Refractive Problems Such as Myopia, Hyperopia, Astigmatism, and Presbyopia, and Eye Diseases, Including Glaucoma, Cataract, Age-Related Macular Degeneration, and Diabetic Retinopathy

Along with a Section on Vision Correction and Refractive Surgeries, Including LASIK and LASEK, a Glossary, and Directories of Resources for Additional Help and Information

Edited by Amy L. Sutton. 543 pages. 2003. 0-7808-0635-2.

ALSO AVAILABLE: *Ophthalmic Disorders Sourcebook, 1st Edition.* Edited by Linda M. Ross. 631 pages. 1996. 0-7808-0081-8.

". . . a solid reference tool for eye care and a valuable addition to a collection."
—*American Reference Books Annual, 2004*

Family Planning Sourcebook

Basic Consumer Health Information about Planning for Pregnancy and Contraception, Including Traditional Methods, Barrier Methods, Hormonal Methods, Permanent Methods, Future Methods, Emergency Contraception, and Birth Control Choices for Women at Each Stage of Life

Along with Statistics, a Glossary, and Sources of Additional Information

Edited by Amy Marcaccio Keyzer. 520 pages. 2001. 0-7808-0379-5.

"Recommended for public, health, and undergraduate libraries as part of the circulating collection."
—*E-Streams, Mar '02*

"Information is presented in an unbiased, readable manner, and the sourcebook will certainly be a necessary addition to those public and high school libraries where Internet access is restricted or otherwise problematic." —*American Reference Books Annual 2002*

"Recommended reference source."
—*Booklist, American Library Association, Oct '01*

"Will prove valuable to any library seeking to maintain a current, comprehensive reference collection of health resources. . . . Excellent reference."
—*The Bookwatch, Aug '01*

SEE ALSO *Pregnancy & Birth Sourcebook*

Fitness & Exercise Sourcebook, 2nd Edition

Basic Consumer Health Information about the Fundamentals of Fitness and Exercise, Including How to Begin and Maintain a Fitness Program, Fitness as a Lifestyle, the Link between Fitness and Diet, Advice for Specific Groups of People, Exercise as It Relates to Specific Medical Conditions, and Recent Research in Fitness and Exercise

Along with a Glossary of Important Terms and Resources for Additional Help and Information

Edited by Kristen M. Gledhill. 646 pages. 2001. 0-7808-0334-5.

***ALSO AVAILABLE:** Fitness & Exercise Sourcebook, 1st Edition.* Edited by Dan R. Harris. 663 pages. 1996. 0-7808-0186-5.

"This work is recommended for all general reference collections."

—*American Reference Books Annual 2002*

"Highly recommended for public, consumer, and school grades fourth through college."

—*E-Streams, Nov '01*

"Recommended reference source." —*Booklist, American Library Association, Oct '01*

"The information appears quite comprehensive and is considered reliable. . . . This second edition is a welcomed addition to the series."

—*Doody's Review Service, Sep '01*

"This reference is a valuable choice for those who desire a broad source of information on exercise, fitness, and chronic-disease prevention through a healthy lifestyle." —*American Medical Writers Association Journal, Fall '01*

"Will prove valuable to any library seeking to maintain a current, comprehensive reference collection of health resources. . . . Excellent reference."

—*The Bookwatch, Aug '01*

Food & Animal Borne Diseases Sourcebook

Basic Information about Diseases That Can Be Spread to Humans through the Ingestion of Contaminated Food or Water or by Contact with Infected Animals and Insects, Such as Botulism, E. Coli, Hepatitis A, Trichinosis, Lyme Disease, and Rabies

Along with Information Regarding Prevention and Treatment Methods, and Including a Special Section for International Travelers Describing Diseases Such as Cholera, Malaria, Travelers' Diarrhea, and Yellow Fever, and Offering Recommendations for Avoiding Illness

Edited by Karen Bellenir and Peter D. Dresser. 535 pages. 1995. 0-7808-0033-8.

"Targeting general readers and providing them with a single, comprehensive source of information on selected topics, this book continues, with the excellent caliber of its predecessors, to catalog topical information on health matters of general interest. Readable and thorough, this valuable resource is highly recommended for all libraries."

—*Academic Library Book Review, Summer '96*

"A comprehensive collection of authoritative information." —*Emergency Medical Services, Oct '95*

Food Safety Sourcebook

Basic Consumer Health Information about the Safe Handling of Meat, Poultry, Seafood, Eggs, Fruit Juices, and Other Food Items, and Facts about Pesticides, Drinking Water, Food Safety Overseas, and the Onset, Duration, and Symptoms of Foodborne Illnesses, Including Types of Pathogenic Bacteria, Parasitic Protozoa, Worms, Viruses, and Natural Toxins

Along with the Role of the Consumer, the Food Handler, and the Government in Food Safety; a Glossary, and Resources for Additional Help and Information

Edited by Dawn D. Matthews. 339 pages. 1999. 0-7808-0326-4.

"This book is recommended for public libraries and universities with home economic and food science programs." —*E-Streams, Nov '00*

"Recommended reference source."

—*Booklist, American Library Association, May '00*

"This book takes the complex issues of food safety and foodborne pathogens and presents them in an easily understood manner. [It does] an excellent job of covering a large and often confusing topic."

—*American Reference Books Annual, 2000*

Forensic Medicine Sourcebook

Basic Consumer Information for the Layperson about Forensic Medicine, Including Crime Scene Investigation, Evidence Collection and Analysis, Expert Testimony, Computer-Aided Criminal Identification, Digital Imaging in the Courtroom, DNA Profiling, Accident Reconstruction, Autopsies, Ballistics, Drugs and Explosives Detection, Latent Fingerprints, Product Tampering, and Questioned Document Examination

Along with Statistical Data, a Glossary of Forensics Terminology, and Listings of Sources for Further Help and Information

Edited by Annemarie S. Muth. 574 pages. 1999. 0-7808-0232-2.

"Given the expected widespread interest in its content and its easy to read style, this book is recommended for most public and all college and university libraries."

—*E-Streams, Feb '01*

"Recommended for public libraries."

—*Reference & User Services Quarterly, American Library Association, Spring 2000*

"Recommended reference source."

—*Booklist, American Library Association, Feb '00*

"A wealth of information, useful statistics, references are up-to-date and extremely complete. This wonderful collection of data will help students who are interested in a career in any type of forensic field. It is a great resource for attorneys who need information about types of expert witnesses needed in a particular case. It also offers useful information for fiction and nonfiction writers whose work involves a crime. A fascinating compilation. All levels." —*Choice, Association of College and Research Libraries, Jan 2000*

"There are several items that make this book attractive to consumers who are seeking certain forensic data. . . . This is a useful current source for those seeking general forensic medical answers."

—*American Reference Books Annual, 2000*

Gastrointestinal Diseases & Disorders Sourcebook

Basic Information about Gastroesophageal Reflux Disease (Heartburn), Ulcers, Diverticulosis, Irritable Bowel Syndrome, Crohn's Disease, Ulcerative Colitis, Diarrhea, Constipation, Lactose Intolerance, Hemorrhoids, Hepatitis, Cirrhosis, and Other Digestive Problems, Featuring Statistics, Descriptions of Symptoms, and Current Treatment Methods of Interest for Persons Living with Upper and Lower Gastrointestinal Maladies

Edited by Linda M. Ross. 413 pages. 1996. 0-7808-0078-8.

". . . very readable form. The successful editorial work that brought this material together into a useful and understandable reference makes accessible to all readers information that can help them more effectively understand and obtain help for digestive tract problems."

— *Choice, Association of College & Research Libraries, Feb '97*

SEE ALSO *Diet & Nutrition Sourcebook, Digestive Diseases & Disorders, Eating Disorders Sourcebook*

Genetic Disorders Sourcebook, 3rd Edition

Basic Consumer Health Information about Hereditary Diseases and Disorders, Including Facts about the Human Genome, Genetic Inheritance Patterns, Disorders Associated with Specific Genes, Such as Sickle Cell Disease, Hemophilia, and Cystic Fibrosis, Chromosome Disorders, Such as Down Syndrome, Fragile X Syndrome, and Turner Syndrome, and Complex Diseases and Disorders Resulting from the Interaction of Environmental and Genetic Factors, Such as Allergies, Cancer, and Obesity

Along with Facts about Genetic Testing, Suggestions for Parents of Children with Special Needs, Reports on Current Research Initiatives, a Glossary of Genetic Terminology, and Resources for Additional Help and Information

Edited by Karen Bellenir. 777 pages. 2004. 0-7808-0742-1.

ALSO AVAILABLE: *Genetic Disorders Sourcebook, 1st Edition.* Edited by Karen Bellenir. 642 pages. 1996. 0-7808-0034-6.

Genetic Disorders Sourcebook, 2nd Edition. Edited by Kathy Massimini. 768 pages. 2001. 0-7808-0241-1.

"Recommended for public libraries and medical and hospital libraries with consumer health collections."

—*E-Streams, May '01*

"Recommended reference source."

—*Booklist, American Library Association, Apr '01*

"Important pick for college-level health reference libraries." —*The Bookwatch, Mar '01*

"Provides essential medical information to both the general public and those diagnosed with a serious or fatal genetic disease or disorder." —*Choice, Association of College and Research Libraries, Jan '97*

Head Trauma Sourcebook

Basic Information for the Layperson about Open-Head and Closed-Head Injuries, Treatment Advances, Recovery, and Rehabilitation

Along with Reports on Current Research Initiatives

Edited by Karen Bellenir. 414 pages. 1997. 0-7808-0208-X.

Headache Sourcebook

Basic Consumer Health Information about Migraine, Tension, Cluster, Rebound and Other Types of Headaches, with Facts about the Cause and Prevention of Headaches, the Effects of Stress and the Environment, Headaches during Pregnancy and Menopause, and Childhood Headaches

Along with a Glossary and Other Resources for Additional Help and Information

Edited by Dawn D. Matthews. 362 pages. 2002. 0-7808-0337-X.

"Highly recommended for academic and medical reference collections." —*Library Bookwatch, Sep '02*

Health Insurance Sourcebook

Basic Information about Managed Care Organizations, Traditional Fee-for-Service Insurance, Insurance Portability and Pre-Existing Conditions Clauses, Medicare, Medicaid, Social Security, and Military Health Care

Along with Information about Insurance Fraud

Edited by Wendy Wilcox. 530 pages. 1997. 0-7808-0222-5.

"Particularly useful because it brings much of this information together in one volume. This book will be a handy reference source in the health sciences library, hospital library, college and university library, and medium to large public library."

—*Medical Reference Services Quarterly, Fall '98*

Awarded "Books of the Year Award"

—*American Journal of Nursing, 1997*

"The layout of the book is particularly helpful as it provides easy access to reference material. A most useful addition to the vast amount of information about health insurance. The use of data from U.S. government agencies is most commendable. Useful in a library or learning center for healthcare professional students."

—*Doody's Health Sciences Book Reviews, Nov '97*

Health Reference Series Cumulative Index 1999

A Comprehensive Index to the Individual Volumes of the Health Reference Series, Including a Subject Index, Name Index, Organization Index, and Publication Index

Along with a Master List of Acronyms and Abbreviations

Edited by Edward J. Prucha, Anne Holmes, and Robert Rudnick. 990 pages. 2000. 0-7808-0382-5.

"This volume will be most helpful in libraries that have a relatively complete collection of the Health Reference Series." —*American Reference Books Annual, 2001*

"Essential for collections that hold any of the numerous *Health Reference Series* titles."
—*Choice, Association of College and Research Libraries, Nov '00*

■

Healthy Aging Sourcebook

Basic Consumer Health Information about Maintaining Health through the Aging Process, Including Advice on Nutrition, Exercise, and Sleep, Help in Making Decisions about Midlife Issues and Retirement, and Guidance Concerning Practical and Informed Choices in Health Consumerism

Along with Data Concerning the Theories of Aging, Different Experiences in Aging by Minority Groups, and Facts about Aging Now and Aging in the Future; and Featuring a Glossary, a Guide to Consumer Help, Additional Suggested Reading, and Practical Resource Directory

Edited by Jenifer Swanson. 536 pages. 1999. 0-7808-0390-6.

"Recommended reference source."
—*Booklist, American Library Association, Feb '00*

SEE ALSO *Physical & Mental Issues in Aging Sourcebook*

■

Healthy Children Sourcebook

Basic Consumer Health Information about the Physical and Mental Development of Children between the Ages of 3 and 12, Including Routine Health Care, Preventative Health Services, Safety and First Aid, Healthy Sleep, Dental Care, Nutrition, and Fitness, and Featuring Parenting Tips on Such Topics as Bedwetting, Choosing Day Care, Monitoring TV and Other Media, and Establishing a Foundation for Substance Abuse Prevention

Along with a Glossary of Commonly Used Pediatric Terms and Resources for Additional Help and Information.

Edited by Chad T. Kimball. 647 pages. 2003. 0-7808-0247-0.

"It is hard to imagine that any other single resource exists that would provide such a comprehensive guide of timely information on health promotion and disease prevention for children aged 3 to 12."
—*American Reference Books Annual, 2004*

"The strengths of this book are many. It is clearly written, presented and structured."
—*Journal of the National Medical Association, 2004*

■

Healthy Heart Sourcebook for Women

Basic Consumer Health Information about Cardiac Issues Specific to Women, Including Facts about Major Risk Factors and Prevention, Treatment and Control Strategies, and Important Dietary Issues

Along with a Special Section Regarding the Pros and Cons of Hormone Replacement Therapy and Its Impact on Heart Health, and Additional Help, Including Recipes, a Glossary, and a Directory of Resources

Edited by Dawn D. Matthews. 336 pages. 2000. 0-7808-0329-9.

"A good reference source and recommended for all public, academic, medical, and hospital libraries."
—*Medical Reference Services Quarterly, Summer '01*

"Because of the lack of information specific to women on this topic, this book is recommended for public libraries and consumer libraries."
—*American Reference Books Annual, 2001*

"Contains very important information about coronary artery disease that all women should know. The information is current and presented in an easy-to-read format. The book will make a good addition to any library." —*American Medical Writers Association Journal, Summer '00*

"Important, basic reference."
—*Reviewer's Bookwatch, Jul '00*

SEE ALSO *Heart Diseases & Disorders Sourcebook, Women's Health Concerns Sourcebook*

■

Heart Diseases & Disorders Sourcebook, 2nd Edition

SEE *Cardiovascular Diseases & Disorders Sourcebook, 3rd Edition*

■

Hepatitis Sourcebook

Basic Consumer Health Information about Hepatitis A, Hepatitis B, Hepatitis C, and Other Forms of Hepatitis, Including Autoimmune Hepatitis, Alcoholic Hepatitis, Nonalcoholic Steatohepatitis, and Toxic Hepatitis, with Facts about Risk Factors, Screening Methods, Diagnostic Tests, and Treatment Options

Along with Information on Liver Health, Tips for People Living with Chronic Hepatitis, Reports on Current Research Initiatives, a Glossary of Terms Related to Hepatitis, and a Directory of Sources for Further Help and Information

Edited by Sandra J. Judd. 597 pages. 2005. 0-7808-0749-9.

Household Safety Sourcebook

Basic Consumer Health Information about Household Safety, Including Information about Poisons, Chemicals, Fire, and Water Hazards in the Home

Along with Advice about the Safe Use of Home Maintenance Equipment, Choosing Toys and Nursery Furniture, Holiday and Recreation Safety, a Glossary, and Resources for Further Help and Information

Edited by Dawn D. Matthews. 606 pages. 2002. 0-7808-0338-8.

"This work will be useful in public libraries with large consumer health and wellness departments."
—*American Reference Books Annual, 2003*

"As a sourcebook on household safety this book meets its mark. It is encyclopedic in scope and covers a wide range of safety issues that are commonly seen in the home." —*E-Streams, Jul '02*

Hypertension Sourcebook

Basic Consumer Health Information about the Causes, Diagnosis, and Treatment of High Blood Pressure, with Facts about Consequences, Complications, and Co-Occurring Disorders, Such as Coronary Heart Disease, Diabetes, Stroke, Kidney Disease, and Hypertensive Retinopathy, and Issues in Blood Pressure Control, Including Dietary Choices, Stress Management, and Medications

Along with Reports on Current Research Initiatives and Clinical Trials, a Glossary, and Resources for Additional Help and Information

Edited by Dawn D. Matthews and Karen Bellenir. 613 pages. 2004. 0-7808-0674-3.

Immune System Disorders Sourcebook, 2nd Edition

Basic Consumer Health Information about Disorders of the Immune System, Including Immune System Function and Response, Diagnosis of Immune Disorders, Information about Inherited Immune Disease, Acquired Immune Disease, and Autoimmune Diseases, Including Primary Immune Deficiency, Acquired Immunodeficiency Syndrome (AIDS), Lupus, Multiple Sclerosis, Type 1 Diabetes, Rheumatoid Arthritis, and Graves Disease

Along with Treatments, Tips for Coping with Immune Disorders, a Glossary, and a Directory of Additional Resources

Edited by Joyce Brennfleck Shannon. 671 pages. 2005. 0-7808-0748-0.

ALSO AVAILABLE: *Immune System Disorders Sourcebook.* Edited by Allan R. Cook. 608 pages. 1997. 0-7808-0209-8.

Infant & Toddler Health Sourcebook

Basic Consumer Health Information about the Physical and Mental Development of Newborns, Infants, and Toddlers, Including Neonatal Concerns, Nutrition Recommendations, Immunization Schedules, Common Pediatric Disorders, Assessments and Milestones, Safety Tips, and Advice for Parents and Other Caregivers

Along with a Glossary of Terms and Resource Listings for Additional Help

Edited by Jenifer Swanson. 585 pages. 2000. 0-7808-0246-2.

"As a reference for the general public, this would be useful in any library." —*E-Streams, May '01*

"Recommended reference source."
—*Booklist, American Library Association, Feb '01*

"This is a good source for general use."
—*American Reference Books Annual, 2001*

Infectious Diseases Sourcebook

Basic Consumer Health Information about Non-Contagious Bacterial, Viral, Prion, Fungal, and Parasitic Diseases Spread by Food and Water, Insects and Animals, or Environmental Contact, Including Botulism, E. Coli, Encephalitis, Legionnaires' Disease, Lyme Disease, Malaria, Plague, Rabies, Salmonella, Tetanus, and Others, and Facts about Newly Emerging Diseases, Such as Hantavirus, Mad Cow Disease, Monkeypox, and West Nile Virus

Along with Information about Preventing Disease Transmission, the Threat of Bioterrorism, and Current Research Initiatives, with a Glossary and Directory of Resources for More Information

Edited by Karen Bellenir. 634 pages. 2004. 0-7808-0675-1.

Injury & Trauma Sourcebook

Basic Consumer Health Information about the Impact of Injury, the Diagnosis and Treatment of Common and Traumatic Injuries, Emergency Care, and Specific Injuries Related to Home, Community, Workplace, Transportation, and Recreation

Along with Guidelines for Injury Prevention, a Glossary, and a Directory of Additional Resources

Edited by Joyce Brennfleck Shannon. 696 pages. 2002. 0-7808-0421-X.

"This publication is the most comprehensive work of its kind about injury and trauma."
—*American Reference Books Annual, 2003*

"This sourcebook provides concise, easily readable, basic health information about injuries. . . . This book is well organized and an easy to use reference resource suitable for hospital, health sciences and public libraries with consumer health collections."
—*E-Streams, Nov '02*

"Practitioners should be aware of guides such as this in order to facilitate their use by patients and their families." —*Doody's Health Sciences Book Review Journal, Sep-Oct '02*

"Recommended reference source."
—*Booklist, American Library Association, Sep '02*

"Highly recommended for academic and medical reference collections." —*Library Bookwatch, Sep '02*

■

Kidney & Urinary Tract Diseases & Disorders Sourcebook, 1st Edition

SEE *Urinary Tract & Kidney Diseases & Disorders Sourcebook, 2nd Edition*

■

Learning Disabilities Sourcebook, 2nd Edition

Basic Consumer Health Information about Learning Disabilities, Including Dyslexia, Developmental Speech and Language Disabilities, Non-Verbal Learning Disorders, Developmental Arithmetic Disorder, Developmental Writing Disorder, and Other Conditions That Impede Learning Such as Attention Deficit/ Hyperactivity Disorder, Brain Injury, Hearing Impairment, Klinefelter Syndrome, Dyspraxia, and Tourette Syndrome

Along with Facts about Educational Issues and Assistive Technology, Coping Strategies, a Glossary of Related Terms, and Resources for Further Help and Information

Edited by Dawn D. Matthews. 621 pages. 2003. 0-7808-0626-3.

ALSO AVAILABLE: *Learning Disabilities Sourcebook, 1st Edition.* Edited by Linda M. Shin. 579 pages. 1998. 0-7808-0210-1.

"The second edition of *Learning Disabilities Sourcebook* far surpasses the earlier edition in that it is more focused on information that will be useful as a consumer health resource."
—*American Reference Books Annual, 2004*

"Teachers as well as consumers will find this an essential guide to understanding various syndromes and their latest treatments. [An] invaluable reference for public and school library collections alike."
— *Library Bookwatch, Apr '03*

Named "Outstanding Reference Book of 1999."
—*New York Public Library, Feb 2000*

"An excellent candidate for inclusion in a public library reference section. It's a great source of information. Teachers will also find the book useful. Definitely worth reading."
—*Journal of Adolescent & Adult Literacy, Feb 2000*

"Readable . . . provides a solid base of information regarding successful techniques used with individuals who have learning disabilities, as well as practical suggestions for educators and family members. Clear language, concise descriptions, and pertinent information for contacting multiple resources add to the strength of this book as a useful tool." —*Choice, Association of College and Research Libraries, Feb '99*

"Recommended reference source."
—*Booklist, American Library Association, Sep '98*

"A useful resource for libraries and for those who don't have the time to identify and locate the individual publications." —*Disability Resources Monthly, Sep '98*

■

Leukemia Sourcebook

Basic Consumer Health Information about Adult and Childhood Leukemias, Including Acute Lymphocytic Leukemia (ALL), Chronic Lymphocytic Leukemia (CLL), Acute Myelogenous Leukemia (AML), Chronic Myelogenous Leukemia (CML), and Hairy Cell Leukemia, and Treatments Such as Chemotherapy, Radiation Therapy, Peripheral Blood Stem Cell and Marrow Transplantation, and Immunotherapy

Along with Tips for Life During and After Treatment, a Glossary, and Directories of Additional Resources

Edited by Joyce Brennfleck Shannon. 587 pages. 2003. 0-7808-0627-1.

"Unlike other medical books for the layperson, . . . the language does not talk down to the reader. . . . This volume is highly recommended for all libraries."
—*American Reference Books Annual, 2004*

■

Liver Disorders Sourcebook

Basic Consumer Health Information about the Liver and How It Works; Liver Diseases, Including Cancer, Cirrhosis, Hepatitis, and Toxic and Drug Related Diseases; Tips for Maintaining a Healthy Liver; Laboratory Tests, Radiology Tests, and Facts about Liver Transplantation

Along with a Section on Support Groups, a Glossary, and Resource Listings

Edited by Joyce Brennfleck Shannon. 591 pages. 2000. 0-7808-0383-3.

"A valuable resource."
—*American Reference Books Annual, 2001*

"This title is recommended for health sciences and public libraries with consumer health collections."
—*E-Streams, Oct '00*

"Recommended reference source."
—*Booklist, American Library Association, Jun '00*

■

Lung Disorders Sourcebook

Basic Consumer Health Information about Emphysema, Pneumonia, Tuberculosis, Asthma, Cystic Fibrosis, and Other Lung Disorders, Including Facts about Diagnostic Procedures, Treatment Strategies, Disease Prevention Efforts, and Such Risk Factors as Smoking, Air Pollution, and Exposure to Asbestos, Radon, and Other Agents

Along with a Glossary and Resources for Additional Help and Information

Edited by Dawn D. Matthews. 678 pages. 2002. 0-7808-0339-6.

"This title is a great addition for public and school libraries because it provides concise health information on the lungs."

—*American Reference Books Annual, 2003*

"Highly recommended for academic and medical reference collections." —*Library Bookwatch, Sep '02*

■

Medical Tests Sourcebook, 2nd Edition

Basic Consumer Health Information about Medical Tests, Including Age-Specific Health Tests, Important Health Screenings and Exams, Home-Use Tests, Blood and Specimen Tests, Electrical Tests, Scope Tests, Genetic Testing, and Imaging Tests, Such as X-Rays, Ultrasound, Computed Tomography, Magnetic Resonance Imaging, Angiography, and Nuclear Medicine

Along with a Glossary and Directory of Additional Resources

Edited by Joyce Brennfleck Shannon. 654 pages. 2004. 0-7808-0670-0.

ALSO AVAILABLE: *Medical Tests, 1st Edition.* Edited by Joyce Brennfleck Shannon. 691 pages. 1999. 0-7808-0243-8.

"Recommended for hospital and health sciences libraries with consumer health collections."

—*E-Streams, Mar '00*

"This is an overall excellent reference with a wealth of general knowledge that may aid those who are reluctant to get vital tests performed."

—*Today's Librarian, Jan 2000*

"A valuable reference guide."

—*American Reference Books Annual, 2000*

■

Men's Health Concerns Sourcebook, 2nd Edition

Basic Consumer Health Information about the Medical and Mental Concerns of Men, Including Theories about the Shorter Male Lifespan, the Leading Causes of Death and Disability, Physical Concerns of Special Significance to Men, Reproductive and Sexual Concerns, Sexually Transmitted Diseases, Men's Mental and Emotional Health, and Lifestyle Choices That Affect Wellness, Such as Nutrition, Fitness, and Substance Use

Along with a Glossary of Related Terms and a Directory of Organizational Resources in Men's Health

Edited by Robert Aquinas McNally. 644 pages. 2004. 0-7808-0671-9.

ALSO AVAILABLE: *Men's Health Concerns Sourcebook, 1st Edition.* Edited by Allan R. Cook. 738 pages. 1998. 0-7808-0212-8.

"This comprehensive resource and the series are highly recommended."

—*American Reference Books Annual, 2000*

"Recommended reference source."

—*Booklist, American Library Association, Dec '98*

■

Mental Health Disorders Sourcebook, 3rd Edition

Basic Consumer Health Information about Mental and Emotional Health and Mental Illness, Including Facts about Depression, Bipolar Disorder, and Other Mood Disorders, Phobias, Post-Traumatic Stress Disorder (PTSD), Obsessive-Compulsive Disorder, and Other Anxiety Disorders, Impulse Control Disorders, Eating Disorders, Personality Disorders, and Psychotic Disorders, Including Schizophrenia and Dissociative Disorders

Along with Statistical Information, a Special Section Concerning Mental Health Issues in Children and Adolescents, a Glossary, and Directories of Resources for Additional Help and Information

Edited by Karen Bellenir. 661 pages. 2005. 0-7808-0747-2.

ALSO AVAILABLE: *Mental Health Disorders Sourcebook, 1st Edition.* Edited by Karen Bellenir. 548 pages. 1995. 0-7808-0040-0.

ALSO AVAILABLE: *Mental Health Disorders Sourcebook, 2nd Edition.*Edited by Karen Bellenir. 605 pages. 2000. 0-7808-0240-3.

"Well organized and well written."

—*American Reference Books Annual, 2001*

"Recommended reference source."

—*Booklist, American Library Association, Jun '00*

■

Mental Retardation Sourcebook

Basic Consumer Health Information about Mental Retardation and Its Causes, Including Down Syndrome, Fetal Alcohol Syndrome, Fragile X Syndrome, Genetic Conditions, Injury, and Environmental Sources

Along with Preventive Strategies, Parenting Issues, Educational Implications, Health Care Needs, Employment and Economic Matters, Legal Issues, a Glossary, and a Resource Listing for Additional Help and Information

Edited by Joyce Brennfleck Shannon. 642 pages. 2000. 0-7808-0377-9.

"Public libraries will find the book useful for reference and as a beginning research point for students, parents, and caregivers."

—*American Reference Books Annual, 2001*

"The strength of this work is that it compiles many basic fact sheets and addresses for further information in one volume. It is intended and suitable for the general public. This sourcebook is relevant to any collection providing health information to the general public."

—*E-Streams, Nov '00*

"From preventing retardation to parenting and family challenges, this covers health, social and legal issues and will prove an invaluable overview."

—*Reviewer's Bookwatch, Jul '00*

Movement Disorders Sourcebook

Basic Consumer Health Information about Neurological Movement Disorders, Including Essential Tremor, Parkinson's Disease, Dystonia, Cerebral Palsy, Huntington's Disease, Myasthenia Gravis, Multiple Sclerosis, and Other Early-Onset and Adult-Onset Movement Disorders, Their Symptoms and Causes, Diagnostic Tests, and Treatments

Along with Mobility and Assistive Technology Information, a Glossary, and a Directory of Additional Resources

Edited by Joyce Brennfleck Shannon. 655 pages. 2003. 0-7808-0628-X.

"... a good resource for consumers and recommended for public, community college and undergraduate libraries."

—*American Reference Books Annual, 2004*

■

Muscular Dystrophy Sourcebook

Basic Consumer Health Information about Congenital, Childhood-Onset, and Adult-Onset Forms of Muscular Dystrophy, Such as Duchenne, Becker, Emery-Dreifuss, Distal, Limb-Girdle, Facioscapulohumeral (FSHD), Myotonic, and Ophthalmoplegic Muscular Dystrophies, Including Facts about Diagnostic Tests, Medical and Physical Therapies, Management of Co-Occurring Conditions, and Parenting Guidelines

Along with Practical Tips for Home Care, a Glossary, and Directories of Additional Resources

Edited by Joyce Brennfleck Shannon. 577 pages. 2004. 0-7808-0676-X.

■

Obesity Sourcebook

Basic Consumer Health Information about Diseases and Other Problems Associated with Obesity, and Including Facts about Risk Factors, Prevention Issues, and Management Approaches

Along with Statistical and Demographic Data, Information about Special Populations, Research Updates, a Glossary, and Source Listings for Further Help and Information

Edited by Wilma Caldwell and Chad T. Kimball. 376 pages. 2001. 0-7808-0333-7.

"The book synthesizes the reliable medical literature on obesity into one easy-to-read and useful resource for the general public."

—*American Reference Books Annual 2002*

"This is a very useful resource book for the lay public."

—*Doody's Review Service, Nov '01*

"Well suited for the health reference collection of a public library or an academic health science library that serves the general population." —*E-Streams, Sep '01*

"Recommended reference source."

—*Booklist, American Library Association, Apr '01*

" Recommended pick both for specialty health library collections and any general consumer health reference collection." — *The Bookwatch, Apr '01*

■

Ophthalmic Disorders Sourcebook, 1st Edition

SEE *Eye Care Sourcebook, 2nd Edition*

■

Oral Health Sourcebook

SEE *Dental Care & Oral Health Sourcebook, 2nd Ed.*

■

Osteoporosis Sourcebook

Basic Consumer Health Information about Primary and Secondary Osteoporosis and Juvenile Osteoporosis and Related Conditions, Including Fibrous Dysplasia, Gaucher Disease, Hyperthyroidism, Hypophosphatasia, Myeloma, Osteopetrosis, Osteogenesis Imperfecta, and Paget's Disease

Along with Information about Risk Factors, Treatments, Traditional and Non-Traditional Pain Management, a Glossary of Related Terms, and a Directory of Resources

Edited by Allan R. Cook. 584 pages. 2001. 0-7808-0239-X.

"This would be a book to be kept in a staff or patient library. The targeted audience is the layperson, but the therapist who needs a quick bit of information on a particular topic will also find the book useful."

—*Physical Therapy, Jan '02*

"This resource is recommended as a great reference source for public, health, and academic libraries, and is another triumph for the editors of Omnigraphics."

—*American Reference Books Annual 2002*

"Recommended for all public libraries and general health collections, especially those supporting patient education or consumer health programs."

—*E-Streams, Nov '01*

"Will prove valuable to any library seeking to maintain a current, comprehensive reference collection of health resources. . . . From prevention to treatment and associated conditions, this provides an excellent survey."

—*The Bookwatch, Aug '01*

"Recommended reference source."

—*Booklist, American Library Association, July '01*

SEE ALSO *Women's Health Concerns Sourcebook*

■

Pain Sourcebook, 2nd Edition

Basic Consumer Health Information about Specific Forms of Acute and Chronic Pain, Including Muscle and Skeletal Pain, Nerve Pain, Cancer Pain, and Disorders Characterized by Pain, Such as Fibromyalgia, Shingles, Angina, Arthritis, and Headaches

Along with Information about Pain Medications and Management Techniques, Complementary and Alternative Pain Relief Options, Tips for People Living with Chronic Pain, a Glossary, and a Directory of Sources for Further Information

Edited by Karen Bellenir. 670 pages. 2002. 0-7808-0612-3.

ALSO AVAILABLE: *Pain Sourcebook, 1st Edition.* Edited by Allan R. Cook. 667 pages. 1997. 0-7808-0213-6.

"A source of valuable information. . . . This book offers help to nonmedical people who need information about pain and pain management. It is also an excellent reference for those who participate in patient education."
—*Doody's Review Service, Sep '02*

"The text is readable, easily understood, and well indexed. This excellent volume belongs in all patient education libraries, consumer health sections of public libraries, and many personal collections."
—*American Reference Books Annual, 1999*

"A beneficial reference." —*Booklist Health Sciences Supplement, American Library Association, Oct '98*

"The information is basic in terms of scholarship and is appropriate for general readers. Written in journalistic style . . . intended for non-professionals. Quite thorough in its coverage of different pain conditions and summarizes the latest clinical information regarding pain treatment." —*Choice, Association of College and Research Libraries, Jun '98*

"Recommended reference source."
—*Booklist, American Library Association, Mar '98*

Pediatric Cancer Sourcebook

Basic Consumer Health Information about Leukemias, Brain Tumors, Sarcomas, Lymphomas, and Other Cancers in Infants, Children, and Adolescents, Including Descriptions of Cancers, Treatments, and Coping Strategies

Along with Suggestions for Parents, Caregivers, and Concerned Relatives, a Glossary of Cancer Terms, and Resource Listings

Edited by Edward J. Prucha. 587 pages. 1999. 0-7808-0245-4.

"An excellent source of information. Recommended for public, hospital, and health science libraries with consumer health collections." —*E-Streams, Jun '00*

"Recommended reference source."
—*Booklist, American Library Association, Feb '00*

"A valuable addition to all libraries specializing in health services and many public libraries."
—*American Reference Books Annual, 2000*

Physical & Mental Issues in Aging Sourcebook

Basic Consumer Health Information on Physical and Mental Disorders Associated with the Aging Process, Including Concerns about Cardiovascular Disease, Pulmonary Disease, Oral Health, Digestive Disorders, Musculoskeletal and Skin Disorders, Metabolic Changes, Sexual and Reproductive Issues, and Changes in Vision, Hearing, and Other Senses

Along with Data about Longevity and Causes of Death, Information on Acute and Chronic Pain, Descriptions of Mental Concerns, a Glossary of Terms, and Resource Listings for Additional Help

Edited by Jenifer Swanson. 660 pages. 1999. 0-7808-0233-0.

"This is a treasure of health information for the layperson." — *Choice Health Sciences Supplement, Association of College & Research Libraries, May 2000*

"Recommended for public libraries."
—*American Reference Books Annual, 2000*

"Recommended reference source."
—*Booklist, American Library Association, Oct '99*

SEE ALSO *Healthy Aging Sourcebook*

Podiatry Sourcebook

Basic Consumer Health Information about Foot Conditions, Diseases, and Injuries, Including Bunions, Corns, Calluses, Athlete's Foot, Plantar Warts, Hammertoes and Clawtoes, Clubfoot, Heel Pain, Gout, and More

Along with Facts about Foot Care, Disease Prevention, Foot Safety, Choosing a Foot Care Specialist, a Glossary of Terms, and Resource Listings for Additional Information

Edited by M. Lisa Weatherford. 380 pages. 2001. 0-7808-0215-2.

"Recommended reference source."
—*Booklist, American Library Association, Feb '02*

"There is a lot of information presented here on a topic that is usually only covered sparingly in most larger comprehensive medical encyclopedias."
—*American Reference Books Annual 2002*

Pregnancy & Birth Sourcebook, 2nd Edition

Basic Consumer Health Information about Conception and Pregnancy, Including Facts about Fertility, Infertility, Pregnancy Symptoms and Complications, Fetal Growth and Development, Labor, Delivery, and the Postpartum Period, as Well as Information about Maintaining Health and Wellness during Pregnancy and Caring for a Newborn

Along with Information about Public Health Assistance for Low-Income Pregnant Women, a Glossary, and Directories of Agencies and Organizations Providing Help and Support

Edited by Amy L. Sutton. 626 pages. 2004. 0-7808-0672-7.

ALSO AVAILABLE: *Pregnancy & Birth Sourcebook, 1st Edition.* Edited by Heather E. Aldred. 737 pages. 1997. 0-7808-0216-0.

"A well-organized handbook. Recommended."
—*Choice, Association of College and Research Libraries, Apr '98*

"Recommended reference source."
—*Booklist, American Library Association, Mar '98*

"Recommended for public libraries."
—*American Reference Books Annual, 1998*

SEE ALSO *Congenital Disorders Sourcebook, Family Planning Sourcebook*

Prostate Cancer Sourcebook

Basic Consumer Health Information about Prostate Cancer, Including Information about the Associated Risk Factors, Detection, Diagnosis, and Treatment of Prostate Cancer

Along with Information on Non-Malignant Prostate Conditions, and Featuring a Section Listing Support and Treatment Centers and a Glossary of Related Terms

Edited by Dawn D. Matthews. 358 pages. 2001. 0-7808-0324-8.

"Recommended reference source."
—*Booklist, American Library Association, Jan '02*

"A valuable resource for health care consumers seeking information on the subject. . . .All text is written in a clear, easy-to-understand language that avoids technical jargon. Any library that collects consumer health resources would strengthen their collection with the addition of the *Prostate Cancer Sourcebook.*"
—*American Reference Books Annual 2002*

Public Health Sourcebook

Basic Information about Government Health Agencies, Including National Health Statistics and Trends, Healthy People 2000 Program Goals and Objectives, the Centers for Disease Control and Prevention, the Food and Drug Administration, and the National Institutes of Health

Along with Full Contact Information for Each Agency

Edited by Wendy Wilcox. 698 pages. 1998. 0-7808-0220-9.

"Recommended reference source."
—*Booklist, American Library Association, Sep '98*

"This consumer guide provides welcome assistance in navigating the maze of federal health agencies and their data on public health concerns."
—*SciTech Book News, Sep '98*

Reconstructive & Cosmetic Surgery Sourcebook

Basic Consumer Health Information on Cosmetic and Reconstructive Plastic Surgery, Including Statistical Information about Different Surgical Procedures, Things to Consider Prior to Surgery, Plastic Surgery Techniques and Tools, Emotional and Psychological Considerations, and Procedure-Specific Information

Along with a Glossary of Terms and a Listing of Resources for Additional Help and Information

Edited by M. Lisa Weatherford. 374 pages. 2001. 0-7808-0214-4.

"An excellent reference that addresses cosmetic and medically necessary reconstructive surgeries. . . . The style of the prose is calm and reassuring, discussing the many positive outcomes now available due to advances in surgical techniques."
—*American Reference Books Annual 2002*

"Recommended for health science libraries that are open to the public, as well as hospital libraries that are open to the patients. This book is a good resource for the consumer interested in plastic surgery."
—*E-Streams, Dec '01*

"Recommended reference source."
—*Booklist, American Library Association, July '01*

Rehabilitation Sourcebook

Basic Consumer Health Information about Rehabilitation for People Recovering from Heart Surgery, Spinal Cord Injury, Stroke, Orthopedic Impairments, Amputation, Pulmonary Impairments, Traumatic Injury, and More, Including Physical Therapy, Occupational Therapy, Speech/ Language Therapy, Massage Therapy, Dance Therapy, Art Therapy, and Recreational Therapy

Along with Information on Assistive and Adaptive Devices, a Glossary, and Resources for Additional Help and Information

Edited by Dawn D. Matthews. 531 pages. 1999. 0-7808-0236-5.

"This is an excellent resource for public library reference and health collections."
—*American Reference Books Annual, 2001*

"Recommended reference source."
—*Booklist, American Library Association, May '00*

Respiratory Diseases & Disorders Sourcebook

Basic Information about Respiratory Diseases and Disorders, Including Asthma, Cystic Fibrosis, Pneumonia, the Common Cold, Influenza, and Others, Featuring Facts about the Respiratory System, Statistical and Demographic Data, Treatments, Self-Help Management Suggestions, and Current Research Initiatives

Edited by Allan R. Cook and Peter D. Dresser. 771 pages. 1995. 0-7808-0037-0.

"Designed for the layperson and for patients and their families coping with respiratory illness. . . . an extensive array of information on diagnosis, treatment, management, and prevention of respiratory illnesses for the general reader."
—*Choice, Association of College and Research Libraries, Jun '96*

"A highly recommended text for all collections. It is a comforting reminder of the power of knowledge that good books carry between their covers."
—*Academic Library Book Review, Spring '96*

"A comprehensive collection of authoritative information presented in a nontechnical, humanitarian style for patients, families, and caregivers."
—*Association of Operating Room Nurses, Sep/Oct '95*

SEE ALSO *Lung Disorders Sourcebook*

Sexually Transmitted Diseases Sourcebook, 2nd Edition

Basic Consumer Health Information about Sexually Transmitted Diseases, Including Information on the Diagnosis and Treatment of Chlamydia, Gonorrhea, Hepatitis, Herpes, HIV, Mononucleosis, Syphilis, and Others

Along with Information on Prevention, Such as Condom Use, Vaccines, and STD Education; And Featuring a Section on Issues Related to Youth and Adolescents, a Glossary, and Resources for Additional Help and Information

Edited by Dawn D. Matthews. 538 pages. 2001. 0-7808-0249-7.

ALSO AVAILABLE: *Sexually Transmitted Diseases Sourcebook, 1st Edition.* Edited by Linda M. Ross. 550 pages. 1997. 0-7808-0217-9.

"Recommended for consumer health collections in public libraries, and secondary school and community college libraries."
—*American Reference Books Annual 2002*

"Every school and public library should have a copy of this comprehensive and user-friendly reference book."
—*Choice, Association of College & Research Libraries, Sep '01*

"This is a highly recommended book. This is an especially important book for all school and public libraries." —*AIDS Book Review Journal, Jul-Aug '01*

"Recommended reference source."
—*Booklist, American Library Association, Apr '01*

"Recommended pick both for specialty health library collections and any general consumer health reference collection." —*The Bookwatch, Apr '01*

■

Skin Disorders Sourcebook, 1st Edition

SEE *Dermatological Disorders Sourcebook, 2nd Edition*

■

Sleep Disorders Sourcebook, 2nd Edition

Basic Consumer Health Information about Sleep and Sleep Disorders, Including Insomnia, Sleep Apnea, Restless Legs Syndrome, Narcolepsy, Parasomnias, and Other Health Problems That Affect Sleep, Plus Facts about Diagnostic Procedures, Treatment Strategies, Sleep Medications, and Tips for Improving Sleep Quality

Along with a Glossary of Related Terms and Resources for Additional Help and Information

Edited by Amy L. Sutton. 567 pages. 2005. 0-7808-0745-6.

ALSO AVAILABLE: *Sleep Disorders Sourcebook, 1st Edition.* Edited by Jenifer Swanson. 439 pages. 1998. 0-7808-0234-9.

"This text will complement any home or medical library. It is user-friendly and ideal for the adult reader."
—*American Reference Books Annual, 2000*

"A useful resource that provides accurate, relevant, and accessible information on sleep to the general public. Health care providers who deal with sleep disorders patients may also find it helpful in being prepared to answer some of the questions patients ask."
—*Respiratory Care, Jul '99*

"Recommended reference source."
—*Booklist, American Library Association, Feb '99*

■

Smoking Concerns Sourcebook

Basic Consumer Health Information about Nicotine Addiction and Smoking Cessation, Featuring Facts about the Health Effects of Tobacco Use, Including Lung and Other Cancers, Heart Disease, Stroke, and Respiratory Disorders, Such as Emphysema and Chronic Bronchitis

Along with Information about Smoking Prevention Programs, Suggestions for Achieving and Maintaining a Smoke-Free Lifestyle, Statistics about Tobacco Use, Reports on Current Research Initiatives, a Glossary of Related Terms, and Directories of Resources for Additional Help and Information

Edited by Karen Bellenir. 621 pages. 2004. 0-7808-0323-X.

■

Sports Injuries Sourcebook, 2nd Edition

Basic Consumer Health Information about the Diagnosis, Treatment, and Rehabilitation of Common Sports-Related Injuries in Children and Adults

Along with Suggestions for Conditioning and Training, Information and Prevention Tips for Injuries Frequently Associated with Specific Sports and Special Populations, a Glossary, and a Directory of Additional Resources

Edited by Joyce Brennfleck Shannon. 614 pages. 2002. 0-7808-0604-2.

ALSO AVAILABLE: *Sports Injuries Sourcebook, 1st Edition.* Edited by Heather E. Aldred. 624 pages. 1999. 0-7808-0218-7.

"This is an excellent reference for consumers and it is recommended for public, community college, and undergraduate libraries."
—*American Reference Books Annual, 2003*

"Recommended reference source."
—*Booklist, American Library Association, Feb '03*

■

Stress-Related Disorders Sourcebook

Basic Consumer Health Information about Stress and Stress-Related Disorders, Including Stress Origins and Signals, Environmental Stress at Work and Home, Mental and Emotional Stress Associated with Depression, Post-Traumatic Stress Disorder, Panic Disorder, Suicide, and the Physical Effects of Stress on the Cardiovascular, Immune, and Nervous Systems

Along with Stress Management Techniques, a Glossary, and a Listing of Additional Resources

Edited by Joyce Brennfleck Shannon. 610 pages. 2002. 0-7808-0560-7.

"Well written for a general readership, the *Stress-Related Disorders Sourcebook* is a useful addition to the health reference literature."
—*American Reference Books Annual, 2003*

"I am impressed by the amount of information. It offers a thorough overview of the causes and consequences of stress for the layperson. . . . A well-done and thorough reference guide for professionals and nonprofessionals alike." —*Doody's Review Service, Dec '02*

Stroke Sourcebook

Basic Consumer Health Information about Stroke, Including Ischemic, Hemorrhagic, Transient Ischemic Attack (TIA), and Pediatric Stroke, Stroke Triggers and Risks, Diagnostic Tests, Treatments, and Rehabilitation Information

Along with Stroke Prevention Guidelines, Legal and Financial Information, a Glossary, and a Directory of Additional Resources

Edited by Joyce Brennfleck Shannon. 606 pages. 2003. 0-7808-0630-1.

"This volume is highly recommended and should be in every medical, hospital, and public library."
—*American Reference Books Annual, 2004*

Substance Abuse Sourcebook

Basic Health-Related Information about the Abuse of Legal and Illegal Substances Such as Alcohol, Tobacco, Prescription Drugs, Marijuana, Cocaine, and Heroin; and Including Facts about Substance Abuse Prevention Strategies, Intervention Methods, Treatment and Recovery Programs, and a Section Addressing the Special Problems Related to Substance Abuse during Pregnancy

Edited by Karen Bellenir. 573 pages. 1996. 0-7808-0038-9.

"A valuable addition to any health reference section. Highly recommended."
—*The Book Report, Mar/Apr '97*

". . . a comprehensive collection of substance abuse information that's both highly readable and compact. Families and caregivers of substance abusers will find the information enlightening and helpful, while teachers, social workers and journalists should benefit from the concise format. Recommended."
—*Drug Abuse Update, Winter '96/'97*

SEE ALSO *Alcoholism Sourcebook, Drug Abuse Sourcebook*

Surgery Sourcebook

Basic Consumer Health Information about Inpatient and Outpatient Surgeries, Including Cardiac, Vascular, Orthopedic, Ocular, Reconstructive, Cosmetic, Gynecologic, and Ear, Nose, and Throat Procedures and More

Along with Information about Operating Room Policies and Instruments, Laser Surgery Techniques, Hospital Errors, Statistical Data, a Glossary, and Listings of Sources for Further Help and Information

Edited by Annemarie S. Muth and Karen Bellenir. 596 pages. 2002. 0-7808-0380-9.

"Large public libraries and medical libraries would benefit from this material in their reference collections."
—*American Reference Books Annual, 2004*

"Invaluable reference for public and school library collections alike." —*Library Bookwatch, Apr '03*

Thyroid Disorders Sourcebook

Basic Consumer Health Information about Disorders of the Thyroid and Parathyroid Glands, Including Hypothyroidism, Hyperthyroidism, Graves Disease, Hashimoto Thyroiditis, Thyroid Cancer, and Parathyroid Disorders, Featuring Facts about Symptoms, Risk Factors, Tests, and Treatments

Along with Information about the Effects of Thyroid Imbalance on Other Body Systems, Environmental Factors That Affect the Thyroid Gland, a Glossary, and a Directory of Additional Resources

Edited by Joyce Brennfleck Shannon. 599 pages. 2005. 0-7808-0745-6.

Transplantation Sourcebook

Basic Consumer Health Information about Organ and Tissue Transplantation, Including Physical and Financial Preparations, Procedures and Issues Relating to Specific Solid Organ and Tissue Transplants, Rehabilitation, Pediatric Transplant Information, the Future of Transplantation, and Organ and Tissue Donation

Along with a Glossary and Listings of Additional Resources

Edited by Joyce Brennfleck Shannon. 628 pages. 2002. 0-7808-0322-1.

"Along with these advances [in transplantation technology] have come a number of daunting questions for potential transplant patients, their families, and their health care providers. This reference text is the best single tool to address many of these questions. . . . It will be a much-needed addition to the reference collections in health care, academic, and large public libraries."
—*American Reference Books Annual, 2003*

"Recommended for libraries with an interest in offering consumer health information." —*E-Streams, Jul '02*

"This is a unique and valuable resource for patients facing transplantation and their families."
—*Doody's Review Service, Jun '02*

Traveler's Health Sourcebook

Basic Consumer Health Information for Travelers, Including Physical and Medical Preparations, Transportation Health and Safety, Essential Information about Food and Water, Sun Exposure, Insect and Snake Bites, Camping and Wilderness Medicine, and Travel with Physical or Medical Disabilities

Along with International Travel Tips, Vaccination Recommendations, Geographical Health Issues, Disease Risks, a Glossary, and a Listing of Additional Resources

Edited by Joyce Brennfleck Shannon. 613 pages. 2000. 0-7808-0384-1.

"Recommended reference source."
—*Booklist, American Library Association, Feb '01*

"This book is recommended for any public library, any travel collection, and especially any collection for the physically disabled."
—*American Reference Books Annual, 2001*

■

Urinary Tract & Kidney Diseases & Disorders Sourcebook, 2nd Edition

Basic Consumer Health Information about the Urinary System, Including the Bladder, Urethra, Ureters, and Kidneys, with Facts about Urinary Tract Infections, Incontinence, Congenital Disorders, Kidney Stones, Cancers of the Urinary Tract and Kidneys, Kidney Failure, Dialysis, and Kidney Transplantation

Along with Statistical and Demographic Information, Reports on Current Research in Kidney and Urologic Health, a Summary of Commonly Used Diagnostic Tests, a Glossary of Related Terms, and a Directory of Resources for Additional Help and Information

Edited by Ivy L. Alexander. 649 pages. 2005. 0-7808-0750-2.

ALSO AVAILABLE: *Kidney & Urinary Tract Diseases & Disorders Sourcebook, 1st Ed.* Edited by Linda M. Ross. 602 pages. 1997. 0-7808-0079-6.

■

Vegetarian Sourcebook

Basic Consumer Health Information about Vegetarian Diets, Lifestyle, and Philosophy, Including Definitions of Vegetarianism and Veganism, Tips about Adopting Vegetarianism, Creating a Vegetarian Pantry, and Meeting Nutritional Needs of Vegetarians, with Facts Regarding Vegetarianism's Effect on Pregnant and Lactating Women, Children, Athletes, and Senior Citizens

Along with a Glossary of Commonly Used Vegetarian Terms and Resources for Additional Help and Information

Edited by Chad T. Kimball. 360 pages. 2002. 0-7808-0439-2.

"Organizes into one concise volume the answers to the most common questions concerning vegetarian diets and lifestyles. This title is recommended for public and secondary school libraries." —*E-Streams, Apr '03*

"Invaluable reference for public and school library collections alike." —*Library Bookwatch, Apr '03*

"The articles in this volume are easy to read and come from authoritative sources. The book does not necessarily support the vegetarian diet but instead provides the pros and cons of this important decision. The *Vegetarian Sourcebook* is recommended for public libraries and consumer health libraries."
—*American Reference Books Annual, 2003*

■

Women's Health Concerns Sourcebook, 2nd Edition

Basic Consumer Health Information about the Medical and Mental Concerns of Women, Including Maintaining Health and Wellness, Gynecological Concerns, Breast Health, Sexuality and Reproductive Issues, Menopause, Cancer in Women, the Leading Causes of Death and Disability among Women, Physical Concerns of Special Significance to Women, and Women's Mental and Emotional Health

Along with a Glossary of Related Terms and Directories of Resources for Additional Help and Information

Edited by Amy L. Sutton. 748 pages. 2004. 0-7808-0673-5.

ALSO AVAILABLE: *Women's Health Concerns Sourcebook, 1st Edition.* Edited by Heather E. Aldred. 567 pages. 1997. 0-7808-0219-5.

"Handy compilation. There is an impressive range of diseases, devices, disorders, procedures, and other physical and emotional issues covered . . . well organized, illustrated, and indexed." —*Choice, Association of College and Research Libraries, Jan '98*

SEE ALSO *Breast Cancer Sourcebook, Cancer Sourcebook for Women, Healthy Heart Sourcebook for Women, Osteoporosis Sourcebook*

■

Workplace Health & Safety Sourcebook

Basic Consumer Health Information about Workplace Health and Safety, Including the Effect of Workplace Hazards on the Lungs, Skin, Heart, Ears, Eyes, Brain, Reproductive Organs, Musculoskeletal System, and Other Organs and Body Parts

Along with Information about Occupational Cancer, Personal Protective Equipment, Toxic and Hazardous Chemicals, Child Labor, Stress, and Workplace Violence

Edited by Chad T. Kimball. 626 pages. 2000. 0-7808-0231-4.

"As a reference for the general public, this would be useful in any library." —*E-Streams, Jun '01*

"Provides helpful information for primary care physicians and other caregivers interested in occupational medicine. . . . General readers; professionals."
—*Choice, Association of College & Research Libraries, May '01*

"Recommended reference source."
—*Booklist, American Library Association, Feb '01*

"Highly recommended." —*The Bookwatch, Jan '01*

Worldwide Health Sourcebook

Basic Information about Global Health Issues, Including Malnutrition, Reproductive Health, Disease Dispersion and Prevention, Emerging Diseases, Risky Health Behaviors, and the Leading Causes of Death

Along with Global Health Concerns for Children, Women, and the Elderly, Mental Health Issues, Research and Technology Advancements, and Economic, Environmental, and Political Health Implications, a Glossary, and a Resource Listing for Additional Help and Information

Edited by Joyce Brennfleck Shannon. 614 pages. 2001. 0-7808-0330-2.

"Named an Outstanding Academic Title." —*Choice, Association of College & Research Libraries, Jan '02*

"Yet another handy but also unique compilation in the extensive Health Reference Series, this is a useful work because many of the international publications reprinted or excerpted are not readily available. Highly recommended." —*Choice, Association of College & Research Libraries, Nov '01*

"Recommended reference source."
—*Booklist, American Library Association, Oct '01*

Teen Health Series

Helping Young Adults Understand, Manage, and Avoid Serious Illness

List price $65 per volume. **School and library price $58 per volume.**

Alcohol Information for Teens

Health Tips about Alcohol and Alcoholism

Including Facts about Underage Drinking, Preventing Teen Alcohol Use, Alcohol's Effects on the Brain and the Body, Alcohol Abuse Treatment, Help for Children of Alcoholics, and More

Edited by Joyce Brennfleck Shannon. 370 pages. 2005. 0-7808-0741-3.

Asthma Information for Teens

Health Tips about Managing Asthma and Related Concerns

Including Facts about Asthma Causes, Triggers, Symptoms, Diagnosis, and Treatment

Edited by Karen Bellenir. 386 pages. 2005. 0-7808-0770-7.

"It is so clearly written and well organized that even hesitant readers will be able to find the facts they need, whether for reports or personal information. . . . A succinct but complete resource."

—*School Library Journal, Sep '05*

Cancer Information for Teens

Health Tips about Cancer Awareness, Prevention, Diagnosis, and Treatment

Including Facts about Frequently Occurring Cancers, Cancer Risk Factors, and Coping Strategies for Teens Fighting Cancer or Dealing with Cancer in Friends or Family Members

Edited by Wilma R. Caldwell. 428 pages. 2004. 0-7808-0678-6.

"Recommended for school libraries, or consumer libraries that see a lot of use by teens."

—*E-Streams, May 2005*

"A valuable educational tool."

—*American Reference Books Annual, 2005*

"Young adults and their parents alike will find this new addition to the *Teen Health Series* an important reference to cancer in teens."

—*Children's Bookwatch, February 2005*

Diet Information for Teens

Health Tips about Diet and Nutrition

Including Facts about Nutrients, Dietary Guidelines, Breakfasts, School Lunches, Snacks, Party Food, Weight Control, Eating Disorders, and More

Edited by Karen Bellenir. 399 pages. 2001. 0-7808-0441-4.

"Full of helpful insights and facts throughout the book. . . . An excellent resource to be placed in public libraries or even in personal collections."

—*American Reference Books Annual 2002*

"Recommended for middle and high school libraries and media centers as well as academic libraries that educate future teachers of teenagers. It is also a suitable addition to health science libraries that serve patrons who are interested in teen health promotion and education."

—*E-Streams, Oct '01*

"This comprehensive book would be beneficial to collections that need information about nutrition, dietary guidelines, meal planning, and weight control. . . . This reference is so easy to use that its purchase is recommended."

—*The Book Report, Sep-Oct '01*

"This book is written in an easy to understand format describing issues that many teens face every day, and then provides thoughtful explanations so that teens can make informed decisions. This is an interesting book that provides important facts and information for today's teens."

—*Doody's Health Sciences Book Review Journal, Jul-Aug '01*

"A comprehensive compendium of diet and nutrition. The information is presented in a straightforward, plain-spoken manner. This title will be useful to those working on reports on a variety of topics, as well as to general readers concerned about their dietary health."

—*School Library Journal, Jun '01*

Drug Information for Teens

Health Tips about the Physical and Mental Effects of Substance Abuse

Including Facts about Alcohol, Anabolic Steroids, Club Drugs, Cocaine, Depressants, Hallucinogens, Herbal Products, Inhalants, Marijuana, Narcotics, Stimulants, Tobacco, and More

Edited by Karen Bellenir. 452 pages. 2002. 0-7808-0444-9.

"A clearly written resource for general readers and researchers alike."

—*School Library Journal*

"The chapters are quick to make a connection to their teenage reading audience. The prose is straightforward and the book lends itself to spot reading. It should be useful both for practical information and for research, and it is suitable for public and school libraries."
—*American Reference Books Annual, 2003*

"Recommended reference source."
—*Booklist, American Library Association, Feb '03*

"This is an excellent resource for teens and their parents. Education about drugs and substances is key to discouraging teen drug abuse and this book provides this much needed information in a way that is interesting and factual." —*Doody's Review Service, Dec '02*

Eating Disorders Information for Teens

Health Tips about Anorexia, Bulimia, Binge Eating, and Other Eating Disorders

Including Information on the Causes, Prevention, and Treatment of Eating Disorders, and Such Other Issues as Maintaining Healthy Eating and Exercise Habits

Edited by Sandra Augustyn Lawton. 337 pages. 2005. 0-7808-0783-9.

Fitness Information for Teens

Health Tips about Exercise, Physical Well-Being, and Health Maintenance

Including Facts about Aerobic and Anaerobic Conditioning, Stretching, Body Shape and Body Image, Sports Training, Nutrition, and Activities for Non-Athletes

Edited by Karen Bellenir. 425 pages. 2004. 0-7808-0679-4.

"This book will be a great addition to any public, junior high, senior high, or secondary school library."
—*American Reference Books Annual, 2005*

Learning Disabilities Information for Teens

Health Tips about Academic Skills Disorders and Other Disabilities That Affect Learning

Including Information about Common Signs of Learning Disabilities, School Issues, Learning to Live with a Learning Disability, and Other Related Issues

Edited by Sandra Augustyn Lawton. 337 pages. 2005. 0-7808-0796-0.

Mental Health Information for Teens

Health Tips about Mental Health and Mental Illness

Including Facts about Anxiety, Depression, Suicide, Eating Disorders, Obsessive-Compulsive Disorders, Panic Attacks, Phobias, Schizophrenia, and More

Edited by Karen Bellenir. 406 pages. 2001. 0-7808-0442-2.

"In both language and approach, this user-friendly entry in the *Teen Health Series* is on target for teens needing information on mental health concerns." —*Booklist, American Library Association, Jan '02*

"Readers will find the material accessible and informative, with the shaded notes, facts, and embedded glossary insets adding appropriately to the already interesting and succinct presentation."
—*School Library Journal, Jan '02*

"This title is highly recommended for any library that serves adolescents and parents/caregivers of adolescents." —*E-Streams, Jan '02*

"Recommended for high school libraries and young adult collections in public libraries. Both health professionals and teenagers will find this book useful."
—*American Reference Books Annual 2002*

"This is a nice book written to enlighten the society, primarily teenagers, about common teen mental health issues. It is highly recommended to teachers and parents as well as adolescents."
—*Doody's Review Service, Dec '01*

Sexual Health Information for Teens

Health Tips about Sexual Development, Human Reproduction, and Sexually Transmitted Diseases

Including Facts about Puberty, Reproductive Health, Chlamydia, Human Papillomavirus, Pelvic Inflammatory Disease, Herpes, AIDS, Contraception, Pregnancy, and More

Edited by Deborah A. Stanley. 391 pages. 2003. 0-7808-0445-7.

"This work should be included in all high school libraries and many larger public libraries. . . . highly recommended."
—*American Reference Books Annual 2004*

"Sexual Health approaches its subject with appropriate seriousness and offers easily accessible advice and information." —*School Library Journal, Feb. 2004*

Skin Health Information for Teens

Health Tips about Dermatological Concerns and Skin Cancer Risks

Including Facts about Acne, Warts, Hives, and Other Conditions and Lifestyle Choices, Such as Tanning, Tattooing, and Piercing, That Affect the Skin, Nails, Scalp, and Hair

Edited by Robert Aquinas McNally. 429 pages. 2003. 0-7808-0446-5.

"This volume, as with others in the series, will be a useful addition to school and public library collections."

—*American Reference Books Annual 2004*

"This volume serves as a one-stop source and should be a necessity for any health collection."

—*Library Media Connection*

Sports Injuries Information for Teens

Health Tips about Sports Injuries and Injury Protection

Including Facts about Specific Injuries, Emergency Treatment, Rehabilitation, Sports Safety, Competition Stress, Fitness, Sports Nutrition, Steroid Risks, and More

Edited by Joyce Brennfleck Shannon. 405 pages. 2003. 0-7808-0447-3.

"This work will be useful in the young adult collections of public libraries as well as high school libraries."

—*American Reference Books Annual 2004*

■

Suicide Information for Teens

Health Tips about Suicide Causes and Prevention

Including Facts about Depression, Risk Factors, Getting Help, Survivor Support, and More

Edited by Joyce Brennfleck Shannon. 368 pages. 2005. 0-7808-0737-5.